S0-BYS-346

PATHOLOGY OF LABORATORY RODENTS & RABBITS

PATHOLOGY OF LABORATORY RODENTS & RABBITS

Second Edition

Dean H. Percy

Stephen W. Barthold

Iowa State University Press

Ames

Dean H. Percy, DVM, MSc, PhD, Dip. ACVP, is Professor Emeritus, Department of Pathobiology, University of Guelph, Ontario, Canada.

Stephen W. Barthold, DVM, PhD, Dip. ACVP, is Professor and Director, Center for Comparative Medicine, University of California, Davis.

© 2001 Iowa State University Press
All rights reserved

Iowa State University Press
2121 South State Avenue, Ames, Iowa 50014

Orders: 1-800-862-6657
Office: 1-515-292-0140
Fax: 1-515-292-3348
Web site: www.isupress.com

Authorization to photocopy items for internal or personal use, or the internal or personal use of specific clients, is granted by Iowa State University Press, provided that the base fee of $.10 per copy is paid directly to the Copyright Clearance Center, 222 Rosewood Drive, Danvers, MA 01923. For those organizations that have been granted a photocopy license by CCC, a separate system of payments has been arranged. The fee code for users of the Transactional Reporting Service is 0-8138-2551-2/2001 $.10.

♾ Printed on acid-free paper in the United States of America

First edition, 1993

Second edition, 2001

Library of Congress Cataloging-in-Publication Data
Percy, Dean H.
  Pathology of laboratory rodents and rabbits / Dean H. Percy, Stephen W. Barthold—2nd ed.
    p. cm.
  Includes bibliographical references (p.) and index.
  ISBN 0-8138-2551-2 (alk. papaer)
  1. Laboratory animals—Diseases. 2. Rodents—Diseases. 3. Rabbits—Diseases. 4. Rodents as laboratory animals. 5. Rabbits as laboratory animals. I. Barthold, Stephen W. II. Title.

SF996.5 .P47 2001
636.932—dc21   00-047256

The last digit is the print number: 9 8 7 6 5 4 3 2 1

CONTENTS

PREFACE

*P*athology of Laboratory Rodents and Rabbits is in its second edition. All sections have been updated to reflect changes in the field of laboratory animal pathology. Mouse pathology has experienced the greatest change and so is emphasized in this edition. The book continues to be designed to serve as a general reference text for veterinary pathologists, laboratory animal veterinarians, students, and others who may require information on the key diagnostic features, differential diagnoses, and significance of diseases that affect commonly used laboratory animals. Infectious diseases are emphasized because of their importance and because there are few other texts that provide an overview of infectious diseases from a diagnostic perspective. The text is not intended to be a comprehensive and detailed source of information on all aspects of laboratory animal pathology. Throughout the text, we refer the reader to other sources of information to assist in that purpose and have placed references at the end of each section so that flow of thought is not interrupted during reading of the text. We have attempted to organize this book in a style that allows easy access to information, but we struggled to organize subject headings and admit to the imperfection of our chosen scheme. Nature doesn't lend itself to orderly presentation of subject material. If the reader can forgive us on that issue, our ultimate purpose is to assist our colleagues in improving the health and welfare of these species that serve such a vital role in biomedical research.

Dean and I have common histories at Yale, common passion for laboratory animal pathology, and common respect for our mentors and colleagues, Drs. T.J. Hulland, H.J. Olander, C. Olson, A.M. Jonas, R.B. Miller, V.E.O. Valli, R.O. Jacoby, and D.G. Brownstein. A number of other individuals have provided considerable effort to this project, including Gary Smith and Tim Sullivan. Many of the photographs featured in this text have been kindly provided by our colleagues in the field of laboratory animal pathology.

In addition to the text, the lives of the authors have changed since the 1993 edition. Dean has joined the ranks of the happily retired from the Ontario Veterinary College and continues to live in Elora, Ontario. He has always been full of wind, but he is putting that attribute to practical use with his love of the bagpipe. I left Yale School of Medicine in 1998 to become Director of the University of California Center for Comparative Medicine in Davis, California. My passion is continuous humiliation while fly-fishing for trout. The greatest reward for writing this book is that the authors have become good friends in addition to colleagues. For this reason, we have enriched the Preface with a figure.

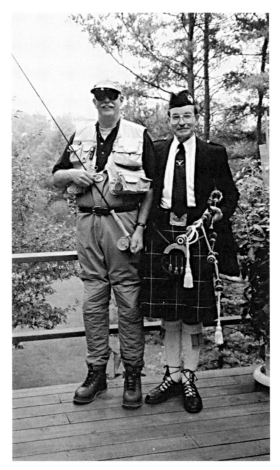

Authors Stephen Barthold (*left*) and Dean Percy (*right*).

Last, but not least, this book is dedicated to the women in our lives, Dean's wife, Connie, and my wife, Bev, who have supported our careers, blessed us with our children, tolerated our idiosyncrasies, and loved us unconditionally. Bev died in 1999, and Dean has been a good enough friend to dedicate this book to her memory.

—Stephen W. Barthold

PATHOLOGY OF LABORATORY RODENTS & RABBITS

MOUSE

Since the last edition of this book, genetically engineered mouse populations have burgeoned beyond the already diverse array of existing mouse strains and stocks. Genetic background has always been the critical factor in disease expression, both spontaneous and infectious, among laboratory mice. The biomedical research community has access to over 3000 inbred, outbred, congenic, recombinant inbred, and other types of mice, each with relatively unique and predictable patterns of disease whose expression is modified by environmental and microbial variables. Contemporary scientists tend to manipulate the mouse genome with little knowledge of (or appreciation for) mouse biology and Mendelian genetics. Issues like genetic drift and subline divergence, which once concerned mouse biologists, pale in comparison with the gross mishandling of mouse genetics in the molecular genomics era. Furthermore, there is a critical need for pathologists with expertise in mouse pathobiology, but paradoxically, the scientific community may not fully appreciate this need.

Many of the strain characteristics (especially cancers) were the reason for creation of specific inbred mouse strains that are used for more general purposes today. It is difficult for a pathologist to command in-depth knowledge of all strains of mice, and in many cases there is little baseline data to utilize, so the pathologist must also be familiar with general patterns of mouse pathology. Recently published books and recommended reading (Maronpot et al. 1999; Mohr et al. 1996) provide comprehensive coverage of spontaneous mouse pathology, based upon the very large data base from C57BL/6 × C3H/He F1 (B6C3F1) hybrids that are used extensively in toxicology, as well as other strains involved in aging research. Our coverage of the esoterica of spontaneous mouse pathology is more superficial, but we pro-vide more thorough coverage of infectious disease and its influence upon immunocompetent and immunodeficient mice.

NOMENCLATURE

The nuances of mouse strain and gene nomenclature are beyond the scope of this book, but the reader is referred to Davisson 1994. In this chapter, we attempt to be as general as possible but mention mouse strains when needed. Common abbreviations used in this text include B6 (C57BL/6), SCID (severe combined immunodeficiency mutation), and nude (athymic, T-cell–deficient mutation).

ANATOMIC FEATURES

There are vast differences in normal anatomy, physiology, and behavior among different strains of mice, many of which actually represent abnormalities arising from homozygosity of recessive or mutant traits in inbred mice. Coat color is an obvious example. For example, 129 and BALB/c mice often lack a corpus callosum due to retarded embryonic formation of the hippocampal commissure. For information about specific strain characteristics, the reader is referred to Michael Festing's (MRC Toxicology Unit, University of Leicester, UK) database, which can be accessed through the Jackson Laboratory web site (http://www. informatics.jax.org/external/festing/mouse/STRAINS.shtml).

Hematology. Hematology is thoroughly reviewed by Bannerman (1983). Mouse erythrocytes are small, with a high reticulocyte count, moderate

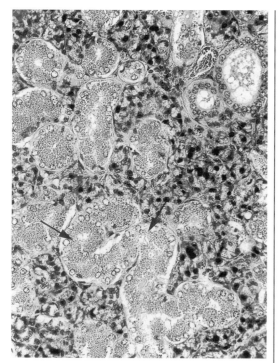

FIG. 1.1—Sections of submandibular (submaxillary) salivary glands from adult male mouse. Note the prominent secretory granules (*arrows*) in the cytoplasm of epithelial cells.

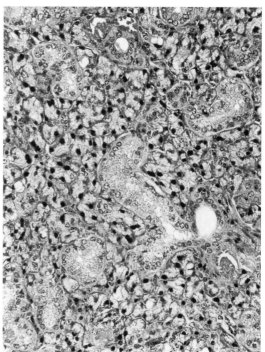

FIG. 1.2—Sections of submandibular salivary gland from sexually mature female. The secretory granules in ductal epithelial cells are less prominent, with fewer granules per unit area, compared with those in males.

polychromasia, and anisocytosis. Mouse leukocytes resemble those of other mammals. Lymphocytes are the predominant circulating leukocyte, and circulating basophils are nonexistent, although tissue mast cells are plentiful. Mature male mice have significantly higher granulocyte counts than do female mice. Mouse granulocytes tend to be hypersegmented in peripheral blood and can have "doughnut" rather than segmented nuclei in tissues. Doughnut nuclei can be visualized as early as the progranulocyte stage in bone marrow and spleen. Mice possess a very high platelet mass, due to high platelet numbers and relatively low mean volume. The spleen is a major hematopoietic organ throughout life in the mouse.

Gastrointestinal System. Incisive foramina, located posterior to the upper incisors, communicate between the roof of the mouth and the anterior nasal cavity. Incisors grow continuously, but cheek teeth do not. Mice have a single set of teeth (no deciduous teeth), and their incisors are pig-

mented due to deposition of iron beneath the enamel layer. Rodents do not have tonsils. The submaxillary salivary glands in sexually mature males reveal increased secretory granules in the cytoplasm of serous cells (Figs. 1.1 and 1.2). The intestine is simple. Mice have a very short (1–2 mm) rectum (the terminal portion of the large bowel that is not enveloped in serosa). Because of this feature, mice are very prone to rectal prolapse, especially if they have colitis. Paneth cells occupy crypt bases in the small intestine (Fig. 1.3). These specialized enterocytes have prominent eosinophilic cytoplasmic granules, which are larger in mice than in rats. Most microflora-associated mice possess prominent gram-positive segmented filamentous bacteria attached to ileal enterocytes (Fig. 1.4). These organisms have not been cultured in the laboratory and are considered to be nonpathogenic. However, they can stimulate the mucosal immune system and IgA production. Pregnant and lactating mice have noticeably thickened bowel walls due to physiological mucosal hyperplasia.

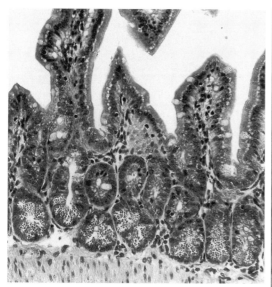

FIG. 1.3—Section of ileum from mouse illustrating the distinct cytoplasmic granules in the enterocytes lining the crypts (Paneth cells), a normal finding in mice.

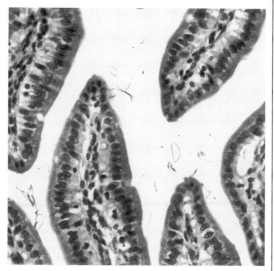

FIG. 1.4—Ileum from mouse demonstrating filamentous bacteria associated with the villi. These organisms are gram-positive and are considered to be a normal finding in this species.

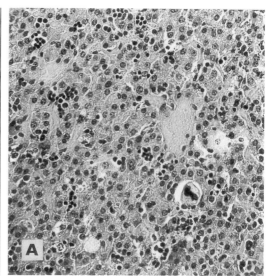

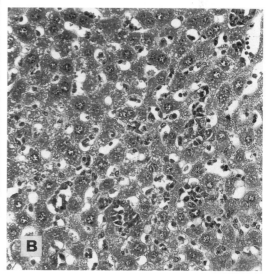

FIG. 1.5—Section of liver from newborn mouse (**A**) and adult mouse (**B**). There are numerous hematopoietic cells in the sinusoidal regions. This is an incidental finding, particularly in young mice.

The liver has variable lobation. Hepatocytes frequently display anisokaryosis, polykarya, karyomegaly, and cytoplasmic invagination into the nucleus. These features are present at all ages but increase with age and disease (see Aging, Degenerative, and Miscellaneous Disorders). Hematopoiesis normally occurs in the infant liver (Fig.1.5) but wanes by weaning age, although islands of hematopoietic cells can be found in hepatic sinusoids of older mice, particularly in disease states (Fig. 1.6). Hepatocytes frequently contain cytoplasmic fat vacuoles. Certain strains, such as BALB mice, normally have diffuse hepatocellular microvesicular fatty change (Fig. 1.7), resulting in grossly pallid livers, compared with

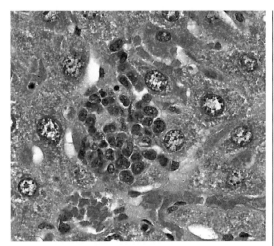

FIG. 1.6—Section of liver from an adult mouse with a suppurative pyelonephritis illustrating marked hepatic myelopoiesis. Note the doughnut-shaped nuclei in the evolving neutrophils.

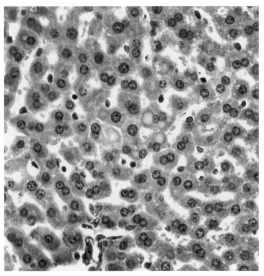

FIG. 1.7—Liver from adult mouse, BALB strain. There are prominent intracytoplasmic vacuoles in a few hepatocytes.

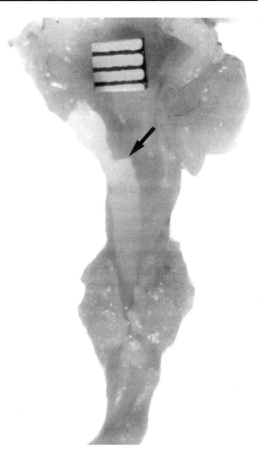

FIG. 1.8—Coagulum (*arrow*) present at the junction of the urinary bladder and urethra in a euthanized male mouse. It is an expelled secretion from the accessory sex glands (copulatory plug). In the absence of any evidence of urinary obstruction, this is considered to be a terminal event and an incidental finding.

the mahogany-colored livers of other mouse strains. One or more foci of hepatic necrosis in the absence of an infectious agent are occasionally observed at necropsy in inbred mice. They are considered to be an incidental finding and are probably ischemic in origin.

Genitourinary System. Female mice have a large clitoris, or genital papillus, with the ure-thral opening near its tip and anterior to the vaginal orifice. Males have redundant testes that readily retract into the abdominal cavity, particularly when they are picked up by the tail. Both sexes have well-developed preputial glands, and males have conspicuous accessory sex glands, including large seminal vesicles, coagulating glands, and prostate. Ejaculation results in formation of a coagulum, or copulatory plug. This frequently occurs agonally; coagulum can be found in urinary bladder or urethra as a normal incidental finding and must not be misconstrued as a calculus or obstruction (Figs. 1.8 and 1.9), but copulatory plugs can and do cause obstructive uropathy. Sexual maturity in males results in

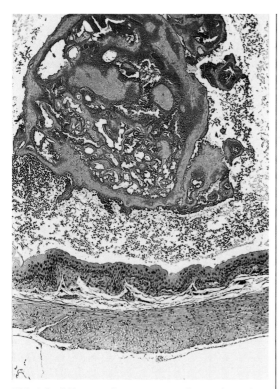

FIG. 1.9—Microscopic appearance of coagulum of accessory sex gland secretions in urinary bladder of male mouse.

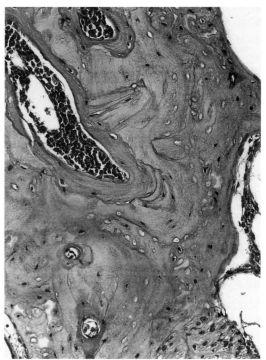

FIG. 1.11—Section of petrous temporal bone from adult mouse, illustrating absence of haversian systems.

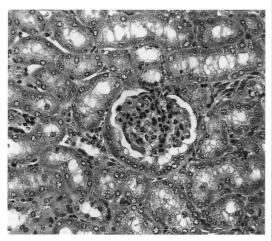

FIG. 1.10—Renal cortex from adult male mouse, illustrating the typical cuboidal epithelium lining the parietal surface of Bowman's capsule.

expression of several sexual dimorphic features, including peripheral blood granulocytosis, salivary gland changes (mentioned previously), and renal changes. In adult males, the parietal layer of Bowman's capsule is lined by cuboidal epithelium, resembling tubular epithelium (Fig. 1.10). This is not absolute, since some glomeruli of male mice are surrounded by squamous epithelium and some glomeruli of female mice are surrounded by cuboidal epithelium. Proteinuria is also normal in mice, with highest levels in sexually mature male mice. Mice are endowed with relatively large numbers of glomeruli per unit area, compared with some species, such as the rat.

Skeletal System. Bones of mice, rats, and hamsters do not have haversian systems (Fig. 1.11), and ossification of epiphyseal plates with age is variable and incomplete, depending upon mouse genotype. Hematopoiesis remains active in long bones throughout life.

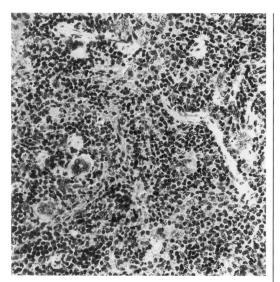

FIG. 1.12—Section of spleen from adult mouse, illustrating the large numbers of hematopoietic cells, including megakaryocytes, in the sinusoids, a common finding throughout life.

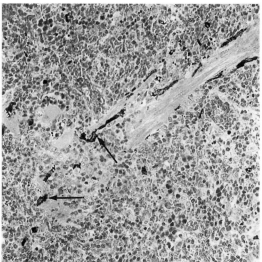

FIG. 1.13—Splenic melanosis in pigmented mouse. Note the pigment-bearing cells (*arrows*) along the splenic trabeculae.

Lymphopoietic System. The thymus does not involute completely in adults. Hassall's corpuscles are indistinct. Islands of ectopic parathyroid tissue can be encountered in the septal or surface connective tissue of the thymus, and conversely, thymic tissue can occur in thyroid and parathyroid glands. Epithelial-lined cysts are also common. The splenic red pulp is an active hematopoietic site throughout life (Fig. 1.12). During disease states and pregnancy, increased hematopoiesis can result in splenomegaly. Lymphocytes tend to accumulate around renal interlobular arteries, salivary gland ducts, urinary bladder submucosa, and other sites, increasing with age. These sites are often involved in generalized lympho-proliferative disorders. Melanosis of the splenic capsule and trabeculae is common in melanotic strains of mice (Fig. 1.13). This must be differentiated from hemosiderin pigment, which tends to accumulate in the red pulp as mice age, particularly in multiparous females. Mast cells can be frequent in the spleen of some mouse strains, such as A strain, but not others.

Respiratory System. The microscopic anatomy of the upper and lower respiratory tract of rodents has been thoroughly reviewed (Kuhn 1985; Popp and Monteiro-Riviere 1985). Cross sections of the nose reveal prominent vomeronasal organs, which are important in pheromone sensing and frequent targets of viral attack. Respiratory epithelium can contain eosinophilic secretory inclusions, which may be especially obvious in some strains, such as B6. The lungs have a single left lobe and four right lobes. Cartilage envelopes are present only in extrapulmonary airways in mice, rats, and hamsters. Thus, primary bronchi are extrapulmonary. Respiratory bronchioles are short or nonexistent. Cardiac muscle surrounds major branches of pulmonary veins in most rodents (Fig. 1.14) and should not be misconstrued as medial hypertrophy. Bronchus-associated lymphoid tissue is normally present only at the hilus of the lung, except in hamsters. Lymphoid accumulations are often encountered on the visceral pleura of mice, within septal clefts. Although not a "normal" finding, focal intra-alveolar hemorrhage is a consistent finding in lungs of mice, regardless of the means of euthanasia.

Endocrine System. The mouse adrenal gland has several notable features. Accessory adrenals, either partial or complete, are very common in the adrenal capsule or surrounding connective tissue. The zona reticularis of the adrenal cortex is not

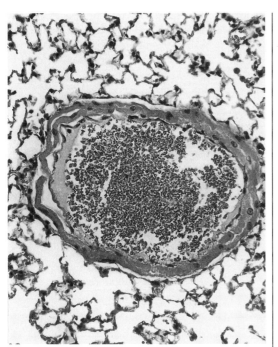

FIG. 1.14—Section of lung from mouse illustrating the extension of cardiac muscle along pulmonary veins, a normal feature in small rodents.

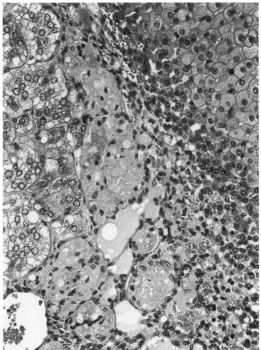

FIG. 1.15—Section of adrenal cortex from young male mouse, illustrating the distinct line of basophilic cells (X zone) at the corticomedullary junction. The medulla is at the left.

discernible from the zona fasciculata. Proliferation of subcortical spindle cells, with displacement of the cortex, is common in mice of all ages. The function of these cells is not known. The most important unique feature of the mouse adrenal is the X zone of the cortex, which surrounds the medulla. The X zone is composed of basophilic cells and appears in mice around 10 d of age. When males reach sexual maturity and females undergo their first pregnancy, the X zone disappears. The zone disappears gradually in virgin females. During involution, the X zone undergoes marked vacuolation (Fig. 1.15) in females but not in males. Residual cells accumulate ceroid. Epithelial cysts are common in the thyroid and pituitary. Thyroid cysts are often lined by ciliated cells.

Other Anatomic Features. Melanosis occurs in several organs, including the anteroventral meninges of the olfactory bulbs, optic nerves, parathyroid glands, heart valves, and spleens of melanotic mouse strains, such as B6 mice. Mice have three pectoral and two inguinal pairs

of mammary glands, with mammary tissue enveloping much of the subcutis, including the neck. Mammary tissue can be found immediately adjacent to salivary glands. Nipple development is hormonally regulated in mice. Mammary elements of males totally involute during development. Remarkably, virgin female mice can be induced to lactate by the presence of other females nursing litters. Mammary glands normally involute between pregnancies, but they do not involute in multiparous FVB mice, which is possibly related to their tendency to develop pituitary adenomas. Brown fat is prominent as a subcutaneous fat pad over the shoulders and is also present in the neck, axillae, and peritoneal tissue.

Developmental Anatomy. The pathologist is being increasingly called upon to evaluate fetal and embryonic pathology in genetically manipulated mice. This requires knowledge of normal placentation and development. Mice have a hemochorial placenta. Excellent references for mouse developmental anatomy have been written by Kaufman, and a resource is available on the web (http://genex.hgu. mrc.ac.uk/).

BIBLIGRAPHPY FOR INTRODUCTION AND ANATOMIC FEATURES

Bannerman, R.M. 1983. Hematology. In *The Mouse in Biomedical Research. III. Normative Biology, Immunology, and Husbandry,* ed. H.F. Foster et al., pp. 293–312. New York: Academic.

Benavides, F., et al. 1997. Evidence of genetic heterogeneity in a BALB/c mouse colony as determined by DNA fingerprinting. Lab. Anim. 32:80–85.

Blumershine, R.V. 1978. Filamentous microbes indigenous to the murine small bowel: A scanning electron microscopic study of their morphology and attachment to the epithelium. Microb. Ecol. 4:95–103.

Cook, M.J. 1983. Anatomy. In *The Mouse in Biomedical Research. III. Normative Biology, Immunology, and Husbandry,* ed. H.F. Foster et al., pp. 102–20. New York: Academic.

Crabtree, C.E. 1941. The structure of Bowman's capsule as an index of age and sex variation in normal mice. Anat. Rec. 79:395–413.

Danse, L.H.J.C., and Crichton, D.N. 1990. Pigment deposition, rat, mouse. In *Monographs on Pathology of Laboratory Animals: Hematopoietic System,* ed. T.C. Jones et al., pp. 226–32. New York: Springer-Verlag.

Davisson, M.T. (chairperson), International Committee on Standardized Genetic Nomenclature for Mice. 1994. Mouse Genome 92:vii–xxxii.

Dunn, T.B. 1970. Normal and pathologic anatomy of the adrenal gland of the mouse, including neoplasms. J. Natl. Cancer Inst. 44:1323–89.

Ebbe, S., and Boudreaux, M.K. 1998. Relationship of megakaryocyte ploidy with platelet number and size in cats, dogs, rabbits and mice. Comp. Hematol. Int. 8:21–25.

Frith, C.H., and Townsend, J.W. 1997. Histology and ultrastructure, salivary glands, mouse. In *Monographs on Pathology of Laboratory Animals: Digestive System,* ed. T.C. Jones et al., pp. 223–30. New York: Springer-Verlag.

Harkema, J.R., and Morgan, K.T. 1996. Normal morphology of the nasal passages of laboratory rodents. In *Monographs on Pathology of Laboratory Animals: Respiratory System,* ed. T.C. Jones et al., pp. 3–17. New York: Springer-Verlag.

Hummel, K.P., et al. 1975. Anatomy. In *Biology of the Laboratory Mouse,* ed. E.L. Green, pp. 247–307. New York: Dover.

Jones, T.C. 1967. Pathology of the liver of rats and mice. In *Pathology of Laboratory Rats and Mice,* ed. E. Cotchin and F.J.C. Roe, pp. 1–17. Oxford: Blackwell.

Kaplan, H.M., et al. 1983. Physiology. In *The Mouse in Biomedical Research. III. Normative Biology, Immunology, and Husbandry,* ed. H.L. Foster et al., pp. 247–92. New York: Academic.

Kaufman, M.H. 1995. *The Atlas of Mouse Development.* Revised edition. New York: Academic.

Kaufman, M.H., and Bard, J.B.L. 1999.*The Anatomical Basis of Mouse Development.* New York: Academic.

Klaasen, H.L.B., et al. 1993. Apathogenic, intestinal, segmented, filamentous bacteria stimulate the mucosal immune system of mice. Infect. Immun. 61:303–6.

Kuhn, C. III. 1985. Structure and function of the lung. In *Monographs on Pathology of Laboratory Animals: Respiratory System,* ed. T.C. Jones et al., 89–98. New York: Springer-Verlag.

Liebelt, A.G. 1986. Unique features of anatomy and ultrastructure, kidney, mouse. In *Monographs on Pathology of Laboratory Animals: Urinary System,* ed. T.C. Jones et al., pp. 24–44. New York. Springer-Verlag.

Maronpot, R.R., et al. (eds.). 1999. *Pathology of the Mouse.* Vienna, IL: Cache River Press.

Mohr, U., et al. (eds.). 1996. *Pathology of the Aging Mouse.* Vols. 1 and 2. Washington, D.C.: ILSI Press.

Plopper, C.G. 1996. Structure and function of the lung. In *Monographs on Pathology of Laboratory Animals: Respiratory System,* ed. T.C. Jones et al., pp. 135–50. New York: Springer-Verlag.

Popp, J.A., and Monteiro-Riviere, N.A. 1985. Macroscopic, microscopic and ultrastructural anatomy of the nasal cavity, rat. In *Monographs on Pathology of Laboratory Animals: Respiratory System,* ed. T.C. Jones et al., pp. 3–10. New York: Springer-Verlag.

Silberberg, M., and Silberberg, R. 1962. Osteoarthritis and osteoporosis in senile mice. Gerontologia 6:91–101.

Staley, M.W., and Trier, J.S. 1965. Morphologic heterogeneity of mouse Paneth cell granules before and after secretory stimulation. Am. J. Anat. 117:365–83.

Sundberg, J.P., et al. 1997. Idiopathic focal hepatic necrosis in inbred mice. In *Monographs on Pathology of Laboratory Animals: Digestive System,* ed. T.C. Jones et al., pp. 213–17. New York: Springer-Verlag.

Wicks, L.F. 1941. Sex and proteinuria in mice. Proc. Soc. Exp. Biol. Med. 48:395–400.

GENETICALLY ENGINEERED LABORATORY MICE

The first transgenic (introduction of ectopic DNA) mouse was created in 1980. This was a random insertion process that remains the most common means of creating transgenic mice, but technology has evolved to successfully target transgenes to specific sites of the genome by homologous recombination for gain of function (knock in mice) or loss of function (knockout or null mice). This process has been embellished with the use of promoters that regulate gene expression or reporter genes that are expressed ubiquitously, in a tissue-specific fashion, or temporally by transcription regulation techniques. The race to associate genes with function and to increase the number of mutant mouse strains has expanded through N-ethyl-n-nitrosourea mutagenesis. Each of these approaches may utilize different strains or hybrids of mice, often arbitrarily chosen by individual scientists, and each poses unique challenges. For example, transgenic mice are often created from FVB/N or F1 hybrids of two inbred strains, whereas targeted mutations are usually created with 129 mice (ES cells) backcrossed onto B6 mice. B6 mice are becoming the gold-standard background genotype in molecular genomics.

Random insertion of transgenes is accomplished through pronuclear microinjection of zygotes. This has generally been achieved using F1 hybrid zygotes of two inbred parental strains of mice to take advantage of hybrid vigor to compensate for the trauma of microinjection and facilitate the process of microinjection by providing large pronuclei. Transgenes become randomly inserted throughout the genome so that each pup within a litter arising from microinjected zygotes is hemizygous for the transgene but is genetically different from its littermate. Thus, gene insertions can lead not only to novel expression of the transgene but also to inadvertent altered function of, or regulation by, flanking genes within the area of insertion. Each founder line of the same transgene represents a unique and nonreproducible genotype. Furthermore, use of F1 hybrids as founders requires filial crosses or backcrosses that result in a randomized assortment of parental genes until such time (20 filial generations or 10 backcrosses) that the line is effectively inbred and congenic to the wild-type strain. This can be circumvented by using inbred founders, such as FVB/N mice (Swiss origin), which are robust and have large pronuclei. FVB mice are prone to seizures with associated neuronal necrosis and suffer from a high prevalence of pituitary adenomas. Others use outbred Swiss mice (CD-1 and CF-1), but their heterozygosity poses problems with uncontrolled modifier genes that may influence phenotype.

In contrast to mice with randomly inserted transgenes, mice with targeted gene mutations should have more predictable outcomes, but this is not always the case. The process of creating these mice usually utilizes placing genetically altered embryonic stem (ES) cells, derived from 129 strain mice, into blastocysts of another strain of mouse to create visibly chimeric progeny that can be easily selected for germline transmission of the 129 genotype. The 129 mouse with the gene alteration is then backcrossed onto a more standard strain of mouse, often the B6 strain, but a wide variety of mouse strains and stocks are used for this purpose.

Effective backcrossing to retain the targeted gene and to delete extraneous 129 genetic material requires nearly 3–4 yr. Few scientists want to wait this long, so homozygous partially backcrossed mice with targeted mutations (−/−) are often compared with wild-type mice (+/+) and heterozygous mice (+/-) that are hybrids with an equivalent degree of backcrossing as controls. In this case, homo- and heterozygosity refer only to the gene of interest, as partially complete backcrosses are literally a hodgepodge of segregating parental genes, even among littermates, and are thus unsuitable control for comparison. Nevertheless, this is an extremely common practice. Furthermore, the value of these animals may preclude any consideration for adequate statistical sampling, let alone consideration of age, sex, and microbial status.

Dependence upon 129 mice for ES cells poses a number of problems. A high frequency (70 percent) of 129 mice have no corpus callosum and other hippocampal abnormalities (as do BALB/c mice). Insufficient backcrossing, with retention of 129 characteristics, results in erroneous reports that selected gene alterations lead to neurologic abnormalities that are, in fact, strain-related traits of 129 mice. A number of other issues relating to 129 mice can impact phenotype of gene alterations. There is considerable genetic variation among different 129 ES cell lines, which is a potential problem for comparing phenotypes of the same gene alteration. Investigators tend to be ignorant of or ignore the history of the 129 sublines that are utilized. Although 129 mice tend to have a low incidence of neoplasia, testicular teratomas are a common characteristic of 129/SvJ mice. Notably, midline teratomas are increasingly recognized among knockout mice derived from 129 ES cells, probably due to insufficient backcrossing. Even in properly backcrossed mutants, modifier genes that flank the target site can be selectively retained along with the gene of interest during backcrossing. This can happen with over 1000 backcross generations, influencing gene expression and phenotype, thereby creating different phenotypes among otherwise genetically identical mice. In the next few years, readily manipulated ES cell lines will be available from B6 and other strains of mice, which may obviate some of these problems.

Gene alteration, either random or targeted, often results in unexpected phenotypes. An example is aryl-hydrocarbon receptor (Ahr) knockout (null) mice (on B6 background). These mice have defective DNA repair and associated immunodeficiency. They also unexpectedly develop cardiomegaly and congestive heart failure. Cardiac disease could be construed as a direct effect of the gene alteration, but immunodeficiency (primary effect) results in susceptibility to a number of opportunistic bacterial infections (secondary effect), which in turn stimulates systemic amyloidosis (tertiary effect). Renal glomerular amyloidosis predisposes these mice to atrial thrombosis (quaternary effect), causing heart failure. Comparison of cardiac disease incidence among null (–/–) mice with wild-type (+/+) or heterozygous (+/–) knockout mice reveals statistically significant differences, with no such disease patterns in age- and sex-matched control mice. Even though this may hold up to scientific and statistical scrutiny, the reality is that B6 mice are prone to late-onset systemic amyloidosis, which has been accelerated in the knockout mice by their immunodeficiency and chronic bacterial infections. Thus, a thorough understanding of the spontaneous pathology of background mouse strains, rather than rigid comparison with controls, may be warranted. Furthermore, phenotypic expression varies with the degree of backcrossing and, in many cases, with the genetic background of the mouse. Different mouse strains carry compensatory genes and other modifiers that can accentuate or mask specific targeted mutations. Markedly different phenotypes have been noted among laboratories that have created Ahr null mice due to the variety of reasons discussed.

Transgenes are usually inserted into the genome with a promoter to enhance expression, to target expression within a specific tissue, or to conditionally express the transgene, but promoters can affect phenotype as much the gene of interest. Promoters are often leaky and can impact upon other types of tissue. The mouse mammary tumor virus (MMTV) long terminal repeat (LTR) promoter and the whey acidic protein (WAP) promoters are often-used promoters in breast cancer biology, to enhance transgene expression within the context of the mammary gland. Such transgenic mice, however, may develop unexpected abnormalities in other tissues, such as tumors of the harderian glands. Conversely, overexpression of transgenes, regardless of their nature, can result in nonspecific abnormalities in normal cell function, as is the case in transgenic mice that develop nonautoimmune diabetes as the result of excessive expression of class II MHC genes in pancreatic beta cells.

Expression of many genes, or deletion of others, can lead to embryonic or fetal death that precludes evaluation of phenotype in adult mice. Thus, pathologists are being increasingly called upon to evaluate developmental defects (see Developmental Anatomy for references). Embryonic/fetal viability is most often influenced by abnormalities in placentation, liver function, or cardiovascular function (including hematopoiesis). Particular attention should be paid to these factors. Depending upon genetic background, lethality can vary. For example, lethality in epidermal growth factor receptor (Egfr) knockout mice occurs at different intervals of development and by different mechanisms, depending upon genetic background. Death occurs in the peri-implantation interval in CF-1 mice due to degeneration of the inner cell mass, midgestation in 129/Sv mice due to placental defects, or postpartum in CD-1 mice due to abnormalities in a variety of organs, all with the identical Egfr null mutation. Gene expression, and therefore circumvention of events such as embryonic lethality, can be controlled temporally and quantitatively by tissue-specific promoters with tetracycline-regulated transcription systems and with *cre/lox* deletion, in which *cre* recombinase can be controlled with transcription techniques. Temporal and quantitative control of transgenes pose new challenges to pathologists when evaluating phenotype.

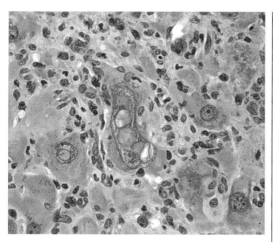

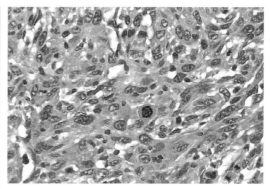

FIG. 1.17—Transponder-induced anaplastic sarcoma from neck of heterozygous p53 $^{+/-}$ mouse (collected from site of transponder implantation).

FIG. 1.16—Liver from transgenic mouse illustrating marked karyomegaly and cytomegaly, an unexpected finding.

Unique pathology can occur that is specific to the transgene, or (more commonly) the transgene can alter background pathology of the mouse strain. Tumor phenotypes found in mice bearing *myc, ras,* and *neu* are distinctive and found only in mice with these transgenes. Notably, mammary carcinomas arising in *neu* (a mutated rat neuroblastoma gene that is the homologue to *c-erbB2* in humans) are comparable to the human mammary tumors. Mammary tumors that arise spontaneously in laboratory mice are primarily influenced by naturally occurring insertion mutagenesis with murine mammary tumor virus, resulting in mouse strain–related patterns of mammary tumors that do not resemble the human condition.

Mice are naturally prone to a variety of hepatocellular changes, including hepatocytomegaly, karyomegaly, polykarya, intranuclear cytoplasmic invaginations, and cytoplasmic inclusions, among others. These changes frequently reach extremes in transgenic mice (Fig. 1.16). Tumors, particularly malignant tumors of mesenchyme, including hemangiosarcomas, lymphangiosarcomas, fibrosarcomas, rhabdomyosarcomas, osteosarcomas, histiocytic sarcomas, and anaplastic sarcomas (Fig. 1.17), are frequent spontaneous lesions in transgenic mice that are relatively rare in wild-type mice. Lymphoreticular tumors, which are quite common and strain-specific tumors in wild-type mice, reach epic pro-

portions in transgenic mice. p53 knockout mice have vast differences in phenotype (spectrum of neoplasia), depending upon whether they are on CD-1, 129/B6, or CF-1 backgrounds.

The emphasis on B6 mice for genetic alteration is fortuitous for the pathologist. B6 mice represent the most commonly utilized inbred strain of mice and the most frequent strain upon which targeted mutations are maintained. The pathologist must beware that B6 mice suffer from a relatively low incidence of neoplasia but develop late-onset amyloidosis (which can be accelerated by immune deficiency, infectious disease, etc.), have a very high incidence of congenital ocular defects (anophthalmia, microophthalmia, cataracts, etc.), have a relatively high incidence of hydrocephalus, develop early-onset deafness (due to inner ear degenerative changes), and are prone to alopecia/dermatitis and hypersensitivity dermatitis. In addition, B6 mice are prone to develop pulmonary alveolar proteinosis, which can be accelerated by genetic mutations, such as the motheaten mouse mutation, and targeted gene disruptions, such as GM-CSF null mice, which are a model for human progressive pulmonary alveolar proteinosis. With rare exceptions, manipulation of the mouse genome (particularly null mutations) results in alteration of mouse phenotypes, rather than something novel.

Many gene alterations have specifically targeted immune response genes or have unintentional effects upon immune response. As already noted with Ahr null mice, when the immune responsiveness of the mouse is altered, opportunistic pathogens become an important factor in phenotype. Perhaps the most overt example of this phenomenon is *Helicobacter colitis*. Mice are commonly infected with a variety of *Helicobacter* species that, given an inappropriate immune response of the host, may lead to proliferative typhlocolitis. This has been erroneously touted as a model of Crohn's disease and/or ulcerative colitis (syndromes that fall under the rubric of inflammatory bowel disease in human pathology). Much has been made about the immune factors involved in this model (which it is not), and little has been made about the etiology (*Helicobacter*). Aside from immune deficiencies, infectious disease can alter phenotype in a number of ways. Many phenotypes disappear when mutant mice are rederived and rid of their adventitious pathogens.

Infectious agents are more important to the laboratory mouse than any other laboratory animal species, not so much because of their ability to cause overt disease (which they do), but because they have significant impact upon the biological response of infected mice to experimental variables. Infectious agents that would otherwise be overlooked or unknown in other species are significant to the mouse biologist because of their potential impact on research results. Furthermore, otherwise insignificant agents, such as *Helicobacter, Pasteurella, Pneumocystis,* paramyxoviruses, and others, are emerging as major pathogens in immunologically deficient strains of mice. Rising populations of mice, being generated by scientists with little appreciation for the nuances of infectious disease, are placing severe strains upon infrastructure, resulting in overcrowding. Unique mutant strains are extensively traded among scientists and often come into animal facilities through the back door. Biological products of mouse origin are not well regulated or monitored, allowing introduction of pathogens, as exemplified by the recent outbreaks of mousepox. Furthermore, mouse pathogens are frequently used as models in biomedical research and continue to be a source of iatrogenic outbreaks in mouse colonies. Financial austerity is being forced upon animal care programs due to the costs of increasing regulations. Infectious disease monitoring and control are often the first to be eliminated or reduced in animal care programs. Thus, infectious diseases are re-emerging among mouse populations due to these various forces.

Consequently, the pathologist must be cognizant of strain-related patterns of spontaneous pathology, general mouse pathology, infectious disease pathology, developmental pathology, comparative pathology (to validate the model), methodology used to create the mice, predicted outcomes of the gene alteration (including effects of the promoter), potential but unexpected outcomes of the gene alteration, and simple Mendelian genetics. The pathologist must also resist capitulation to the pressure to document a desired phenotype or to underemphasize an undesired phenotype. There is no better person to be the gatekeeper of reality in the world of functional genomics than the comparative pathologist.

BIBLIOGRAPHY FOR GENETICALLY ENGINEERED LABORATORY MICE

Blackshear, P., et al. 1999. Extragonadal teratocarcinoma in chimeric mice. Vet. Pathol. 36:457–60.

Blanchard, K.T., et al. 1999. Transponder-induced sarcoma in the heterozygous $p53^{+/-}$ mouse. Toxicol. Pathol. 27:519–27.

Cardiff, R.D., and Wellings, S.R. 1999. The comparative pathology of human and mouse mammary glands. J. Mammary Gland Biol. Neoplasia 4:105–22.

Donehower, L.A., et al. 1995. Effects of genetic background on tumorigenesis in p53-deficient mice. Mol. Carcinog. 14:16–22.

Fernandez-Salguero, P.M., et al. 1997. Lesions of aryl-hydrocarbon receptor-deficient mice. Vet. Pathol. 34:605–14.

Gerlai, R. 1996. Gene-targeting studies of mammalian behavior: Is it the mutation or the background genotype? Trends Neurosci. 19:177–81.

Goelz, M.F., et al. 1998. Neuropathologic findings associated with seizures in FVB mice. Lab. Anim. Sci. 48:34–37.

Harvey, M., et al. 1993. Genetic background alters the spectrum of tumors that develop in p53-deficient mice. FASEB 7:938–43.

Hulcrantz, M., and Li, H.S. 1993. Inner ear morphology in CBA/Ca and C57Bl/6J mice in relationship to noise, age and phenotype. Eur. Arch. Oro-Rhino-Laryngol. 250:257–64.

Kistner, A., et al. 1996. Deoxycycline-mediated quantitative and tissue-specific control of gene expression in transgenic mice. PNAS USA 93:10933–38.

Lahvis, G.P., and Bradfield, C.A. 1998. Ahr null alleles: Distinctive or different? Biochem. Pharmacol. 56:781–87.

Livy, D.V., and Wahlsten, D. 1997. Retarded formation of the hippocampal commisure in embryos from mouse strains lacking a corpus callosum. Hippocampus 7:2–14.

Lo, D., et al. 1988. Diabetes and tolerance in transgenic mice expressing class II MHC molecules in pancreatic beta cells. Cell 53:159–68.

McNamara, R.K., et al. 1998. Effect of reduced myristoylated alanine-rich C kinase substrate expression on hippocampal mossy fiber development and spatial learning in mutant mice: Transgenic rescue and interactions with gene background. Proc. Natl. Acad. Sci. USA 95:14517–22.

Sauer, B. 1994. Site-specific recombination: Developments and applications. Curr. Opin. Biotechnol. 5:521–27.

Simpson, E.M., et al. 1997. Genetic variation among 129 substrains importance for targeted mutagenesis in mice. Nat. Genet. 16:19–27.

Smith, G.S., et al. 1973. Lifespan and incidence of cancer and other diseases in selected long-lived inbred mice and their F1 hybrids. J. Natl. Cancer Inst. 50:1195–1213.

Smith, R.S., et al. 1994. Microphthalmia and associated abnormalities in inbred black mice. Lab. Anim. Sci. 44:551–60.

Threadgill, D.W., et al. 1995. Targeted disruption of mouse EGF receptor: Effect of genetic background on mutant phenotype. Science 269:230–34.

Transgenic and knockout animals as models of human disease. 1999. Immunological Reviews 169. (Multiple-author publication).

Zsengeller, Z.K., et al. 1998. Adenovirus-mediated granulocyte-macrophage colony-stimulating factor improves lung pathology of pulmonary alveolar proteinosis in granulocyte-macrophage colony-stimulating factor- deficient mice. Hum. Gene Ther. 9:2101–9.

VIRAL INFECTIONS

Laboratory mice are host to a large spectrum of viral agents. For practical purposes, this list can be abbreviated considerably for a number of reasons. Several agents have been essentially eliminated from contemporary mouse colonies by modern husbandry practices, including mouse adenovirus type 1 (FL strain), K virus, polyoma virus, mouse cytomegalovirus (MCMV), mouse thymic virus (MTV), lactate dehydrogenase virus (LDV), horizontally transmissible murine leukemia virus (MuLV), and murine mammary tumor virus (MMTV). They may, however, reappear, since most have been retained or are still being used experimentally. The actual prevalence of the herpesviruses and lactate dehydrogenase elevating virus (LDV) is not known, since these agents are not routinely monitored by serological methods, but they are probably rare. Ectromelia virus and lymphocytic choriomeningitis virus, although significant agents, are also relatively rare, but periodically re-emerge. Furthermore, some of the common viruses seldom produce discernible pathology, including minute virus of mice (MVM) and reovirus, even in immunodeficient mice. Thus, the list of agents likely to cause lesions that will be encountered by the diagnostic pathologist is relatively short. This text emphasizes those agents, but all are discussed because of the expanding use of immunologically deficient mice, burgeoning (and overcrowded) mouse populations, inadequate microbial control practices, and the re-emergence of rare infectious agents. The dynamics of mouse housing have changed dramatically. Increasing numbers of scientists are creating genetically altered mice, with minimal or no awareness of infectious disease issues, and animal programs are cutting operating costs (microbial control) to meet the opposing pressures of cost-efficiency and government regulations.

Disease expression is significantly influenced by age, genotype, and immune status. Under most circumstances, even the most pathogenic murine viral agents cause minimal clinical disease. However, under select circumstances, the same agents can have devastating consequences. Infant mice less than 2 wk of age are highly susceptible to viral disease and lesions but are often protected by maternal antibody during this period of vulnerability. Genotype, as already discussed, is also an important factor in host susceptibility. Immune status can be influenced by maternally derived passive immunity, which usually wanes around 4–6 wk of age; actively acquired immunity, which can be virus strain–specific or short-lived; and genetic or induced immunologic aberrations caused by spontaneous mutations, targeted gene alterations, x-irradiation, corticosteroids, etc. Investigation of host-virus epizootiology by the astute clinician must encompass these three major factors as well as population dynamics and husbandry practices. This is an important component of murine diagnostics.

Most viral infections in immunocompetent mice are acute, or short-term, and lesions are often subtle. Animals submitted for necropsy should be carefully selected to provide maximal opportunity for diagnosis. Live, clinically ill animals should be selected, since they would be most likely to have active lesions. Diagnosis of viral infections in a rodent colony should not be solely dependent upon gross and microscopic pathology. A very useful adjunct is viral serology, but this should not be used alone for diagnosis. Mice are likely to be seronegative if actively infected with cytolytic viruses, such as mouse hepatitis virus (MHV), and seroconvert during recovery. Conversely, mice can be seropositive yet actively infected with a second strain of the same agent, as is the case with MHV. Young mice can be seropositive due to passively derived maternal antibody, but not infected or exposed to the virus in question. Some virus infections, such as Sendai viral pneumonia, do not become clinically evident until the mouse develops immunity to the viruses (therefore seroreactivity would be expected in clinically ill mice). These examples underscore that seroconversion to an agent does not imply a cause and effect relationship with disease, unless epizootiology, pathology, and serology are considered collectively.

DNA VIRAL INFECTIONS

Adenoviral Infections. Mice are host to two distinct adenoviruses, mouse adenovirus type 1 (MAV-1, or FL) and mouse adenovirus type 2 (MAV-2 or K87), which can be differentiated from one another by both serology and pathology. These agents partially cross-react serologically, depending on method, in a one-sided relationship with antiserum to MAV-2 cross-reacting with MAV-1, but not conversely. Adenoviruses are nonenveloped DNA viruses that replicate in the nucleus and produce characteristic intranuclear inclusions.

EPIZOOTIOLOGY AND PATHOGENESIS. MAV-1, previously known as mouse adenovirus FL, was first discovered as a contaminating cytopathic agent during an attempt to establish Friend leukemia (FL) virus in tissue culture. Naturally occurring clinical disease or lesions due MAV-1 have not been described, but experimental inoculation of suckling mice with MAV-1 by a variety of routes results in viremia and a fatal, multisystemic infection within 10 d. Inoculation of weanling or adult mice also results in multisystemic

infection with prolonged viruria, with mortality in some strains of mice. Infection is transmitted by direct contact through urine, feces, and nasal secretions. Serological surveys have indicated that the MAV-1 was at one time found in 11 percent of mouse colonies tested, but it is now rare in North America and Europe. MAV-2 was initially isolated from feces of an otherwise healthy mouse. In contrast to MAV-1, MAV-2 appears to be principally enterotropic, regardless of route of inoculation and is excreted in feces. Following oral inoculation of 4-wk-old or younger mice, MAV-2 is excreted in feces for 3 or more weeks with peak infection between 7 and 14 d. Mice apparently recover. Clinical signs are usually absent in experimentally or naturally infected mice, but runting can occur. Clinically normal nude mice have been found to be infected. The prevalence of MAV-2 infection is unknown, since serological monitoring with MAV-2 antigen has not been routinely done. It has been reported in Japan, Europe, and North America. Seroconversion of rats to MAV-2 has been noted, but they are not susceptible to experimental inoculation, suggesting that they are host to a related, but different, adenovirus (see Chap. 2).

PATHOLOGY. Mice experimentally inoculated with MAV-1 develop runting, dehydration, thymic involution, and grossly evident foci of necrosis in liver, spleen, and other organs. Gastrointestinal tracts can be empty, with segmental inflammation of the distal duodenum and jejunum. Hemorrhagic foci occur in the central nervous system of some mouse strains. Nude mice and SCID mice develop hemorrhagic lesions in the duodenum and wasting disease when inoculated with MAV-1. Gross lesions of MAV-2 infection are not evident, except that juvenile mice may be runted.

Mice experimentally inoculated with MAV-1 develop type A intranuclear inclusions in foci of necrosis that occur in multiple organs, including brown fat, myocardium, adrenal gland (Fig. 1.18), spleen, brain, pancreas, liver, intestine, salivary glands, and kidney. Central nervous system lesions consist of focal hemorrhage, necrosis, and gliosis. Endothelial cell necrosis is prominent in these foci. In some mice, severe mucosal epithelial necrosis with hemorrhage is apparent in the duodenum and jejunum. Generalized lymphoid necro-

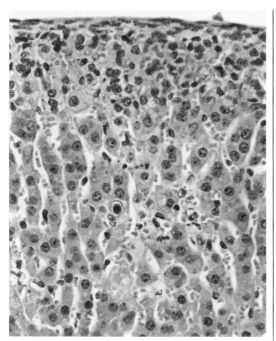

FIG. 1.18—Adrenal cortex from mouse experimentally infected with mouse adenovirus, MAD-1 (FL strain). There is necrosis with mononuclear cell infiltration in the superficial cortex. A single intranuclear inclusion is present in the zona reticularis region.

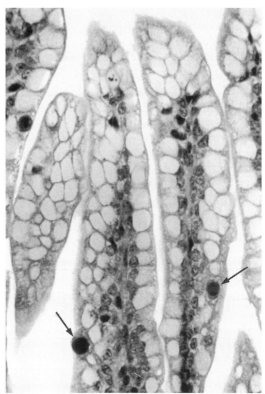

FIG. 1.19—Section of small intestine from mouse subclinically infected with mouse adenovirus MAD-2 (K87). Note the distinct intranuclear inclusion bodies (*arrows*) in a few enterocytes lining the villi.

sis, probably nonspecific, is a common lesion in mice with multisystemic infection. Central nervous system lesions can be manifest as rigid tails, hypermetria, paraphimosis, ataxia, and urinary bladder distention. Adult nude mice inoculated with MAV-1 develop inclusions in endothelial and mucosal cells of the duodenum. Lesions have not been described in naturally infected mice. Hemorrhagic enteric lesions, without overt inclusions, are prominent in oronasally infected SCID mice, along with disseminated infection of multiple tissues, including central nervous system. Thus, MAV-1 has some degree of enterotropism, which is particularly manifest in immunodeficient mice. Experimental inoculation of C.B-17-*scid* mice can induce Reye's-like syndrome (see Reye's-Like Syndrome).

Mice naturally or experimentally infected with MAV-2 develop intranuclear inclusions in mucosal epithelial cells of the small intestine, especially in the distal segments, and the cecum. Inclusions are most plentiful in infant mice but can be found in smaller numbers in the mucosa of adult mice as well. Similar inclusions have been noted in nude mice without other detectable lesions. Typically, inclusion-bearing nuclei are often located in the apical portions of cells, rather than in their normal basal location (Fig. 1.19). Such nuclei must be differentiated from mitotic cells and intraepithelial lymphocytes.

DIAGNOSIS. Adenovirus inclusions are often quite obvious and pathognomonic, especially when found in intestinal epithelium, but they may not always be apparent, even in experimental infections. Success at finding MAV-2 inclusions is maximized in infant mice. Both MAV-1 and MAV-2 viruses are amenable to in vitro culture. Using the indirect immunofluorescence assay, serological testing is probably the most effective means of screening mouse populations for MAV. Since MAV-1 is virtually nonexistent and serological cross-reactivity between MAV-1 and MAV-2 strains is one-way, MAV-2 antigen should be used. Nevertheless, murine serological testing continues to frequently employ MAV-1 antigen, so that MAV-2 infection will continue to be overlooked. *Differential diagnoses:* Multisystemic infections that produce intranuclear inclusions, such as polyoma virus and cytomegalovirus, both of which are also rare, must be differentiated for MAV-1. Intestinal mucosal MAV-2 inclusions are pathognomonic and not induced by any other known agent.

SIGNIFICANCE. Enhanced susceptibility to experimental coliform pyelonephritis in adenovirus-infected mice has been reported. However, MAV-1 can now be relegated to historical interest. MAV-2 is innocuous, even in infant and nude mice.

Herpesviral Infections

MOUSE THYMIC VIRAL (MTV) INFECTION. MTV is a herpesvirus, based on morphological criteria, but it is biologically and antigenically distinct from another herpesvirus of mice, murine cytomegalovirus. Detailed information about this virus is generally lacking, since in vitro methods of propagation have not been identified and little experimental work has been performed. Synonyms include thymic necrosis virus, thymic agent, and mouse T lymphotropic virus (MTLV). The latter term is unfortunate, as it emphasizes a naturally unimportant feature of the virus (its primary tropism is for salivary glands).

EPIZOOTIOLOGY AND PATHOGENESIS. MTV was first discovered during early studies on the etiology of mammary tumor viruses. Inoculation of newborn mice less than 10 d of age resulted in thymic necrosis. This feature of the virus has been emphasized in subsequent studies, but MTV infects salivary glands as its primary target. Outcome of experimental infection is strikingly age-dependent and also influenced by mouse genotype. Intraperitoneal inoculation of newborn mice results in acute thymic necrosis, which is visible grossly as diminished thymic mass, within 14 d. Although largely an experimental

phenomenon, thymic necrosis has been encountered in infant mice from naturally infected mouse colonies. CD4+ T cells are the specific cellular target for MTV, although virus replication also occurs in thymic epithelial cells and macrophages. Older mice do not develop thymic necrosis. Mice of all ages develop infection of salivary glands, with persistent virus shedding in saliva for several months or more. The mode of MTV transmission is therefore presumed to be via the saliva. MTV has also been isolated from mammary tissue of an infected mother and from mammary tumor extracts, suggesting another probable route of transmission. Vertical (in utero) transmission has not been documented. The current prevalence of MTV in mouse colonies is unknown, but earlier serological surveys indicated that 4 of 15 commercial mouse colonies tested were positive. It is very common among wild mouse populations.

PATHOLOGY. MTV infection of infant mice results in the formation of intranuclear inclusion bodies and necrosis of thymocytes and, to a lesser extent, cells in lymph nodes and spleens. During recovery, there is granuloma formation. Lesions in salivary glands have not been noted.

DIAGNOSIS. Diagnosis of active infections in infant mice can be made by confirmation of thymic necrosis with characteristic intranuclear inclusions. Definitive diagnosis can be made by immunofluorescence of affected thymic tissue or infant mouse bioassay. *Differential diagnoses* include agents that cause thymic necrosis in infant mice, such as coronavirus or stress. Confirmation of infection in mice without thymic lesions is more problematic. Saliva or salivary glands from suspect mice can be inoculated into infant mice as a bioassay, but in vitro propagation is currently not feasible. Serologic tests include complement fixation, serum neutralization (mouse bioassay), and immunofluorescence, but mice infected as neonates may not seroconvert. MTV does not share antigenic cross-reactivity with murine cytomegalovirus.

SIGNIFICANCE. The major concern of MTV infection is the variety of immunosuppressive effects that can be of prolonged duration in infected mice. MTV is a frequent contaminant of murine cytomegalovirus stocks, which are prepared from salivary glands. MTV can experimentally induce autoimmune disease in selected strains of mice, via nonspecific activation and expansion of self-reactive T cells.

MOUSE CYTOMEGALOVIRAL (MCMV) INFECTION. MCMV is a mouse-specific cytomegalovirus. Cytomegaloviruses (CMVs) belong to the betaherpesvirus group of the herpesvirus family. Cytomegaloviruses cause cytomegalic inclusion disease, characterized by enlarged cells bearing both intranuclear and intracytoplasmic inclusions, particularly in salivary glands. They have also been termed salivary gland viruses for this reason. MCMV has been studied extensively as an animal model of human CMV infection, but significant biological differences exist. For reviews on MCMV see Lussier (1975) and Osborne (1982).

EPIZOOTIOLOGY AND PATHOGENESIS. MCMV lesions are common in the salivary glands, and virus can be isolated from salivary glands or saliva in a majority of wild mice but not in laboratory mice. The true prevalence of MCMV infection among laboratory mice is unclear, since serological surveillance is not generally practiced. In situ DNA hybridization techniques have revealed MCMV DNA in tissues of many "specific-pathogen-free" laboratory mice, in the absence of virus detectable by other means. A great deal of emphasis has been placed on disease resulting from experimental inoculation, with clear-cut effects of virus strain, dose, route of inoculation, and host factors (age, genotype). Virus is transmitted oronasally by direct contact and is excreted in saliva, tears, and urine. Following experimental inoculation of infant mice, viremia and multisystemic dissemination occur within 1 wk. Maternally derived antibody is protective in newborn mice and probably plays a significant role in protecting young mice from overt disease under natural conditions. In utero transmission does not appear to take place in naturally infected mice. Intranasal or oral inoculation of young adult mice causes subclinical pulmonary infection, viremia, and dissemination, with virus replicating in alveolar macrophages and monocytes.

Mice develop alveolar septal thickening and edema. Salivary glands are preferentially infected regardless of host age and other factors, and natural infections are localized to salivary glands. Salivary gland infection occurs later than infection of other tissues and persists for many months in this site after virus is cleared from other organs. Persistent salivary gland infections can result in chronic replication and excretion as well as latent infections without virus replication. MCMV latency can also occur in macrophages, B lymphocytes, and reproductive tissues, but not brain, thymus, liver, or kidney. Experimental immunosuppression of chronically or latently infected mice can reactivate virus, with dissemination. Immunocompromised mice are particularly susceptible to experimental infections with MCMV, producing disseminated lesions with mortality. Spontaneous disseminated cytomegalic inclusion disease has been reported in an aging laboratory mouse.

PATHOLOGY. Overt disease and disseminated lesions do not usually occur in naturally infected mice. The most frequently encountered lesions occur in the submandibular (submaxillary) salivary glands and, rarely, in the parotid glands. Eosinophilic intranuclear and intracytoplasmic inclusions are present in acinar epithelial cells with cytomegaly and lymphoplasmacytic infiltration of interstitium (Fig. 1.20 A and B). During the acute disseminated phase in experimentally inoculated infant mice, focal necrosis, cytomegaly, inclusions, and inflammation occur in many tissues, including salivary glands, lacrimal glands, brain, liver, spleen, thymus, lymph nodes, peritoneum, lung, skin, kidney, bowel, pancreas, adrenal, skeletal and cardiac muscle, cartilage, and brown fat. Arteritis of the pulmonary artery and aorta (at the base of the heart) has been documented during experimental MCMV infection in B6 and BALB/c mice, but no virus was confirmed within the lesions. Spontaneous arteritis, which is unrelated to MCMV, must be ruled out. Only a single case of spontaneous disseminated infection with MCMV has been reported, involving an aged laboratory mouse. Oronasal inoculation of SCID mice results in severe disseminated disease, with many inclusions in salivary gland tissue.

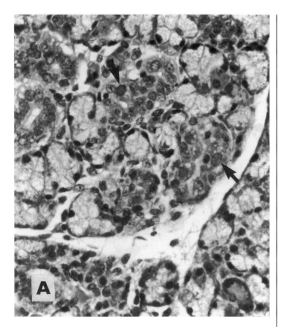

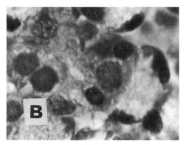

FIG. 1.20—Section of submaxillary (submandibular) salivary gland from animal infected with mouse cytomegalovirus. Intranuclear inclusions (*arrows*) are present in some ductal epithelial cells at a low magnification (**A**) and a higher magnification (**B**).

DIAGNOSIS. Lesions in salivary glands are typical of cytomegalovirus but are not always present in infected animals. Virus can be isolated from saliva or salivary gland and grown in cell culture. In situ DNA hybridization has also been used to detect nonproductive, latent infection of tissues. A variety of serological methods have been developed, including enzyme-linked immunosorbent assay (ELISA), but have not been generally applied as a surveillance method. *Differential diagnosis* for sialoadenitis with inclusion bodies must include polyoma virus. Other viruses that infect salivary glands include reovirus 3, mouse thymic virus, and mammary tumor virus.

SIGNIFICANCE. MCMV seldom causes overt disease in naturally infected mice. MCMV has a number of immunosuppressive effects due to B-cell, T-cell, macrophage, and interferon aberrations. Persistent infections can lead to immune complex glomerulitis and antinuclear antibodies. MCMV has also been shown to have a synergistic effect with *Pseudomonas aeruginosa*. Immunosuppression of naturally infected mice can precipitate disseminated disease.

Papovaviral Infections

K VIRAL INFECTION. Mouse K virus was initially discovered by Lawrence Kilham (thus the K) following intracerebral inoculation of infant mice with tissue extracts from an adult mouse during experiments on the mammary tumor virus. K virus is a papovavirus of the genus *Polyomavirus* but is distinctly different from polyoma virus of mice, which is the namesake of the genus. It should also not be confused with rat parvovirus, which is often called Kilham rat virus. For all practical purposes, K virus is of historical interest and occurs rarely, if at all, in contemporary laboratory mouse colonies.

EPIZOOTIOLOGY AND PATHOGENESIS. K virus appears to be spread by the orofecal route. When orally inoculated into neonatal mice, the virus initially replicates in intestinal capillary endothelium, then disseminates hematogenously to other organs, including liver, lung, spleen, and adrenals, where it replicates in vascular endothelium of these tissues. At 6–15 d after inoculation, there is a sudden onset of dyspnea, due to pulmonary vascular edema and hemorrhage, resulting in rapid death. Pulmonary disease does not occur when older mice are inoculated, with complete resistance evolving between 12 and 18 d of age. Older mice apparently mount an early and effective immune response that prevents the viremic phase of infection. Regardless of age, mice remain persistently infected. Infection of nude mice results in disease similar to that seen in suckling mice. In naturally infected colonies, clinical signs are absent, with dams conferring passive immunity to litters during the susceptible neonatal period.

PATHOLOGY. Gross lesions are restricted to lungs of neonatal mice. Microscopically, intranuclear inclusions are present in vascular endothelium of jejunum, ileum, lung, and liver. Inclusions are poorly discernible and require optimal fixation. Pulmonary lesions consist of congestion, edema, hemorrhage, atelectasis, and septal thickening. Livers of neonatal mice can have sinusoidal leukocytic infiltration and nuclear ballooning of cells lining sinusoids.

DIAGNOSIS. Recognition of diagnostic lesions is difficult at best and is most likely in neonatally infected mice. Immunohistochemistry of infected tissues greatly enhances sensitivity of detecting infected tissues including brain. Serological surveillance can be carried out by a variety of methods. *Differential diagnosis* of multisystemic infection with intranuclear inclusions should include polyoma virus of mice, adenovirus, and MCMV.

SIGNIFICANCE. There is minimal significance. K virus is pathogenic in experimentally infected adult nude mice, but its natural prevalence is so low that infection of immunodeficient mice is unlikely.

POLYOMA VIRAL INFECTION. Polyoma virus of mice is a papovavirus, which has been extensively studied as an oncogenic virus that induces many (*poly*–) types of tumor (*-oma*). Under experimental conditions, it is oncogenic in several different species. It is the type species of the *Polyomavirus* genus of Papovaviridae, to which a number of similar viruses (SV40, BK, JC, etc.) belong. Polyoma virus of mice, originally termed the Stewart-Eddy (SE) polyoma virus and the parotid tumor virus, was initially discovered by Ludwig Gross when newborn mice developed salivary gland tumors following inoculation with filtered extracts of mouse leukemia tissue. The oncogenic activity for which this virus is so well-known is a laboratory phenomenon, requiring parenteral inoculation of mice with high titers of virus within the first 24 hr of life. The relevance of polyoma virus to the laboratory mouse has been resurrected with the common use of polyoma middle T (PyV-MT) transgene.

EPIZOOTIOLOGY AND PATHOGENESIS. Polyoma virus is an environmentally stable virus that is shed primarily in urine, and infection is most efficiently acquired intranasally. Infection of a mouse population requires a continuous source of exposure, which is provided by the repeatedly utilized nesting sites of wild mice. The virus fails to survive under laboratory mouse husbandry conditions and is therefore quite rare in contemporary mouse colonies. Oronasal inoculation of neonatal mice results in virus replication in the nasal mucosa, submaxillary salivary glands, and lungs, followed by viremic dissemination to multiple organs, including kidneys. Mortality can be high at this stage. By day 12, the virus is cleared from most sites but persists in the lung and especially kidney for months. Infection of older mice is more rapidly cleared, with inefficient virus excretion for short periods. Thus, under natural conditions, maternal antibody from immune dams, coupled with the low level of environmental contamination in a laboratory mouse facility, precludes successful infection of neonatal mice and survival of the virus in the population. If mice are experimentally inoculated parenterally with high doses of virus at less than 24 hr of age, tumors arise in multiple sites, particularly salivary glands. Transplacental transmission does not seem to occur naturally, but virus can be reactivated in the kidneys of adult mice during pregnancy if they were infected as neonates. Since polyoma virus is a widely used experimental virus, contamination of laboratory mice can take place, but consequences are limited, for the reasons just cited. Accidental infection of nude mice has caused multisystemic wasting disease, with paralysis and development of multiple tumors, particularly of uterus and bone.

PATHOLOGY. Under natural conditions, lesions are not likely to be encountered, except in nude mice. Nude mice develop multifocal necrosis and inflammation, followed by tumor formation in multiple tissues reminiscent of experimentally inoculated neonatal mice. Intranuclear inclusions can be observed with difficulty in cytolytic lesions. Nude mice also develop infection of oligodendroglia with demyelination, similar to progressive multifocal leukoencephalopathy in humans. Cytopathic and proliferative changes are especially apparent in bronchial, renal pelvic, and ureteral epithelium. Paralysis is due to vertebral tumors as well as demyelination. If polyoma virus gains access to immune-deficient mice, it is likely to behave in a similar manner, but its rarity and inefficient transmission have limited the chances of natural exposure.

DIAGNOSIS. The presence of polyoma virus in immunocompetent mouse populations is best detected serologically. *Differential diagnoses* of nude mice with wasting disease include primarily mouse hepatitis virus, *Pneumocystis carinii,* Sendai virus, and pneumonia virus of mice. Microscopic lesions containing intranuclear inclusion bodies must be differentiated from lesions caused by K virus, adenovirus, and MCMV.

SIGNIFICANCE. The major significant feature of polyoma virus is its usefulness as a research tool. Its significance in laboratory mouse populations is minimal, except that its polytropism can result in contamination of transplantable tumors and cell lines, which in turn have served as inadvertent sources of contamination of mouse stocks.

Parvoviral Infections: Minute Virus of Mice (MVM) and Mouse Parvovirus (MPV). Laboratory mice are frequently infected with autonomously replicating parvoviruses of two different serotypes: MVM and MPV. Genome sequences encoding for nonstructural proteins of these two serotypes are almost identical, but capsid-encoding gene sequences are divergent. MVM was given its name because of its small size, typical of the parvovirus family to which it belongs. MVM was originally discovered as an inadvertent contaminant of a stock of mouse adenovirus, although it is not an adeno-associated parvovirus. MPV, which for a brief period was referred to as mouse orphan parvovirus (MOPV), was discovered as a contaminant of murine T-cell clones. MVM has a number of closely related strains, including MVM-p (prototype), MVM-i (immunosuppressive), and MVM-c (Cutter). MPV also has different strains, including MPV-1a. A hamster parvovirus (HaPV) has been recently described, with close genetic homology to MPV.

EPIZOOTIOLOGY AND PATHOGENESIS. MVM and MPV are common viral agents among laboratory mice but are virtually never associated with either natural disease or lesions. Both types of virus target small intestine and lymphoid tissue, and MVM also replicates preferentially in kidney. Infant mice are more permissive hosts for MVM infection, whereas MPV infection is equally or more efficient in adult mice. Under experimental conditions, MVM produces an acute, self-limiting infection, but MPV infection tends to be persistent within lymphoid tissue. MVM was a very common contaminant of transplantable tumors and leukemia virus stocks. Many isolates or strains have been obtained from such material, as well as other mouse tissues. The propensity of MPV to infect lymphoid tissue in adult mice heralded its discovery in T cells. The lymphotropism of parvoviruses should be a concern for immunologists, but the propensity of MPV to infect adult mice accentuates its importance in modifying immune response. Parvoviruses replicate in rapidly dividing tissues (including lymphoid tissues undergoing antigenic stimulation) and are dependent upon the S phase of the host cell cycle for replicative function. However, growth is limited to certain differentiated cell types, which bear viral receptors. Neonatal mice can be protected from infection by maternal antibody. Mice resist reinfection with the homotypic virus but are fully susceptible to infection with the heterotypic serotype.

PATHOLOGY. Experimental inoculation of infant mice with MVM results in proliferation of virus in multiple tissues, including the subventricular zone, subependymal zone of the olfactory bulb, and the dentate gyrus of the hippocampus. These are the three main germinal centers of the cerebrum in postbirth neurogenesis. MVM also targets the cerebellum, with infection of cells in the outer granular layer, but replication and destruction are confined to cells that have already undergone mitosis and have migrated to the internal granular layer, resulting in cerebellar hypoplasia. Disease in neonatal mice is virus strain– and mouse genotype–dependent. Infection of adult mice results in erythrocyte-associated viremia. In pregnant mice, virus replication may occur in various tissues, including placenta and fetus, without histological evidence of lesions. MVM has been shown to have a strong association with erythroid cells, but not granulocytes, in infant mice. Paradoxically, experimental intranasal inoculation of MVM into adult SCID mice results in severe and eventually fatal leukopenia due to virus replication in primordial hematopoietic cells, with severe depletion of granulomacrophaghic cells and compensatory erythropoiesis in the bone marrow. There are no lesions described in mice naturally infected with MVM. Likewise, MPV infection is clinically innocuous, but active infection of adult mice can cause significant anomalies in immune function.

DIAGNOSIS. MVM and MPV infection of a mouse is usually diagnosed by seroconversion rather than clinical signs or lesions. Methods such as hemagglutination inhibition (HAI) or virion-based ELISA, which target virus capsid antigens, are serotype-specific, whereas indirect fluorescent antibody (IFA), which utilizes infected cells as the antigen, will detect seroconversion to noncapsid antigens of both serotypes. Recombinant noncapsid antigens are now available for serodetection of cross-reacting parvovirus antibodies.

SIGNIFICANCE. MVM can be a troublesome contaminant of many different mouse tissues, including tumors. MVM can induce oncolysis as well as immunosuppressive effects, but these effects are minimal. On the other hand, MPV causes significant immune perturbations in naturally infected adult mice.

Poxviral Infection: Ectromelia Viral Infection; Mousepox. No virus of laboratory mice conjures up an image of ruin like ectromelia virus. Some of this reputation is justified, but most is human in origin. Ectromelia virus is a large DNA virus of the poxvirus family and *Orthopoxvirus* genus, to which vaccinia, variola, monkeypox, cowpox, and others also belong. Orthopoxviruses share antigenic cross-reactivity, but each is a distinct species. Unlike many viral infections of laboratory mice, the disease was discovered before the agent. Marchal (1930) reported an epizootic disease with high mortality in adult mice and termed it "infectious ectromelia," because of the frequency of limb amputation (ectromelia) in surviving mice. Frank Fenner has performed the seminal work on pathogenesis of the agent "ectromelia virus," which causes the disease "mousepox," although the terms are often erroneously interchanged. Outbreaks in the United States stimulated renewed interest in the pathogenesis of mousepox.

EPIZOOTIOLOGY AND PATHOGENESIS. The origin of ectromelia virus remains an enigma, since it has never been found in wild populations of *Mus musculus*. Although laboratory mice have been freely disseminated to all parts of the world, ectromelia virus seems to be enzootic only in Europe and Asia. In the past, outbreaks in the United States have been due to introduction of infected mice or mouse products from Europe. In more recent outbreaks of mousepox, the source of the virus was traced to commercial mouse sera either collected from mice in the United States or imported from China. Strains of virus vary in virulence but are serologically indistinguishable from one another. Ectromelia virus does not seem to be highly contagious. It can be experimentally transmitted via a number of routes, but the primary means of natural transmission is probably through cutaneous trauma, which requires direct contact. Epizootiological studies in a large mouse breeding population have indicated that only a few cages of mice were infected at any one time and that transmission was facilitated by handling. Young mice suckling immune dams were protected by maternal antibody from disease but not from infection. Since rate of exposure was low, virus-naive mice remained susceptible when maternal antibody waned within 4 wk. The hypothetical model of infection involves invasion (through skin), local replication, liberation to regional lymph nodes, primary viremia, and then replication in spleen and liver. Between 3 and 4 d after exposure, a secondary viremia ensues, inducing replication of virus in skin, kidney, lung, intestine, and other organs. There is increasing evolution of lesions (disease) days 7–11, including cutaneous rash. This scenario differs markedly between mouse genotypes. Susceptible mouse strains, such as C3H, A, DBA, SWR, and BALB/c, die acutely with minimal opportunity for virus excretion. Many mouse strains develop illness but survive long enough to develop cutaneous lesions with maximal opportunity for virus shedding. Others, such as B6 mice, are remarkably resistant to disease but allow virus replication and excretion. Thus, a textbook mousepox epizootic requires a select combination of introduction, suitable mouse strains for transmission, and the presence of susceptible strains for disease expression. Immunosuppression will exacerbate disease in mildly or subclinically infected mice. For these reasons, classic outbreaks of high mortality are often not seen. Immunologically competent mice recover completely from infection and do not generally serve as carriers. Therefore, rederivation of virus-free stock can be achieved from immune mice. Immunodeficient mice cannot clear virus and are likely to be highly susceptible to fatal disease.

PATHOLOGY. Expression of lesions is dependent upon factors discussed above. Clinical signs range from subclinical infection to sudden death. External lesions during the acute phase of infection in susceptible surviving mice include conjunctivitis, alopecia, cutaneous erythema and erosions, and swelling and dry gangrene of extremities. Internally, livers can be swollen, friable, and mottled with multiple pinpoint white to coalescing hemorrhagic foci. Spleens, lymph nodes, and Peyer's patches are enlarged, with patchy pale or hemorrhagic areas. Intestinal hemorrhage, particularly in the upper small intestine, is common. Microscopic lesions consist of focal coagulative necrosis in liver, spleen, lymph nodes, Peyer's patches, and thymus, as well as other organs (Fig. 1.21). Multiple basophilic to eosinophilic intracytoplasmic inclusion bodies (1.5–6 μm) are evident in infected cells, especially hepatocytes at the periphery of necrotic foci. These inclusions are poorly discernible with routine staining but can be enhanced by doubling hematoxylin-staining time. Lymphoid tissue can be hyperplastic and/or focally necrotic, with occasional eosinophilic cytoplasmic inclusion bodies (type A pox inclusions or Marchal bodies). Erosive enteritis, often in association with Peyer's patches, is common, with type A inclusions in enterocytes. Skin lesions consist of focal epidermal hyperplasia, with hypertrophy and ballooning of epithelial cells and formation of prominent

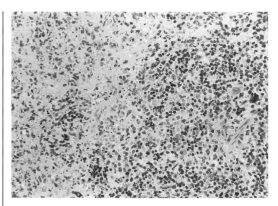

FIG. 1.21—Section of spleen from mouse experimentally infected with ectromelia virus (mousepox). There is extensive splenic necrosis, with karyorrhexis and karyolysis of lymphoid tissue.

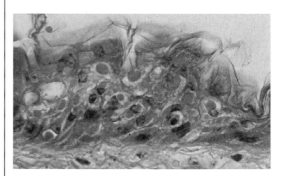

FIG. 1.22—Skin from a mouse infected with ectromelia virus (mousepox). Note epidermal hyperplasia and intracytoplasmic inclusions.

large type A inclusions (Fig. 1.22). Later, skin lesions become erosive and inflammatory in character. Inclusions, inflammation, and erosion are also found in conjunctiva, vagina, and nasal mucosa. The conjunctival mucosa is a preferred area to search for inclusion bodies. Recovered mice often have fibrosis of the spleen and can have amputated tails and digits.

DIAGNOSIS. The variable clinical signs and lesions can be problematic, but careful selection of clinically ill mice will enhance an accurate diagnosis. The complex of liver, spleen, and epithelial lesions bearing typical inclusions is pathognomonic. Splenic fibrosis in recovered mice is also a unique feature of this disease. Confirmation can be achieved by electron microscopic identification of the strikingly large poxvirus particles, immunohistochemistry, or virus isolation. Serology is a useful diagnostic adjunct in recovered mice and is an important surveillance tool for monitoring mouse populations. However, serologic testing is likely to be of little value during the early stages of the disease. Vaccination is variably practiced and can interfere with interpretation of serology results. It should also be noted that vaccination may protect mice from severe disease but still allow active infection. *Differential diagnoses* must include agents that cause hepatitis in adult mice, such as MHV, Tyzzer's disease, salmonellosis, and others. Skin lesions must be differentiated from bite wounds, alopecia, hypersensitivity, and other forms of dermatitis. Gangrene and amputation of digits or tail can also occur due to trauma or "ringtail."

SIGNIFICANCE. Mousepox is an exceptional virus disease of mice, since it can cause high mortality in adult mice. The polytropic nature of the virus and often subclinical but active nature of the infection can allow ready contamination of mouse tissues and biological products and serves as a major mode of spread between laboratories. The drastic measures that have been taken to eliminate ectromelia virus from mouse colonies, particularly in the United States, are clearly disruptive to research.

RNA VIRAL INFECTIONS

Arenaviral Infection: Lymphocytic Choriomeningitis Viral (LCMV)Infection. LCMV was named for its ability to produce lymphocytic choriomeningitis upon intracerebral inoculation of mice and monkeys. This is not a major feature of natural infection. LCMV belongs to the family Arenaviridae, named because of the granular-appearing (from the Latin *arenosus* "sandy") ribosomes within virions. Virions are highly pleomorphic, ranging in diameter from 50 to 300 nm, and bud from the cell membrane without cytolysis. LCMV has been studied extensively as a model system of immune-mediated disease, virus persistence, and immune tolerance, resulting in emphasis on aspects of infection that are not necessarily relevant to natural infection. More recently, LCMV has been used as a model of non-cytolytic viral disruption of differentiated cell function, resulting in disease without lesions (a claim that has not involved pathologists).

EPIZOOTIOLOGY AND PATHOGENESIS. There are several laboratory-modified strains of LCMV that vary in pathogenicity but are serologically similar. Some laboratory-adapted strains have been selected to be more virulent ("aggressive") and neurotropic, while wild-type isolates are generally less virulent ("docile") and viscerotropic. The natural host for LCMV is the wild mouse, but it can naturally infect a variety of mammals, including hamsters, guinea pigs, cotton rats, chinchillas, canids, and primates, including humans. Newborn rats can be infected experimentally, but this species seems to be refractory to natural infection. Among mice, the highly labile virus can be transmitted by direct contact with nasal secretions as well as urine and saliva. However, in utero infection is the major means of transmission within infected mouse populations. LCMV is rare among contemporary laboratory mice and occurs sporadically among wild mouse populations.

The course of LCMV infection is dependent upon virus strain, mouse age, and genotype, as well as upon route of inoculation. Since the virus is generally not directly cytolytic, disease is the result of host immune response to infected cells. Infection of fetal or neonatal mice results in a state of immune tolerance to LCMV, with multisystemic, persistent, subclinical infection. Eventually, tolerance breaks down, resulting in chronic illness, with lymphocytic infiltrates occurring in multiple tissues and immune complex glomerulonephritis ("late disease"). Runting occurs in mice infected in utero or as neonates due to the direct, nonlytic effect of virus upon endocrine tissue function. Prior to onset of illness, mice transmit virus, especially by the in utero route. Infection of immunocompetent, older mice is inconsequential, since they mount an efficient immune response that clears the infection without a carrier state. Effective immunity is through cell-mediated immunity. Experimental inoculation of LCMV into neonatal mice results in minimal acute disease with persistence, while inoculation of immunocompetent, older mice causes severe immune-mediated disease several days after inoculation, including lymphocytic choriomeningitis if inoculated intracerebrally. Experimental infections of infant mice with LCMV have been shown to cause alterations in differentiated cell function, such as endocrinopathies, but this has not been noted under natural conditions.

PATHOLOGY. Clinical signs of natural LCMV infection are minimal but can include runting in infant mice and chronic wasting in older mice if infection is occurring in utero within the colony. Microscopic lesions are likewise nonspecific and most likely to be found in persistently infected aged mice, which can have vasculitis and lymphocytic infiltration in multiple tissues, including brain, liver, adrenal, kidney, and lung. Some mice can develop immune complex glomerulonephritis. Acute disease is largely an experimental phenomenon but can include necrotizing hepatitis and a generalized lymphoid depletion. Although natural infection of nude mice has been documented, pathology was not described.

DIAGNOSIS. Definitive diagnosis of LCMV infection cannot be based on pathology. Serology is also problematic, since horizontal infection among adult mice is inefficient and likely to cause seroconversion among a very few mice within a population. Mice infected in utero or as neonates are immune-tolerant to LCMV and do not efficiently seroconvert, or circulating antibody is complexed with antigen in late infections. Thus, serological testing must be applied to a large sample size and can be enhanced by cohousing adult sentinel mice with mice suspected to be persistently infected. As adults, mice will seroconvert to LCMV when exposed. LCMV can be confirmed in suspect tissues with a variety of bioassay approaches, such as mouse antibody production (MAP) testing, that is, inoculation of immunized and nonimmune adult mice. Serology engages the hazards of growing the virus for antigen, but recent development of recombinant nucleoprotein antigen may circumvent this problem. LCMV is the only virus of mice currently recognized that will kill adults but not neonates when inoculated intracerebrally, which can be a useful diagnostic bioassay. *Differential diagnoses* for runting in infant mice include a number of other viral infections. Chronic illness in older mice must be differentiated from generalized lymphoprolifer-ative disorders, amyloidosis, glomerulonephritis, and chronic renal disease of aging mice.

SIGNIFICANCE. The overwhelming significant feature of LCMV is its zoonotic potential. This is enhanced when infections involve laboratory hamsters (see Chap. 3), and infection of nude mice has been associated with transmission to humans. It can be predicted that T cell–deficient mice will amplify LCMV infection. LCMV is an unacceptable agent in laboratory animal facilities, and its eradication should be aggressively effected. The polytropic nature of LCMV and its wide host range allow this virus to readily infect transplantable tumors and cell lines, which can serve as a source of contamination for mouse colonies. The effects of LCMV on the immune system are well documented.

Arteriviral Infection: Lactate Dehydrogenase–Elevating Viral (LDV) Infection. LDV is currently classified as an arterivirus, which is a floating genus of Coronaviridae. LDV was originally discovered as a contaminant of a transplantable tumor that caused significant elevation of lactate dehydrogenase (LDH) in serum of inoculated mice. LDV is inefficiently transmitted among mice and can be easily eradicated, but it paradoxically is seldom tested for and remains one of the most (if not the most) frequent contaminants of murine transplantable tumors.

EPIZOOTIOLOGY AND PATHOGENESIS. The prevalence of LDV among contemporary mouse colonies is unknown, since serological surveillance seldom includes this agent. LDV is highly specific to the mouse and also has a very restricted cell tropism for a specific subset of macrophages and neural tissue. The primary means of natural transmission is through bite wounds among fighting mice, but recent studies also suggest that it can be a sexually transmitted infection. In the absence of fighting or mating, LDV is inefficiently transmitted by direct contact, even though virus is excreted in feces, urine, milk, saliva, and semen. Different strains, or quasispecies, of LDV exist, including LDV-P, which tends to be persistent and evade antibody neutralization, and LDV-C, which is susceptible to antibody neutralization but tends to be neuropathogenic. Persistent infection with mixed LDV populations favors LDV-P. The most important means of transmission is through experimental inoculation of mice with biological products derived from infected mice. Viremia peaks within 12 to 24 hr after infection and then drops but persists for the lifetime of the mouse, complexed with antibody. LDV infects macrophages and monocytes without overt lesions. In addition to elevations in LDH enzyme, several other enzymes are also significantly elevated. Enzyme elevations are believed to be due to diminished enzyme clearance function of the infected reticuloendothelial system rather than to direct effects of the virus, but these mechanisms are unclear. LDV establishes a lifelong infection that is maintained by replication of virus in a renewable subpopulation of macrophages. Virus infection of macrophages is rapidly cytocidal, thereby releasing large amounts of virus into the circulation. Host immunity and exhaustion of the target cell population attenuate the level of viremia and results in immune complex formation, but not elimination of infection. Immune complex disease does not develop in chronically infected mice.

Specific strains of mice, most notably C58 and AKR mice, develop a paralytic syndrome, age-dependent poliomyelitis (ADPM). ADPM requires suppressed host immunity as the result of old age, immunodeficiency, or chemical immunosuppression. It also requires interaction with ecotropic murine leukemia virus (MuLV). Susceptible mouse strains possess N-ecotropic MuLV and are homozygous at the Fv-1 locus. Ecotropic MuLV is expressed in glial cells and neurons of the central nervous system. Increased susceptibility with age is associated with increased expression of MuLV, and such expression can be accelerated by immunodeficiency. MuLV infection of anterior horn neurons renders these cells susceptible to cytolytic infection with LDV, thereby resulting in ADPM. Possession of a single replication-competent ecotropic MuLV provirus by Fv-1 mice is sufficient to render mice susceptible to ADPM by LDV. In utero infection of CE/J mice (which are devoid of endogenous ecotropic MuLV) with an infectious MuLV provirus clone rendered these mice susceptible to ADPM, whereas provirus-uninfected littermates

remained ADPM resistant when co-infected with LDV.

PATHOLOGY. No clinical signs or lesions have been seen in naturally infected mice. Experimentally inoculated mice develop transient splenomegaly, necrosis of T-cell areas of lymphoid tissues, pyknosis of reticuloendothelial cells, and leukopenia within 72 hr after inoculation. Central nervous system disease in experimentally infected, immunosuppressed C58 and AKR mice consists of mononuclear leukocytic infiltrates in the ventral, and to a lesser extent dorsal, horns of the spinal cord, scattered neuronolysis, and perivasculitis. C57 mice infected with LDV develop mild to moderate nonsuppurative leptomeningitis, myelitis, and occasionally radiculitis without clinical signs.

DIAGNOSIS. Serological methods for LDV have not been generally used because of difficulties with antigen-antibody complexes and low avidity of antibody for antigen. LDV replicates in vitro but causes no cytopathic effect. The old standard for LDV diagnosis has been measurement of plasma lactate dehydrogenase in mice given serial dilutions of test material, but this has given way to polymerase chain reaction (PCR), which can discriminate between different strains of LDV by restriction enzyme analysis of the amplicons. *Differential diagnoses* include any agent that causes enzyme elevations, but other enzyme elevations are not as high or persistent. Although not likely, there is the potential that neurologic LDV disease can emerge in immunodeficient or genetically altered mice that are inadvertently exposed to this oddly common virus. Neurologic LDV lesions must be distinguished from spinal cord lesions induced by mouse encephalomyelitis virus (MEV) and MHV.

SIGNIFICANCE. LDV usually causes no clinical disease or lesions but significantly alters macrophage function and immune response, rendering infected mice useless for immunological research. LDV can be a contaminant of murine biological products, including transplantable tumors. Indeed, LDV remains one of the most common murine agents to contaminate transplantable tumors, including hybridomas. LDV can be eliminated from transplantable tumors by growth in vitro, or by passage in athymic rats, both of which lack the necessary mouse macrophage subpopulations needed to sustain infection.

Coronaviral Infection: Mouse Hepatitis Viral (MHV) Infection. MHV is a coronavirus with numerous antigenically and genetically related strains that vary considerably in their virulence and organotropism. The name MHV was given to a group of virus isolates with similar biological behavior, although it is now known that many MHV strains are not hepatotropic. The misleading name is probably here to stay. MHV shares antigenic cross-reactivity with human coronavirus OC43, bovine coronavirus, rat coronavirus, and hemagglutinating encephalomyelitis virus of swine, but not with other coronaviruses. MHV, however, is biologically distinct from these other agents. Although the role of these related viruses is often questioned in unexplained MHV outbreaks, there is no evidence that MHV comes from anywhere else but mice and the human factors associated with their husbandry.

EPIZOOTIOLOGY AND PATHOGENESIS. MHV is highly contagious by the oronasal route and prevalent in laboratory and wild mouse populations throughout the world. Under select circumstances, it can cause significant disease. Despite its prevalence and potential pathogenicity, clinical MHV disease is not common. This is due to the interaction of different MHV strains on host variables, which include age, genotype, and immune status. MHV strains appear to possess primary tropism for upper respiratory or enteric mucosa. Those strains with respiratory tropism initially replicate in nasal mucosa and then tend to disseminate to a variety of other organs because of their polytropic nature. Infection of mice with virulent polytropic MHV strains, infection of mice less than 2 wk of age, infection of genetically susceptible strains of mice, or infection of immunocompromised mice favors dissemination of virus from the nose by viremia and lymphatics throughout the body. Virus then secondarily replicates in endothelium and parenchyma, causing disease of brain, liver, lymphoid organs, bone marrow, and other sites. Infection of brain by viremic dissemination occurs primarily in neonatal, but not older, mice. However, infection of adult mouse brain can occur by extension of virus along olfactory neural pathways, even in the absence of dissemination to other organs. After approximately 5–7 d, immune-mediated clearance of virus begins, with no persistence or carrier state beyond 3–4 wk after oronasal inoculation. Infection of post–weaning-age mice is usually subclinical, particularly in natural infections caused by generally nonvirulent strains of virus. The obvious exception is nude or SCID mice, which cannot clear the virus and develop progressively severe disease. They can die acutely or develop chronic wasting disease if infected with relatively avirulent strains of MHV.

In contrast, enterotropic MHV strains tend to selectively infect intestinal mucosal epithelium, with minimal or no dissemination to other organs, even in immunodeficient mice. All ages and strains of mice are susceptible to infection, but disease is age-related. Infection of neonatal mice results in severe necrotizing enterocolitis with high mortality within 48 hr after inoculation. Before MHV was known to be the causative agent, the unclassified agent of high mortality and enteritis in infant mice was known as lethal intestinal virus of infant mice (LIVIM). Mortality and lesion severity diminish rapidly with advancing age at inoculation. Adult mice develop minimal lesions, but replication of equal or higher titers of virus occurs, compared with neonates. The severity of intestinal disease is associated with age-related intestinal mucosal proliferative kinetics, rather than immune-related susceptibility. To underscore this point, disease is minimal in nude or SCID mice infected as adults. Recovery from enterotropic MHV is immune-mediated and requires functional T cells. Again, no persistent carrier state seems to occur in recovered, immunocompetent mice, but chronic infections occur in nude and SCID mice. Enterotropic MHV infections are often complicated by other opportunistic pathogens, including *Escherichia coli* and *Spironucleus muris.*

A number of generalizations can be made about the MHV complex that provides insight into its epizootiology. Mice are susceptible to infection at any age and allow virus replication and excretion, but disease generally occurs in mice less than

2 wk of age or in immunocompromised mice. Disease severity is mouse genotype-dependent, but this effect is specific to the infecting MHV strains. In other words, mouse genotypes that are susceptible to disease caused by one MHV strain may be resistant to disease caused by another strain, but all mice are susceptible to productive infection. Passive immunity from immune dams readily protects infant mice from MHV infection, allowing them to acquire active infections later when they are resistant to disease. Infection is acute, with no carrier state in immunocompetent mice. Recovered immune mice are resistant to reinfection with the same MHV strain but are susceptible to repeated infections with different strains of MHV. Finally, MHV is highly mutable, and new strains of virus are constantly evolving, particularly when subjected to immune selective pressure.

PATHOLOGY. The majority of natural MHV infections are subclinical, with mild or no discernible lesions. In susceptible mouse strains, particularly immunodeficient mice, there may be wasting with prominent multifocal hepatic necrosis evident at necropsy (Figs. 1.23 and 1.24). Susceptible mice actively infected with respiratory (polytropic) MHV strains have acute necrosis with syncytia in liver (Fig.1.25), splenic red pulp,

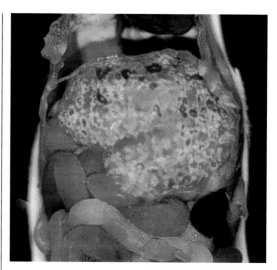

FIG. 1.24—Severe multifocal coalescing hepatic necrosis in a SCID mouse naturally infected with MHV.

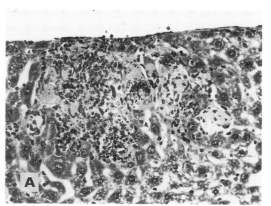

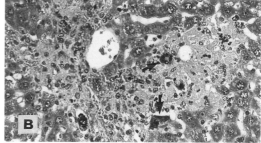

FIG. 1.25—Focal hepatitis in mice with MHV infection. Note prominent debris (**A**) and the syncytia associated with the lesions (*arrows*) in **B.**

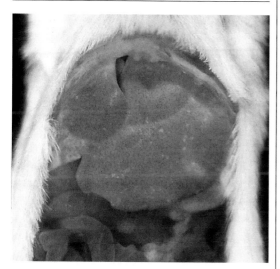

FIG. 1.23—Multifocal hepatitis in BALB/c mouse infected with MHV (JHM strain).

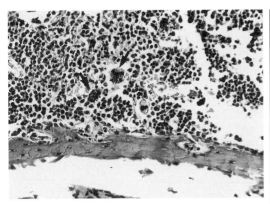

FIG. 1.26—Bone marrow from mouse with MHV infection. There is destruction of hematopoietic cells, and syncytial giant cells (*arrows*) are scattered in the area.

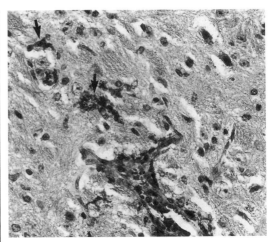

FIG. 1.27—Section of brain, hippocampal region, from a case of MHV-associated encephalitis. There are foci of hypercellularity, with multinucleate giant cell formation (*arrows*).

and lymphoid tissue in spleen, lymph nodes, and gut-associated lymphoid tissue and bone marrow (Fig. 1.26). Neonatally infected mice can have vascular-oriented necrotizing encephalitis with spongiosis and demyelination in the brain stem. Lesions in peritoneum, bone marrow, thymus, and other tissues can be variably present. Mice can develop nasoencephalitis due to localized infection of olfactory nerves, olfactory bulbs, and olfactory tracts of the brain, with meningoencephalitis and demyelination. This pattern of infection occurs regularly after intranasal inoculation of many MHV strains but is a relatively rare event by natural exposure. Hallmark lesions include virus-induced syncytia arising from endothelium, parenchyma, or leukocytes in target organs, including central nervous system (Fig. 1.27). These cells often display nuclear pyknosis, with dense basophilic bodies. Lesions are transient and seldom fully developed in adult immunocompetent mice, but they are fully manifest in immunocompromised mice. In such animals, vascular endothelial syncytia and hematopoietic involvement are particularly apparent. Immunodeficient mice can develop chronic, nodular hepatitis and splenomegaly due to compensatory hematopoiesis. Highly unusual presentations can occur in mice with specific gene defects. Granulomatous serositis, without hepatitis or intestinal lesions, was found in interferon-gamma knockout mice. MHV antigen was present within the serosal macrophages of these mice.

Lesions due to enterotropic MHV depend primarily upon age of the host. Neonatal mice in naive mouse colonies can experience massive outbreaks of high mortality. These mice have segmentally distributed areas of villus attenuation, enterocytic syncytia (balloon cells), and mucosal necrosis (Fig. 1.28). Eosinophilic intracytoplasmic inclusions are present but are not as diagnostic as syncytia. Mesenteric lymph nodes usually contain lymphocytic syncytia, and mesenteric vessels may contain endothelial syncytia. Surviving mice develop compensatory intestinal mucosal hyperplasia. Lesions are most likely to be found in the terminal small intestine, cecum, and ascending colon. Lesions are progressively milder with increasing age at the time of exposure. Adult mice usually have minimal lesions, except for enterocytic syncytia in surface mucosa, particularly in cecum and ascending colon (Fig. 1.29). Immunodeficient mice develop similar but progressive lesions, depending upon age at inoculation. Natural enterotropic MHV infection has been described in adult nude mice with chronic hyperplastic typhlocolitis and mesenteric lymphadenopathy, but other agents, such as *Helicobacter*, may have been involved. More typically, intestinal lesions in immunodeficient mice are remarkably mild with minimal hyperplasia.

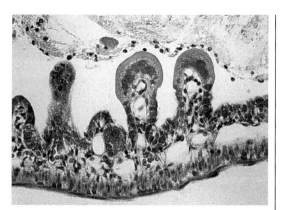

FIG. 1.28—Small intestine of neonatal mouse infected with enterotropic MHV. Villi are markedly attenuated, with prominent multinucleated syncytia.

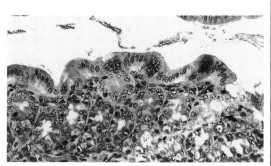

FIG. 1.29—Section of colon from nude mouse with chronic MHV infection. Syncytia are present on the mucosal surface.

Enterotropic MHV strains do not generally disseminate, but hepatitis and encephalitis can occur with some virus strains in certain mouse genotypes.

DIAGNOSIS. Diagnosis during the acute stage of infection can be made by visualization of characteristic lesions with syncytia in target tissues, but clinical signs and lesions can be highly variable for reasons discussed above. Active infection can be confirmed by immunohistochemistry or by virus isolation. Recovered mice may have perivascular lymphocytic infiltrates in the lung and microgranulomas in the liver. In general, respiratory strains of MHV are polytropic and grow in a number of established cell lines in vitro, but enterotropic MHV strains are far more restrictive and fastidious in vitro. Virus in suspect tissue can be confirmed by a variety of bioassay methods, such as MAP testing or infant or nude mouse inoculation. Amplification by passage in immunodeficient mice will increase the likelihood of in vitro isolation from infected tissue. Recently, PCR has been utilized to detect MHV in feces or tissue of infected mice. PCR has equivalent sensitivity as infant mouse bioassays but is more rapid. PCR must be utilized with caution and with adequate controls and appropriate means of verification (sequencing the amplicons), as false-positive results are known to occur with some primer sets. Thus, the practicality of PCR as a universal means for surveillance is limited. Serology is the most useful means of surveillance for retrospective infection in a colony. Seropositive mice are poor candidates for pathology workup, since they are likely to be recovered, but on occasion they can be actively infected with a second strain of virus. Nude mice can develop antibody that can be detected by IFA or ELISA, although their antibody response is unpredictable. There is little merit in attempting to identify MHV strains serologically, since all strains are broadly cross-reactive and antigenic relatedness does not predict virulence or organotropism. *Differential diagnoses* include salmonellosis, Tyzzer's disease, and mousepox in adult mice, as well as reovirus, cytomegalovirus, and adenovirus in infant mice. Mice with enteritis must be differentiated from epizootic diarrhea of infant mice (EDIM), salmonellosis, Tyzzer's disease, and reovirus infection. Demyelinating lesions must be differentiated from those caused by mouse encephalomyelitis virus, LDV in immunosuppressed mice, or polyoma virus in immunodeficient mice.

SIGNIFICANCE. The polytropic potential, ubiquity, and contagiousness of MHV make it the most probable virus to interfere with biological responses of mice and the likelihood of contamination of transplantable tumors and cell lines. A number of research effects have been documented, particularly immunomodulation. Infection of immunodeficient mice or the tumors generated in them, including hybridomas, can be troublesome.

Paramyxoviral Infections

PNEUMONIA VIRUS OF MICE (PVM) INFECTION. PVM was originally discovered following serial blind lung passages in mice, which ultimately produced an agent capable of causing pneumonia. The name PVM does not therefore reflect the natural, avirulent behavior of the virus in mice. PVM is a member of the paramyxovirus family, genus *Pneumovirus,* to which respiratory syncytial viruses also belong. PVM is not antigenically related to these viruses.

EPIZOOTIOLOGY AND PATHOGENESIS. PVM is a highly labile virus with a low degree of contagion, requiring close contact between mice. In spite of its name, PVM naturally infects a variety of rodents, including mice, rats, cotton rats, gerbils, guinea pigs, and rabbits. PVM infection occurs in laboratory rodents throughout the world. Clinical disease caused by natural infections with PVM has never been reported, except in immunodeficient mice. Intranasal inoculation of immunocompetent mice results in bronchiolar desquamation and inflammation, followed by nonsuppurative perivascular and interstitial inflammation, which peaks within 2 wk and undergoes resolution within 3 wk. Despite these experimental results, natural isolates of PVM are typically apathogenic. The low pathogenicity of PVM allows immunodeficient mice to develop progressively severe interstitial pneumonia with wasting syndrome without succumbing acutely. In these mice, PVM antigen is confined to alveolar type II cells and occasionally bronchiolar epithelial cells. SCID mice that were naturally infected with *Pneumocystis carinii,* then inoculated with a normally apathogenic isolate of PVM, developed more severe pneumocystis pneumonia and higher pneumocystis cyst counts, whereas PVM-infected, but Pneumocystis-free, SCID mice survived for 2 mo despite high PVM titers in lung. Thus, PVM-related pneumonia in immunodeficient mice is often complicated by *Pneumocystis,* and vice-versa, since both are common agents in mouse colonies.

PATHOLOGY. Clinical signs of disease and gross lesions are absent in natural infections of immunocompetent mice. Microscopic lesions in intranasally inoculated experimental mice consist of mild necrotizing rhinitis, necrotizing bronchiolitis, and nonsuppurative interstitial pneumonia. Infiltrating leukocytes include neutrophils, but lymphocytes and macrophages predominate.

Residual perivascular infiltrates of lymphocytes and plasma cells can persist for several weeks after virus is cleared. Immunodeficient mice manifest chronic wasting with cyanosis and dyspnea. Lungs are dark, fleshy, and firm and do not collapse. Microscopically, alveolar septa are thickened with edema and infiltrating macrophages and leukocytes, and alveolar spaces are collapsed and filled with fibrin, blood, macrophages, and large polygonal mononuclear cells, representing detached alveolar type II cells (Fig. 1.30).

DIAGNOSIS. Most PVM infections are detected retrospectively by seroconversion. Because PVM is not highly contagious, infection within a colony of mice can be focal, and the number of seropositive mice can be small. Seropositive mice often have mild perivascular lymphoplasmacytic infiltrates. *Differential diagnoses* for pulmonary disease and wasting syndrome in immunodeficient mice include Sendai virus and *Pneumocystis carinii* infections, which also cause progres-

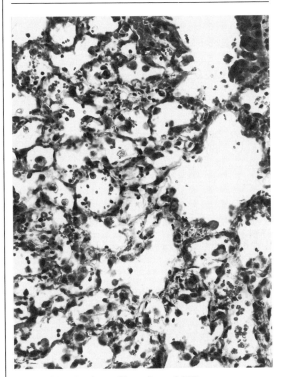

FIG. 1.30—Section of lung from SCID mouse infected with PVM. There is marked alveolitis, characterized by hypercellularity of alveolar septa and mobilization of alveolar macrophages.

sive pulmonary disease. PVM lesions are similar to Sendai viral lesions microscopically, but PVM tends not to induce bronchiolar hypertrophy like Sendai virus and can be differentiated by immunohistochemistry, virus isolation, or MAP testing of suspect tissues. Nude mice do not seroconvert to PVM.

SIGNIFICANCE. PVM appears to have no adverse effect on mice under natural conditions, except in immunodeficient mice. Interspecies transmission may occur.

SENDAI VIRAL INFECTION. Sendai virus is a parainfluenza 1 virus that is closely related to other parainfluenza 1 viruses of human origin. It is named after Sendai, Japan, where it was first isolated from laboratory mice inoculated with human lung suspensions and later isolated from naturally infected mice. In some circles, the host of origin is still controversial.

EPIZOOTIOLOGY AND PATHOGENESIS. Sendai virus is a labile but highly contagious virus that is contact-transmitted by aerosol. In addition to laboratory mice, it is infectious to laboratory rats and hamsters. Guinea pigs seroconvert to Sendai virus, but it is suspected, although not proven, that this is caused by another, related parainfluenza 1 virus. Humans seroconvert to Sendai virus due to infection with related parainfluenza 1 viruses. Sendai virus infects mice throughout the world and is one of the more common infectious disease agents of laboratory mouse populations. It certainly stands out as the virus that is most likely to cause clinical disease in adult, immunocompetent mice. Reports of Sendai virus in mouse colonies in the United States have been rare in recent years, but Sendai virus is still prevalent in Europe and Asia.

Mice develop a descending infection of respiratory epithelium, which is abrogated by a cellmediated immune response that clears the infection, but also generates disease. The level to which the infection extends is determined by mouse genotype–related differences in mucociliary clearance and kinetics of immune response. Certain strains of mice, such as DBA/2, and infant mice (which are immunodeficient) are exquisitely susceptible to severe disease. These animals have a strong but delayed immune response to the virus, allowing infection to extend deep into the lung, but then mount a zealous response that results in severe disease. Other mouse strains, such as B6 mice, often have subclinical infections because of their rapid immune response, which precludes lower respiratory tract infection. Due to waning immune competence, aged mice develop more severe Sendai viral pneumonia. Infection is acute, with no persistent carrier state, except in immunedeficient mice. Sendai virus causes little direct damage to target cells, which include conducting airway epithelium, as well as type II and, to a lesser extent, type I alveolar epithelium. The severe necrotizing and inflammatory lesions typical of this infection are immune-mediated. Peak virus titers occur within 3–6 d, and virus is cleared by 8–12 d. The acute phase of Sendai viral pneumonia occurs in 8–12 d, when immunological attack is under way.

Sendai viral infection is also associated with a number of infectious paraphenomena in mice and rats. It can predispose to the development of bacterial otitis media and interna, as well as precipitate mycoplasma-associated lower respiratory disease in previously subclinically infected mice. Outbreaks of vestibular disease and pneumonia due to *Mycoplasma* or other bacteria can often be associated with recent activity of Sendai virus within the population.

PATHOLOGY. Severely affected mice are dyspneic and have plum-colored consolidation of sharply demarcated foci, anteroventral lung, or entire lung lobes (Fig. 1.31). These consolidated areas may turn gray in surviving mice. Microscopic changes during the acute phase of disease consist of segmental, necrotizing inflammation of nasal and airway epithelium (Fig. 1.32), as well as foci of interstitial pneumonia associated with terminal airways. Infiltrating cells vary with stage of infection but include neutrophils, lymphocytes, and macrophages (Fig. 1.33). Alveolar spaces may be filled with fibrin, leukocytes, and necrotic cells, with atelectasis. Prior to immune-mediated necrosis, bronchiolar epithelium may be hypertrophic and hyperplastic, contain virus-induced syncytia, and possess poorly organized intracytoplasmic eosinophilic inclusions representing accumulation of viral nucleocapsid material.

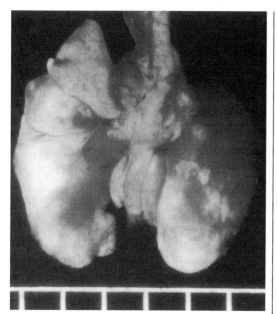

FIG. 1.31—Lungs from DBA mouse infected with Sendai virus. Note the dark areas around the hilus of both lungs consistent with congestion and early consolidation.

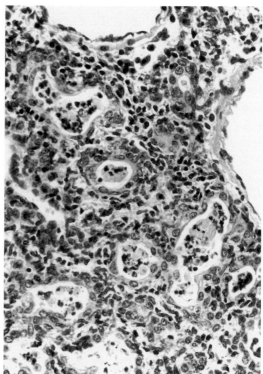

FIG. 1.33—Lung from DBA mouse with Sendai virus infection, illustrating a marked proliferative alveolitis with mononuclear cell infiltration in the interstitial regions. Note the cellular debris within alveoli.

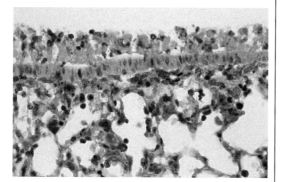

FIG. 1.32—Lung from DBA mouse with Sendai viral infection. Note the acute necrotizing bronchitis with underlying lymphocytic infiltration.

Intranuclear inclusions have been reported in nude mice. These virus-related changes are most apt to be seen in immature or immunologically deficient mice, since they are rapidly obscured by immune-mediated necrosis. During resolution, sloughed airway epithelium is replaced by proliferating hyperplastic epithelium, which may undergo transient but marked nonkeratinizing squamous metaplasia. Alveoli become lined by cuboidal epithelium or filled with metaplastic squamous epithelium. Increased lymphoid cells populate the bronchial tree, adventitia of adjacent blood vessels, and alveolar septa. All of these changes completely resolve by the third or fourth week. Severely affected but surviving mice can have focal alveolar fibrotic scarring (Fig. 1.34).

T-cell immunodeficient mice develop progressive pulmonary consolidation with wasting. Because they cannot mount an effective immune response, necrotizing changes are minimal, and airway epithelium is typically markedly hypertrophic and hyperplastic (Fig. 1.35). The mice develop progressively severe, diffuse alveolitis, similar to progressive PVM pneumonia in immunodeficient mice.

DIAGNOSIS. The clinical and microscopic features of Sendai viral pneumonia in immunocompetent adult mice are diagnostic and can be confirmed by seroconversion, which generally occurs

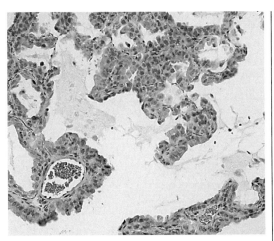

FIG. 1.34—Lung from mouse in the reparative phase postexposure to Sendai virus. Note the cuboidal metaplasia of pneumocytes lining alveolar septa.

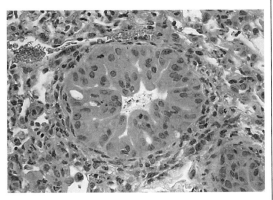

FIG. 1.35—Lung from SCID mouse infected with Sendai virus. Note the marked hypertrophy and hyperplasia of bronchial/bronchiolar epithelial cells that occur in the absence of immune-mediated necrosis.

coincidentally with clinical disease. *Differential diagnoses* include other causes of respiratory disease, such as *Mycoplasma* and *Corynebacterium kutscheri*. Mild respiratory tract lesions can also occur with PVM or MHV. Immunodeficient mice can develop wasting disease with progressive pneumonia, which must be differentiated from pneumonia caused by PVM or *Pneumocystis carinii*. Sendai virus and PVM lesions in nude and SCID mice are similar, although in SCID mice, bronchial and bronchiolar lesions are more extensive with Sendai virus infection (see Pneumonia Virus of Mice [PVM] Infection).

SIGNIFICANCE. Sendai virus can cause overt disease and mortality in genetically susceptible and immune-deficient mice, predispose to bacterial respiratory infections, cause transient infertility, affect the immune response, and delay wound healing. Sendai infections may also alter the incidence of pulmonary neoplasms in experimental carcinogenesis studies. The virus's periodic frequency in mouse facilities and its direct and indirect effects render this agent a major concern.

Picornaviral Infection: Mouse Encephalomyelitis Viral (MEV) Infection; Mouse Polio. MEV is commonly referred to as mouse poliovirus or Theiler's virus, after its initial discoverer, Max Theiler. There are numerous strains of MEV that infect mice, including TO (Theiler's original), GDVII, FA, and DA, among others. Some of these strains have been studied extensively as models for viral encephalitis and demyelination, resulting in emphasis of the neurological disease, which is only rarely a component of natural infection. MEV strains are closely related antigenically, but they can be differentiated by serum neutralization and differ in pathogenicity. MEV is a cardiovirus of the family Picornaviridae and is serologically related to encephalomyocarditis virus (EMC). EMC has a less-selective host range, can infect wild mice, but is not known to infect laboratory mice. MEV and EMC can be differentiated by serum neutralization.

EPIZOOTIOLOGY AND PATHOGENESIS. MEV is largely regarded as a mouse virus, but serum antibody reactivity to MEV has also been detected in sera from rats and guinea pigs. At least one rat agent (MHG) has been isolated from naturally infected rats that is experimentally pathogenic in both rats and mice and is closely related antigenically to the MEV group. Hamsters are susceptible to experimental infection with MEV. MEVs are enteric viruses that induce virtually no adverse intestinal effects. Virus excretion from the intestine is highly variable among mice, but it is often prolonged and intermittent. Transmission is apparently inefficient, often with only a small percentage of seropositive mice within a population. In utero infection does not occur. Infected mice develop a transient viremia that is limited by host immune response. Occasionally, virus gains access to the central nervous system. Vascular endothelial cells appear to serve as a conduit for entry into the brain. Virulent strains of virus, such as GDVII or FA, induce severe fatal encephalitis, regardless of route of inoculation. Most other strains are less virulent and can cause biphasic disease, consisting initially of acute poliomyelitis, followed later by late-onset demyelinating disease. Virus can persist in the central nervous system for over a year, but virus titers decline markedly, and residual virus is restricted to white matter, where it replicates in macrophages, leukocytes, astrocytes, and oligo-dendrocytes. Immune attack on infected white matter results in demyelination and motor dys-function, with gait disorders, tremors, ataxia, extensor spasm, urinary incontinence, and other signs. The neurological manifestations of MEV are grossly overemphasized because of their experimental value. Under natural conditions, usually only 1 in 1000–10,000 infected immuno-competent mice develops clinical signs of the nervous system, and this is invariably flaccid paralysis associated with the acute, poliomyelitis phase. However, in immunodeficient mice, expo-sure to MEV may result in high morbidity and mortality.

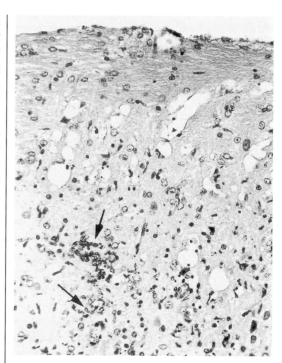

FIG. 1.36—Cervical spinal cord from young adult mouse with acute mouse encephalomyelitis virus infection. There is a nonsuppurative poliomyelitis, with focal microgliosis (*arrows*).

PATHOLOGY. Lesions are not present in the intes-tine. During the acute central nervous system (poliomyelitis) phase, the virus attacks neurons and glia of the hippocampus, thalamus, brain stem, and spinal cord. Neuronolysis, neuronopha-gia, microgliosis, nonsuppurative meningitis, and perivasculitis are typical changes seen microscop-ically (Fig. 1.36). These changes are most preva-lent in the brain stem and ventral horns of the spinal cord. In the experimentally produced dis-ease, during the demyelinating phase, foci of demyelination are present in the white matter of the spinal cord, brain stem, and cerebellum. Demyelinating lesions are not a likely component of natural infections. Acute myositis and focal myocarditis were observed in mice inoculated intraperitoneally with the DA strain of MEV, emphasizing the polytropism of the virus.

The naturally occurring disease is much more devastating in immunodeficient mice, with high morbidity and mortality. In SCID mice, lesions are characterized by marked vacuolation and enlargement of affected neurons, particularly in the brain stem and ventral horn region of the spinal cord (Fig. 1.37). Vacuolation of adjacent astrocytes and oligodendrocytes, with minimal to no inflammatory cell response, are other features of the disease in SCID mice. Similar changes have been observed in the gray and white matter of nude mice postinoculation with MEV.

DIAGNOSIS. MEV infection is usually diagnosed serologically. Seropositive mice should be con-sidered to be actively infected with virus. Diag-nosis can also be achieved by neurological signs and lesions in the small percentage of infected mice that develop central nervous system disease. MEV is not very contagious, requiring large sam-ple sizes to accurately detect infection within a colony. Because of its low contagious potential, MEV can be eliminated from a colony of immunocompetent mice over time by test-and-

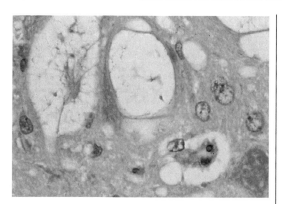

FIG. 1.37—Sections of brain from SCID mouse naturally infected with mouse encephalomyelitis virus. Note the marked cytoplasmic vacuolation of neurons and cells in the neuropil. (Courtesy N. Rozengurt)

slaughter at the cage level, if appropriate safeguards are taken against contamination of mice in adjacent cages. *Differential diagnoses* for neurological disease include trauma, neoplasia, otitis, MHV, LDV and in immunodeficient mice, polyoma virus.

SIGNIFICANCE. MEV has been an inadvertent contaminant of clinical specimens, including mouse serum, inoculated into mice. Most strains of MEV display low virulence and are thus nearly innocuous. Extensive and distinctive lesions have been observed in the CNS of immunodeficient mice postexposure to MEV. The increasing usage of immunodeficient mice and the common occurrence of MEV in mouse colonies will likely result in more frequent observance of this syndrome. Selected strains of MEV have been used to produce demyelinating disease in laboratory mice.

Reoviral Infection. The name reovirus (respiratory enteric orphan virus) was proposed for a group of viruses associated with respiratory and enteric infections in humans. Reoviruses have since been isolated from a wide variety of mammals, birds, reptiles, insects, and other species. Mammalian reoviruses are divided into three serotypes, based upon hemagglutination inhibition and neutralization tests. They are commonly referred to as reovirus 1, reovirus 2, and reovirus 3, although they actually represent a spectrum of viruses that are antigenically cross-reactive by other serological methods. Reovirus 3 has been associated with natural infections in laboratory rodents and as a pathogen in mice. A number of reovirus 3 strains have been studied experimentally.

EPIZOOTIOLOGY AND PATHOGENESIS. Reovirus seroconversion is a frequent finding in mouse colonies. Reoviruses are transmitted by the orofecal and aerosol routes, as well as through arthropod vectors. Transmission among mice seems to occur primarily by direct contact among young mice. Contact transmission between adult mice is inefficient. Mice of all ages are susceptible to experimental infection by a variety of routes, but only mice infected as neonates develop disease. Following oral inoculation of neonatal mice, virus enters through the upper intestine and disseminates to multiple organs. Experimental studies have shown that reovirus 1 replicates in intestinal epithelium, but reovirus 3 does not. Reovirus 3 replication occurs in multiple organs of neonatal mice in the absence of significant lesions, until around day 10–12, when mice become clinically ill and develop lesions in multiple tissues, followed by recovery. This suggests an immune-mediated mechanism for development of lesions during the process of recovery, but this mechanism has not been defined. Pups can develop steatorrhea secondary to liver and pancreatic lesions. Pups born to immune dams do not develop disease.

PATHOLOGY. Disease and lesions occur only in infant mice from colonies previously unexposed to reovirus. At around 2 wk of age, mice can be runted, jaundiced, and uncoordinated and have matted hair (caused by steatorrhea). Surviving mice can remain runted and have transient dorsal alopecia. The most significant microscopic lesion is acute diffuse encephalitis that has a vascular distribution. Mice also develop focal necrotizing myocarditis, variable necrosis of lymphoid tissue, focal necrotizing hepatitis, portal hepatitis, acinar pancreatitis, and sialodacryoadenitis.

DIAGNOSIS. Reovirus infection is usually documented in a mouse population serologically, in the absence of obvious disease, although outbreaks of disease can occur among neonates.

Virus can be isolated from infected tissues, or antigen can be visualized by immunohistochemistry. Lesions are nonspecific. *Differential diagnoses* of neonatal disease with steatorrhea include mouse hepatitis virus, epizootic diarrhea of infant mice (EDIM) virus, and salmonella infections.

SIGNIFICANCE. Reoviruses are not generally significant pathogens in laboratory mice. Many of the lesions attributed to reovirus in the historic literature are likely due to other murine viruses, such as MHV. Reoviruses frequently contaminate transplantable tumors.

Rotaviral Infection: Epizootic Diarrhea of Infant Mice (EDIM). EDIM virus is a group A rotavirus that shares a common inner capsid antigen with other group A rotaviruses of humans, nonhuman primates, cattle, sheep, horses, pigs, dogs, cats, turkeys, chickens, and rabbits. Each of these viruses is relatively host-specific, but interspecies infection can be shown experimentally with high doses of virus. Rotaviruses belong to the family Reoviridae but are distinct from reovirus (above).

EPIZOOTIOLOGY AND PATHOGENESIS. EDIM virus is highly contagious and prevalent among both laboratory and wild mice, but disease manifestations are relatively rare. Rotaviruses are shed copiously in feces, and transmission is by the orofecal route. Clinical disease ranges from inapparent to severe, depending primarily upon age. All ages of mice are susceptible to infection; however, disease is limited to mice less than 2 wk of age. Virus selectively infects terminally differentiated enterocytes of villi and surface mucosa of the small and large intestine, respectively. These cells are most plentiful and widespread in the neonatal bowel and diminish in number, distribution, and degree of terminal differentiation as mucosal proliferative kinetics accelerate with acquisition of intestinal microflora. Infection does take place in older mice, but the target cell population is limited in number and to small intestine. Thus, functional disturbances tend not to be noted in older mice. Regardless of age at infection, recovery from diarrhea occurs at 14–17 d of age. Active immunity plays a role in resolu-tion of infection but not susceptibility. Infection of SCID mice follows the same age-related pattern of disease as immunocompetent mice. Both humoral and cellular immunity are involved in resolution of infection, with persistent shedding of virus in B-cell–deficient mice. Pups born to and suckling immune dams are protected against EDIM during their period of disease susceptibility. Typically, clinical signs of EDIM occur in naive breeding populations, but once infection is enzootic within the colony, EDIM disease is no longer apparent, although EDIM virus remains. The duration of EDIM virus infection in an individual mouse is variable, depending upon the mouse genotype.

PATHOLOGY. Infection is often clinically silent, but clinically affected mice can be runted and pot-bellied, with loose, mustard-colored feces staining the perineum. Steatorrhea with oily hair may also be apparent. The bowel is flaccid and distended with fluid and gas, but mice continue to suckle. Some deaths can occur due to obstipation caused by fecal caking around the anus. In infant mice, EDIM virus causes hydropic change and vacuolation of enterocytes at the tips of villi and large intestinal surface mucosa. Some nuclei may be pyknotic. Acidophilic intracytoplasmic inclusions have been described but are not diagnostic. In addition, the lamina propria is edematous and lymphatics are dilated, although inflammation is minimal. These changes are difficult to discern under the best of circumstances and are not apparent in mice older than 14 d of age. Remarkably, mice can manifest significant diarrhea with minimal microscopic lesions. Malabsorption and osmotic diarrhea, with overgrowth of *Escherichia coli,* appear to be major components of the disease process.

DIAGNOSIS. EDIM can be diagnosed presumptively on the basis of age, clinical signs, and lesions. *Differential diagnoses* include enterotropic MHV, MAV, reovirus, salmonellosis, and Tyzzer's disease. Vacuolation and intracytoplasmic inclusions must be differentiated from absorption vacuoles of the neonatal enterocytic apical tubular system that occur in the distal small intestine and contain solitary eosinophilic globules. Definitive diagnosis can be achieved by electron microscopy of intestinal mucosa or feces. Rotavirus antigen can be detected in feces by ELISA. This can be accomplished with commercially available rotavirus diagnostic kits, but false-positive reactions can occur with certain mouse diets. Careful controls are therefore advised. Serology for EDIM virus antibody is useful for surveillance and retrospective confirmation of infection.

SIGNIFICANCE. EDIM can be clinically significant, but its effects are transient. Clinical signs of EDIM disappear rapidly, once the virus has become enzootic within the breeding colony and pups are protected by maternal antibody through their early age of susceptibility. Infected infant mice often have severe transient thymic necrosis, probably stress-related, that can potentially cause immunologic aberrations. EDIM has been studied as an animal model for rotaviral infections in other species.

Retroviral Infection. Although retroviruses play a significant role in disease pathogenesis in mice, they are seldom considered in the same way as other viruses. This is because most of them are incorporated in the mouse genome as proviruses and transmitted genetically as inherited Mendelian characteristics. In many respects, they represent specific characteristics of different mouse strains. They are known as the murine leukemia viruses (MuLVs) and the murine mammary tumor viruses (MMTV-s). This section provides a brief summary of retroviruses in mice; the major lesions they induce (tumors) are described in the Neoplasms sections of this chapter. MMTV long terminal repeats (LTRs) are now commonly incorporated as transgenes for tissue-specific promoters in genetically engineered mice.

EPIZOOTIOLOGY AND PATHOGENESIS. MuLVs possess two replication strategies. Endogenous MuLVs are integrated into the host genome (provirus) and depend upon their chromosomally integrated state for transmission. Exogenous MuLVs behave like conventional, transmissible viruses. Both endogenous and exogenous MuLVs are genetically, morphologically, and antigenically homologous. All wild and laboratory mice harbor multiple copies of endogenous MuLV in their genomes. Today, exogenous MuLVs occur only in wild mice, but several laboratory MuLV isolates (Gross, Friend, Moloney, and Rauscher LVs) obtained in the early years of tumor biology are more closely related to exogenous MuLV. Endogenous MuLVs have integrated into the mouse genome randomly, and once integrated, they have remained stable. No two endogenous genomes are known to be located in the same chromosomal site among different mouse strains. Although endogenous MuLVs are transmitted genetically, they are expressed in somatic cells, and this expression is mouse strain–, age-, and tissue-specific. When expressed, they have a tendency for recombination or transduction with host genes to produce new variants that produce disease. Endogenous MuLVs have three categories of host-range polymorphism. Ecotropic viruses can infect mouse cells but not cells of other species. Xenotropic viruses can infect cells of other species but not those of mice. Amphotropic (or polytropic) viruses can infect both mouse and xenogeneic cells. Tropism is also restricted to tissue types and mouse genotype. For example, B (BALB)-ecotropic viruses can only infect mice that are homozygous at the Fv-1^b locus and N (NIH)-ecotropic viruses at the Fv-1^n locus.

The significance of these characteristics is best provided by example. AKR mice develop a high prevalence of thymic lymphomas at 6–12 mo of age. They carry an endogenous nononcogenic ectotropic MuLV that is expressed in multiple tissues at birth. They also carry an endogenous nononcogenic xenotropic MuLV that is expressed in thymus at 6 mo of age. At 6 mo, the concomitant expression of these viruses allows recombinant viruses to be expressed that are polytropic and oncogenic, capable of infecting cells and causing neoplasia. BALB/c mice develop a late-onset lymphoma. They carry nononcogenic, N-ecotropic, and xenotropic viruses that form recombinants that are oncogenic and B-ecotropic, resulting in disease. Each mouse genotype possesses its own set of circumstances, with varying degrees of MuLV expression and disease that are mouse strain–, age-, tissue-, and cell type–specific. Not all outcomes are neoplastic. MuLV reintegrations can occur randomly in both germ cells and somatic cells, with varied results, including most often no effect, or altered coat color and consistency, central nervous system disease (see Arteriviral Infection: Lactate Dehydrogenase–Elevating Viral [LDV] Infection), premature graying, etc. Another group of viruses, called murine sarcoma viruses (MuSV), have undergone similar recombination and/or transduction, incorporating portions of the host genome. These viruses are missing components of their own genome and are unable to replicate on their own (defective) without the assistance of another, non-defective MuLV (helper) virus.

Likewise, MMTVs are both endogenous and exogenous in nature. Exogenous MMTV is transmitted in the milk, and to a lesser extent saliva, as a conventional virus, inducing mammary neoplasia. This virus, which is known as the MMTV-S (standard), the "milk factor," or the Bittner agent, has been eliminated from modern mouse populations by cesarean rederivation or foster nursing, unless intentionally maintained for experimental purposes. All strains of laboratory mice possess endogenous MMTV provirus in their genome, and expression of disease (mammary tumors) is virus-, mouse strain–, age-, and cell type-specific. Disease expression is not always mammary. A common "lymphoma" of SJL mice, a follicular center (B-cell) polyclonal lymphoproliferative disease, is due to expression of *Mtv-29* (an MMTV provirus in SJL mice) superantigen that stimulates T cells to produce cytokines, which in turn stimulate B cells and B-cell lymphomas. Endogenous MMTVs, because of their intimate association with the genome, are now given gene designations according to standardized mouse gene nomenclature (*Mtv-1, -2, -8, -11*, etc.). MMTV-S is not included in this nomenclature, because it is not a provirus. The MuLVs are less well characterized and have not benefited from such classification.

PATHOLOGY. See the Neoplasms sections of this chapter.

DIAGNOSIS. Diagnosis of MuLV or MMTV is not necessary, since all mice are infected or have at least some provirus sequences within their genome. Electron microscopic examination of normal and neoplastic mouse tissues frequently reveals C-type (MuLV), A-type, and B-type (MMTV) particles as an incidental finding. Certain specific disease entities are known to be caused by these viruses, but the relationship of retroviruses to disease expression in mice is complex and largely undefined.

SIGNIFICANCE. MuLVs and MMTVs are an integral and important part of mouse biology and inseparable features of the laboratory mouse. They become significant when they induce life-limiting disease and are valuable models for retrovirus pathogenesis.

BIBLIOGRAPHY FOR VIRAL INFECTIONS

Adenoviral Infection

Barthold, S.W. 1997. Adenovirus infection, intestine, mouse, rat. In *Monographs on Pathology of Laboratory Animals: Digestive System*, ed. T.C. Jones et al., pp. 389–92. New York: Springer-Verlag.

Cohen, B.J., and deGroot, F.G. 1976. Adenovirus infection in athymic (nude) mice. Lab. Anim. Sci. 26:955–56.

Ginder, D.R. 1964. Increased susceptibility of mice infected with mouse adenovirus to *Escherichia coli*–induced pyelonephritis. J. Exp. Med. 120:1117–28.

Guida, J.D., et al. 1995. Mouse adenovirus type 1 causes a fatal hemorrhagic encephalomyelitis in adult C57BL/6 but not BALB/c mice. J. Virol. 69:7674–81.

Hartley, J.W., and Rowe, W.P. 1960. A new mouse adenovirus apparently related to the adenovirus group. Virology 11:645–47.

Hashimoto, K., et al. 1966. An adenovirus isolated from feces of mice. I. Isolation and identification. Jap. J. Microbiol. 10:115–25.

Heck, F.C., Jr., et al. 1972. Pathogenesis of experimentally-produced mouse adenovirus infection in mice. Am. J. Vet. Res. 33:841–46.

Kring, S.C., et al. 1995. Susceptibility and signs associated with mouse adenovirus type 1 infection of adult outbred Swiss mice. J. Virol. 69:8084–88.

Leuthans, T.N., and Wagner, J.E. 1983. A naturally occurring intestinal mouse adenovirus infection associated with negative serologic findings. Lab. Anim. Sci. 33:270–72.

Lussier, G., et al. 1987. Serological relationship between mouse adenovirus strains FL and K87. Lab. Anim. Sci. 37:55–57.

Margolis, G., et al. 1974. Experimental adenovirus infection of the mouse adrenal gland. I. Light microscopic observations. Am. J. Pathol. 75:363–72.

Parker, J.C., et al. 1966. Prevalence of viruses in mouse colonies. Natl. Cancer Inst. Monogr. 20:25–36.

Pirofski, L., et al. 1991. Murine adenovirus infection of SCID mice induces hepatic lesions that resemble human Reye's syndrome. Proc. Natl. Acad. Sci. 88:4358–62.

Smith, A.L., and Barthold, S.W. 1987. Factors influencing susceptibility of laboratory rodents to infection with mouse adenovirus strains K87 and FL. Arch. Virol. 95:143–48.

Sugiyama, T., et al. 1967. An adenovirus isolated from the feces of mice. II. Experimental infection. Jap. J. Microbiol. 11:33–42.

Takeuchi, A., and Hashimoto, K. 1976. Electron microscope study of experimental enteric adenovirus infection in mice. Infect. Immun. 13:569–80.

Vander Veen, J., and Mes, A. 1974. Serological classification of two mouse adenoviruses. Arch. Virol. 45:386–87.

———. 1973. Experimental infection with mouse adenovirus in adult mice. Arch. Virol. 42:235–41.

Wigand, R., et al. 1977. Biological and biophysical characteristics of mouse adenovirus, strain FL. Arch. Virol. 54:131–42.

Winters, A.L., and Brown, H.K. 1980. Duodenal lesions associated with adenovirus infection in athymic "nude" mice. Proc. Soc. Exp. Biol. Med. 164:280–86.

Mouse Thymic Viral (MTV) Infection

Athanassious, R., et al. 1993. Ultrastructural study of mouse thymus virus replication. Acta Virol. 37:175–80.

Cohen, P.L., et al. 1975. Immunologic effects of neonatal infection with mouse thymic virus. J. Immunol. 115:706–10.

Cross, S.S., et al. 1979. Biology of mouse thymic virus, a herpesvirus of mice, and the antigenic relationship to mouse cytomegalovirus. Infect. Immun. 26:1186–95.

Cross, S.S., et al. 1976. Neonatal infection with mouse thymic virus. Differential effects on T cells mediating the graft-versus-host reaction. J. Immunol. 117:635–38.

Morse, H.C., III, et al. 1976. Neonatal infection with mouse thymic virus: Effects on cells regulating the antibody response to type III pneumococcal polysaccharide. J. Immunol. 116:1613–17.

Morse, S.S. 1987. Mouse thymic necrosis virus: A novel murine lymophotropic agent. Lab. Anim. Sci. 37:717–25.

Morse, S.S., and Valinsky, J.E. 1989. Mouse thymic virus (mTLV): A mammalian herpesvirus cytolytic for CD4+ (L3T4+) T lymphocytes. J. Exp. Med. 169:591–96.

Morse, S.S., et al. 1999. Virus and autoimmunity: Induction of autoimmune disease in mice by mouse T lymphotropic virus (MTLV) destroying CD4+ T cells. J. Immunol. 162:5309–16.

Parker, J.C., et al. 1973. Classification of mouse thymic virus as a herpesvirus. Infect. Immun. 7:305–8.

Rowe, W.P., and Capps, W.I. 1961. A new mouse virus causing necrosis of the thymus in newborn mice. J. Exp. Med. 113:831–44.

Wood, B.A., et al. 1981. Neonatal infection with mouse thymic virus: Spleen and lymph node necrosis. J. Gen. Virol. 57:139–47.

Mouse Cytomegalovirus (MCMV) Infection

Brautigam, A.R., et al. 1979. Pathogenesis of murine cytomegalovirus infection: The macrophage as a permissive cell for cytomegalovirus infection, replication and latency. J. Gen. Virol. 44:349–59.

Brody, A.R., and Craighead, J.E. 1974. Pathogenesis of pulmonary cytomegalovirus infection in immunosuppressed mice. J. Infect. Dis. 129:677–89.

Chen, H.C., and Cover, C.E. 1988. Spontaneous disseminated cytomegalic inclusion disease in an ageing laboratory mouse. J. Comp. Pathol. 98:489–93.

Cheung, K.-S., et al. 1980. Murine cytomegalovirus: Detection of latent infection by nucleic acid hybridization technique. Infect. Immun. 27:851–54.

Dangler, C.A., et al. 1995. Murine cytomegalovirus-associated arteritis. Vet. Pathol. 32:127–33.

Gardner, M.B., et al. 1974. Induction of disseminated virulent cytomegalovirus infection by immunosuppression of naturally chronically infected wild mice. Infect. Immun. 10:966–69.

Hamilton, J.R., and Overall, J.C., Jr. 1978. Synergistic infection with murine cytomegalovirus and *Pseudomonas aeruginosa* in mice. J. Infect. Dis. 137:775–82.

Hudson, J.B. 1979. The murine cytomegalovirus as a model for the study of viral pathogenesis and persistent infections. Arch. Virol. 62:1–29.

Jordan, M.C. 1978. Interstitial pneumonia and subclinical infection after intranasal inoculation of murine cytomegalovirus. Infect. Immun. 21:275–80.

Klotman, M.E., et al. 1990. Detection of mouse cytomegalovirus nucleic acid in latently infected mice by in vitro enzymatic amplification. J. Infect. Dis. 161:220–25.

Lussier, G. 1975. Murine cytomegalovirus (MCMV). Adv. Vet. Comp. Med. 10:223–47.

McCordock, H.A., and Smith, M.G. 1963. The visceral lesions produced in mice by the salivary gland virus of mice. J. Exp. Med. 63:303–10.

Mannini, A., and Medearis, D.N., Jr. 1961. Mouse salivary gland virus infections. Am. J. Hyg. 73:329–43.

Medearia, D.N., Jr. 1964. Mouse cytomegalovirus infection: Attempts to produce intrauterine infections. Am. J. Hyg. 80:113–20.

Mims, C.A., and Gould, J. 1979. Infection of salivary glands, kidneys, adrenals, ovaries and epithelia by murine cytomegalovirus. J. Med. Microbiol. 12:113–22.

Olding, L.B., et al. 1976. Pathogenesis of cytomegalovirus infection: Distribution of viral products, immune complexes and autoimmunity during latent murine infection. J. Gen. Virol. 33:267–80.

Osborne, J.E. 1982. Cytomegalovirus and other herpesviruses. In *The Mouse in Biomedical Research. II. Diseases,* ed. H.L. Foster, et al., pp. 267–92. New York: Academic.

Reynolds, R.P., et al. 1993. Experimental murine cytomegalovirus infection in severe combined immunodeficient mice. Lab. Anim. Sci. 43:291–95.

K Viral Infection

Fisher, E.R., and Kilham, L. 1953. Pathology of a pneumotropic virus recovered from C3H mice carrying the Bittner milk agent. Arch. Pathol. 55:14–19.

Greenlee, J.E. 1981. Effect of host age on experimental K virus infection in mice. Infect. Immun. 33:297–303.

———. 1979. Pathogenesis of K virus infection in newborn mice. Infect. Immun. 26:705–13.

Kilham, L., and Murphy, H.W. 1953. A pneumotropic virus isolated from C3H mice carrying the Bittner milk agent. Proc. Soc. Exp. Biol. Med. 82:133–37.

Kraus, G.E., et al. 1968. Uber Vorkommen, Diagnostik und Pathologie latenter Infektionen mit Kilhamvirus in Laboratoriums Mausen. Arch. Exp. Veterinaermed. 22:1203–10.

Margolis, G., et al. 1976. Oxygen tension and the selective tropism of K virus for mouse pulmonary endothelium. Am. Rev. Respir. Dis. 114:4–51.

Mokhtarian, F., and Shah, K.V. 1983. Pathogenesis of K papovavirus infection in athymic nude mice. Infect. Immun. 41:434–36.

———. 1980. Role of antibody response in recovery from K papovavirus infection in mice. Infect. Immun. 29:1169–79.

Polyoma Viral Infection

Allison, A.C. 1980. Immune responses to polyoma virus and polyoma virus–induced tumors. In *Viral Oncology,* ed. G. Klein, pp. 481–87. New York: Raven.

Buffet, R.F., and Levinthal, J.D. 1962. Polyoma virus infection in mice. Arch. Pathol. 74:513–26.

Dawe, C.J. 1979. Tumors of the salivary and lachrymal glands, nasal fossa and maxillary sinuses. In *Pathology of Tumours in Laboratory Animals. II. Tumours of the Mouse,* ed. V.S. Turusov. Lyon: IARC Scientific Publications.

Dubensky, T.W., et al. 1984. Detection of DNA and RNA virus genomes in organ systems of whole mice: Patterns of mouse organ infection by polyomavirus. J. Virol. 50:779–83.

Eddy, B.E. 1982. Polyomavirus. In *The Mouse in Biomedical Research. II. Diseases,* ed. H.L. Foster et al., pp. 293–311. New York: Academic.

Gross, L. 1970. The parotid tumor (polyoma) virus. In *Oncogenic Viruses,* ed. L. Gross, 2d ed., pp. 651–750. London: Pergamon.

McCance, D.J., and Mims, C.A. 1979. Reactivation of polyomavirus in kidneys of persistently infected mice during pregnancy. Infect. Immun. 25:998–1002.

McCance, D.J., et al. 1983. A paralytic disease in nude mice associated with polyoma virus infection. J. Gen. Virol. 64:57–67.

Rowe, W.P. 1961. The epidemiology of mouse polyoma virus infection. Bacteriol. Rev. 25:18–31.

Sebesteny, A., et al. 1980. Demyelination and wasting associated with polyomavirus infection in nude (nu/nu) mice. Lab. Anim. Sci. 14:337–45.

Stanton, M.F., et al. 1959. Oncogenic effect of tissue culture preparations of polyomavirus on fetal mice. J. Natl. Cancer Inst. 23:1441–75.

Stewart, S.E. 1960. The polyoma virus. Adv. Virus Res. 7:61–90.

Vandeputte, M., et al. 1974. Induction of polyoma tumors in athymic nude mice. Int. J. Cancer. 14:445–50.

Parvoviral Infection

Besselsen, D.G., et al. 1996. Molecular characterization of newly recognized rodent parvoviruses. J. Gen. Virol. 77:899–911.

Bonnard, G.D., et al. 1976. Immunosuppressive activity of a subline of the mouse EL-4 lymphoma. Evidence for minute virus of mice causing the inhibition. J. Exp. Med. 143:187–205.

Collins, M.J., Jr., and Parker, J.C. 1972. Murine virus contaminants of leukemia viruses and transplantable tumors. J. Natl. Cancer Inst. 49:1139–43.

Crawford, L.V. 1966. A minute virus of mice. Virology 29:605–12.

Hanson, G.M., et al. 1999. Humoral immunity and protection of mice challenged with homotypic or heterotypic parvovirus. Lab. Anim. Sci. 49:380–84.

Harris, R.E., et al. 1974. Erythrocyte association and interferon production of minute virus of mice. Proc. Soc. Exp. Biol. Med. 145:1288–92.

Jacoby, R.O., et al. 1996. Special topic overview: Rodent parvovirus infections. Lab. Anim. Sci. 46:370–80

Kilham, L., and Margolis, G. 1971. Fetal infections of hamsters, rats, and mice induced with the minute virus of mice (MVM). Teratology 4:43–62.

———. 1970. Pathogenicity of minute virus of mice (MVM) for rats, mice and hamsters. Proc. Soc. Exp. Biol. Med. 133:1447–52.

McKisic, M.D., et al. 1998. Mouse parvovirus infection potentiates allogeneic skin graft rejection and induces syngeneic graft rejection. Transplantation 65:1436–46.

McKisic, M.D., et al. 1996. Mouse parvovirus infection potentiates rejection of tumor allografts and modulates T cell effector functions. Transplantation 61:292–99.

McMaster, G.K., et al. 1981. Characterization of an immunosuppressive parvovirus related to minute virus of mice. J. Virol. 38:317–26.

Parker, J.C., et al. 1970. Minute virus of mice. II. Prevalence, epidemiology, and occurrence as a contaminant of transplanted tumors. J. Natl. Cancer Inst. 45:305–10.

Ramairez, J.C., et al. 1996. Parvovirus minute virus of mice strain I multiplication and pathogenesis in the newborn mouse brain are restricted to proliferative areas and to migratory cerebellar young neurons. J. Virol. 70:8109–16.

Riley, L.K., et al. 1996. Expression of recombinant parvovirus NS1 protein by a baculovirus and application to serologic testing of rodents. J. Clin. Microbiol. 34:440–44.

Segovia, J.C., et al. 1999. Severe leukopenia and dysregulated erythropoiesis in SCID mice persistently infected with the parvovirus minute virus of mice. J. Virol. 73:1774–84.

Smith, A.L., et al. 1988. Acute and chronic effects of minute virus of mice (MVM) infection of neonatal inbred mice. Lab. Anim. Sci. 38:488.

Poxviral Infection

Allen, A.M., et al. 1981. Pathology and diagnosis of mousepox. Lab. Anim. Sci. 31:599–608.

Bhatt, P.N., and Jacoby, R.O. 1987a. Effect of vaccination on the clinical response, pathogenesis and transmission of mousepox. Lab. Anim. Sci. 37:610–14.

———. 1987b. Mousepox in inbred mice innately resistant or susceptible to lethal infection with ectromelia virus. 1. Clinical responses. Lab. Anim. Sci. 37:11–15.

Dick, E.J., et al. 1996. Mousepox outbreak in a laboratory mouse colony. Lab. Anim. Sci. 46:602–11.

Fenner, F. 1981. Mousepox (infectious ectromelia): Past, present, and future. Lab. Anim. Sci. 31:553–59.

Lipman, N.S., et al. 1999. Mousepox: A threat to US mouse colonies. Lab. Anim. Sci. 49:229.

Marchal, J. 1930. Infectious ectromelia: A hitherto undescribed virus disease of mice. J. Pathol. Bacteriol. 33:713–18.

New, A.E. 1981. Ectromelia (mousepox) in the United States. Proceedings of seminar, 31st annual meeting, American Association for Laboratory Animal Science. Lab. Anim. Sci. 31:549–622.

Wallace, G.W., and Buller, R.M.L. 1985. Kinetics of ectromelia virus (mousepox) transmission and clinical response in C57BL/6J, BALB/cByJ and AKR/J inbred mice. Lab. Anim. Sci. 35:41–46.

Arenaviral Infection

Buchmeier, M.J. 1980. The virology and immunobiology of lymphocytic choriomeningitis virus infection. Adv. Immunol. 30:275–331.

Butz, E.A., and Southern, P.J. 1994. Lymphocytic choriomeningitis virus-induced immune dysfunction: Induction of and recovery from T-cell anergy in acutely infected mice. J. Virol. 68:8477–80.

Christofferson, P.J., et al. 1976. Immunological unresponsiveness of nude mice to LCM virus infection. Acta Pathol. Microbiol. Scand. {C} 84:520–23.

Dalton, A.J., et al. 1968. Morphological and cytochemical studies on lymphocytic choriomeningitis virus. J. Virol. 2:1465–78.

Dykewicz, C.A., et al. 1992. Lymphocytic choriomeningitis outbreak associated with nude mice in a research institute. J. Am. Med. Assoc. 267:1349–53.

Findlay, G.M., and Stern, R.O. 1936. Pathological changes due to infection with the virus of lymphocytic choriomeningitis. J. Pathol. Bacteriol. 43:327–38.

Gossmann, J., et al. 1995. Murine hepatitis caused by lymphocytic choriomeningitis virus II. Cells involved in pathogenesis. Lab. Invest. 72:559–70.

Homberger, F.R., et al. 1995. Enzyme-linked immunosorbent assay for detection of antibody to lymphocytic choriomeningitis virus in mouse sera, with recombinant nucleoprotein as antigen. Lab. Anim. Sci. 45:493–96.

Lilly, R.D., and Armstrong, C. 1945. Pathology of lymphocytic choriomeningitis in mice. Arch. Pathol. 40:141–52.

Oldstone, M.B.A., and Dixon, F.J. 1970. Pathogenesis with persistent lymphocytic choriomeningitis viral infection. II. Relationship of tissue injury in chronic lymphocytic choriomeningitis disease. J. Exp. Med. 131:1–19.

———. 1969. Pathogenesis of chronic disease associated with persistent lymphocytic choriomeningitis viral infection. I. Relationship of antibody production to disease in neonatally infected mice. J. Exp. Med. 129:483–505.

Oldstone, M.B.A., et al. 1982. Virus-induced alterations in homeostasis: Alterations in differentiated functions of infected cells in vivo. Science 218:1125–27.

Rai, S., et al. 1996. Murine infection with lymphocytic choriomeningitis virus following gastric inoculation. J. Virol. 70:7213–18.

Thomsen, A.R., et al. 1982. Lymphocytic choriomeningitis virus-induced immunosuppression: Evidence for viral interference with T-cell maturation. Infect. Immun. 37:981–86.

Traub, E. 1936. The epidemiology of lymphocytic choriomeningitis in white mice. J. Exp. Med. 64:183–200.

vander Zeijst, B.A.M., et al. 1983. Persistent infection of some standard cell lines by lymphocytic choriomeningitis virus: Transmission of infection by an intracellular agent. J. Virol. 48:249–61.

Volkert, M., and Lundstedt, C. 1971. Tolerance and immunity to the lymphocytic choriomeningitis virus. Ann. N.Y. Acad. Sci. 181:183–95.

Arteriviral Infection

Anderson, G.W., et al. 1995a. C58 and AKR mice of all ages develop motor neuron disease after lactate dehydrogenase-elevating virus infection but only if antiviral immune responses are blocked by chemical or genetic means or as a result of old age. J. Neurovirol. 1:244–52.

———. 1995b. Infection of central nervous system cells by ecotropic murine leukemia virus in C58 and AKR mice and in in utero-infected CE/J mice predisposes mice to paralytic infection by lactate dehydrogenase-elevating virus. J. Virol. 69:308–19.

———. 1995c. Lactate dehydrogenase-elevating virus replication persists in liver, spleen, lymph node, and testis tissues and results in accumulation of viral RNA in germinal centers, concomitant with polyclonal activation of B cells. J. Virol. 69:5177–85.

Cafruny, W.A., et al. 1999. Regulation of immune complexes during infection of mice with lactate dehydrogenase-elevating virus: studies with interferon-gamma gene knockout and tolerant mice. Viral Immunol. 12:163–73.

Chen, Z., et al. 1999. Selective antibody neutralization prevents neuropathogenic lactate dehydrogenaase-elevating virus from causing paralytic disease in immunocompetent mice. J. Neurovirol. 5:200–208.

Goto, K., et al. 1998. Detection and typing of lactate dehydrogenase-elevating virus RNA from transplantable tumors, mouse livers, and cell lines, using polymerase chain reaction. Lab. Anim. Sci. 48:99–102.

Nicklas, W., et al. 1993. Contamination of transplantable tumors, cell lines, and monoclonal antibodies with rodent viruses. Lab. Anim. Sci. 43:296–300.

Rowson, K.E.K., and Mahy, B.W.J. 1975. Lactic dehydrogenase virus. Virol. Monogr. 13:1–121.

Snodgrass, M.J., et al. 1972. Changes induced by lactic dehydrogenase virus in thymus and thymus-dependent areas of lymphatic tissue. J. Immunol. 108:877–92.

Van den Broek, M.F., et al. 1997. Lactate dehydrogenase-elevating virus (LDV): Lifelong coexistence of virus and LDV-specific immunity. J. Immunol. 159:1585–88.

Coronaviral Infection

Bailey, O.T., et al. 1949. A murine virus (JHM) causing disseminated encephalomyelitis with extensive destruction of myelin. II. Pathology. J. Exp. Med. 90:195–221.

Barthold, S.W. 1988. Olfactory neural pathway in mouse hepatitis virus nasoencephalitis. Acta Neuropathol. 76:502–6.

———. 1986. Mouse hepatitis virus biology and epizootiology. In Viral and Mycoplasmal Infections of Laboratory Rodents: Effects on Biomedical Research, ed. P.N. Bhatt et al., pp. 571–601. New York: Academic.

———. 1985a. Mouse hepatitis virus infection, liver, mouse. In Monographs on Pathology of Laboratory Animals. III. Digestive System, ed. T.C. Jones et al., pp. 134–39. New York: Springer-Verlag.

———. 1985b. Research complications and state of knowledge of rodent coronaviruses. In Complications of Viral and Mycoplasmal Infections in Rodents to Toxicology Research and Testing, ed. T.E. Hamm, pp. 53–89. Washington, D.C.: Hemisphere.

Barthold, S.W., and Smith, A.L. 1989. Virus strain specificity of challenge immunity to coronavirus. Arch. Virol. 104:187–96.

———. 1987. Response of genetically susceptible and resistant mice to intranasal inoculation with mouse hepatitis virus. Virus Res. 7:225–39.

Barthold, S.W., et al. 1985. Enterotropic mouse hepatitis virus infection in nude mice. Lab. Anim. Sci. 35:613–18.

———. 1983. Enterotropic coronovirus (MHV) in mice: Influence of host age and strain on infection and disease. Lab. Anim. Sci. 43:276–84.

———. 1982. Epizootic coronaviral typhlocolitis in suckling mice. Lab. Anim. Sci. 32:376–83.

Biggers, D.C., et al. 1964. Lethal intestinal virus in mice (LIVIM): An important new model for study of the response of the intestinal mucosa to injury. Am. J. Pathol. 45:413–27.

Boorman, G.A., et al. 1982. Peritoneal macrophage alterations caused by naturally occurring mouse hepatitis virus. Am. J. Pathol. 106:11–117.

Carrano, V.A., et al. 1984. Alteration of viral respiratory infections in mice by prior infection with mouse hepatitis virus. Lab. Anim. Sci. 34:573–76.

Croy, B.A., and Percy, D.H. 1993. Viral hepatitis in scid mice. Lab. Anim. Sci. 43:193–94.

France, M.P., et al. 1999. Granulomatous peritonitis and pleuritis in interferon gamma gene knockout mice naturally infected with mouse hepatitis virus. Aust. Vet. J. 77:600–604.

Gustafsson, E., et al. 1996. Maternal antibodies protect immunoglobulin deficient mice from mouse hepatitis virus (MHV)-associated wasting syndrome. Am. J. Reprod. Immunol. 36:33–39.

Homberger, F.R., and Barthold, S.W. 1992. Passively acquired challenge immunity to enterotropic coronavirus in mice. Archiv. Virol. 126:35–43.

Homberger, F.R., et al. 1998. Prevalence of enterotropic and polytropic mouse hepatitis virus in enzootically infected mouse colonies. Lab. Anim. Sci. 48:50–54.

———. 1992. Duration and strain-specificity of immunity to enterotropic mouse hepatitis virus. Lab. Anim. Sci. 42:347–51.

———. 1991. Detection of rodent coronaviruses in tissues and cell cultures using polymerase chain reaction. J. Clin. Microbiol. 29:2789–93.

Pneumonia Virus of Mice (PVM) Infection

Berthiaume, L., et al. 1974. Comparative structure, morphogenesis and biological characteristics of the respiratory syncytial (RS) virus and the pneumonia virus of mice (PVM). Arch. Virusforsch. 45:39–51.

Bray, M.V., et al. 1993. Exacerbation of Pneumocystis carinii pneumonia in immunodeficient (scid) mice by concurrent infection with pneumovirus. Infect. Immun. 61:1586–88.

Carthew, P., and Sparrow, S. 1980a. A comparison in germ-free mice of the pathogenesis of Sendai virus and mouse pneumonia virus infections. J. Pathol. 130:153–58.

———. 1980b. Persistence of pneumonia virus of mice and Sendai virus in germ-free (nu/nu) mice. Br. J. Pathol. 61:172–75.

Horsfall, F.L., and Curnen, E.C. 1946. Studies on pneumonia virus of mice (PVM). II. Immunological evidence of latent infection with the virus in numerous mammalian species. J. Exp. Med. 83:43–64.

Horsfall, F.L., and Hahn, R.G. 1940. A latent virus in normal mice capable of producing pneumonia in its natural host. J. Exp. Med. 71:391–408.

Richter, C.B., et al. 1988. Fatal pneumonia with terminal emaciation in nude mice caused by pneumonia virus of mice. Lab. Anim. Sci. 38:255–61.

Weir, E.C., et al. 1988. Respiratory disease and wasting in athymic mice infected with pneumonia virus of mice. Lab. Anim. Sci. 38:133–37.

Sendai Viral Infection

Brownstein, D.G. 1996. Sendai virus infection, lung, mouse, and rat. In *Monographs on Pathology of Laboratory Animals: Respiratory System,* ed. T.C. Jones et al., pp. 308–16. New York: Springer-Verlag.

———. 1987. Resistance/susceptibility to lethal Sendai virus infection genetically linked to a mucociliary transport polymorphism. J. Virol. 61:1670–71.

———. 1986. Sendai virus. In *Viral and Mycoplasmal Infections of Laboratory Rodents: Effects on Biomedical Research,* ed. P.N. Bhatt et al., pp. 37–61. New York: Academic.

Brownstein, D.G., and Weir, E.C. 1987. Immunostimulation in mice infected with Sendai virus. Am. J. Vet. Res. 48:1692–98.

Brownstein, D.G., and Winkler, S. 1986. Genetic resistance to lethal Sendai virus pneumonia: Virus replication and interferon production in C57/6J and DBA/2J mice. Lab. Anim. Sci. 36:126–29.

Brownstein, D.G., et al. 1981. Sendai virus infection in genetically resistant and susceptible mice. Am. J. Pathol. 105:156–63.

Ishida, N., and Homma, M. 1978. Sendai virus. Adv. Virus Res. 23:349–83.

Jacoby, R.O., et al. 1994. Sendai viral pneumonia in aged BALB/c mice. Exp. Gerontol. 29:89–100.

Jakob, G. 1981. Interactions between Sendai virus and bacterial pathogens in the murine lung: A review. Lab. Anim. Sci. 31:170–77.

Kay, M.M.B. 1978. Long term subclinical effects of parainfluenza (Sendai) infection on immune cells of aging mice. Proc. Soc. Exp. Biol. Med. 158:326–31.

Kenyon, A.J. 1983. Delayed wound healing in mice associated with viral alteration of macrophages. Am. J. Vet. Res. 44:652–56.

Parker, J.C., and Richter, C.B. 1982. Viral diseases of the respiratory system. In *The Mouse in Biomedical Research. II. Diseases,* ed. H.L. Foster et al., pp. 109–34. New York: Academic.

Peck, R.M., et al. 1983. Influence of Sendai virus on carcinogenesis in strain A mice. Lab. Anim. Sci. 33:154–56.

Roberts, N.J. 1982. Different effects of influenza virus, respiratory syncytial virus, and Sendai virus on human lymphocytes and macrophages. Infect. Immun. 35:1142–46.

Picornaviral Infection

Abzug, M.J., et al. 1989. Demonstration of a barrier to transplacental passage of murine enteroviruses in late gestation. J. Infect. Dis. 159:761–65.

Brownstein, D., et al. 1989. Duration and patterns of transmission of Theiler's mouse encephalomyelitis virus infection. Lab. Anim. Sci. 39:299–301.

Gomez, R.M., et al. 1996. Theiler's mouse encephalomyelitis virus-induced cardiac and skeletal muscle disease. J. Virol. 70:8926–33.

Jacoby, R.O. 1988. Encephalomyelitis, Theiler's virus, mouse. In *Monographs on Pathology of Laboratory Animals: Nervous System,* ed. T.C. Jones et al., pp. 175–79. New York: Springer-Verlag.

Lipton, H.L., and Rozhon, E.J. 1986. The Theiler's murine encephalomyelitis viruses. In *Viral and Mycoplasmal Infections of Laboratory Animals: Effects on Biomedical Research,* ed. P.N. Bhatt et al., pp. 253–75. New York: Academic.

Pevear, D.C., et al. 1987. Analysis of the complete nucleotide sequence of the picornavirus Theiler's mouse encephalomyelitis virus indicated that it is closely related to cardioviruses. J. Virol. 61:1507–16.

Rozengurt, N. and Sanchez, S. 1993. A spontaneous outbreak of Theiler's encephalomyelitis in a colony of severe combined immunodeficient mice in the UK. Lab. Anim. 27:229–34.

———. 1992. Vacuolar neuronal degeneration in the ventral horns of SCID mice in naturally occurring Theiler's encephalomyelitis. J. Comp. Path. 107:389–98.

Zurbriggen, A., and Fujinami, R.S. 1988. Theiler's virus infection in nude mice: Viral RNA in vascular endothelial cells. J. Virol. 62:3589–96.

Reoviral Infection

Barthold, S.W., et al. 1993. Infectivity, disease patterns, and serologic profiles of reovirus serotypes 1, 2, and 3 in infant and weanling mice. Lab. Anim. Sci. 43:425–30.

Bennette, J.G., et al. 1967a. Characteristics of a newborn runt disease induced by neonatal infection with an oncolytic strain of reovirus type 3 (REO3MH). I. Pathological investigations in rats and mice. Br. J. Exp. Pathol. 48:251–66.

———. 1967b. Characteristics of a newborn runt disease induced by neonatal infection with an oncolytic strain of reovirus type 3 (REO3MH). II. Immunological aspects of the disease in mice. Br. J. Exp. Pathol. 48:267–84.

Branski, D., et al. 1980. Reovirus type 3 infection in a suckling mouse: The effects on pancreatic structure and enzyme content. Pediatr. Res. 14:8–11.

Cook, I. 1963. Reovirus type 3 infection in laboratory mice. Aust. J. Exp. Biol. 41:651–59.

Joske, R.A., et al. 1966. Murine infection with reovirus. IV. Late chronic disease and the induction of lymphoma after reovirus type 3 infection. Br. J. Exp. Pathol. 47:337–46.

Papadimitriou, J.M. 1968. The biliary tract in acute murine reovirus 3 infection. Light and electron microscopic study. Am. J. Pathol. 52:595–611.

Papadimitriou, J.M., and Walters, M.N.-I. 1967. Studies on the exocrine pancreas. II. Ultrastructural investigation of reovirus pancreatitis. Am. J. Pathol. 51:387–403.

Phillips, P.A., et al. 1969. Chronic obstructive jaundice induced by reovirus type 3 in weanling mice. Pathology 1:193–203.

Stanley, N.F. 1974. The reovirus murine models. Prog. Med. Virol. 18:257–72.

Stanley, N.F., et al. 1966. The association of murine lymphoma with reovirus type 3 infection. Proc. Soc. Exp. Biol. Med. 121:90–93.

———. 1964. Murine infections with reovirus: II. The chronic disease following reovirus type 3 infection. Br. J. Exp. Pathol. 45:142–49.

———. 1954. Studies on the hepatoencephalomyelitis virus (HEV). Aust. J. Exp. Biol. 32:543–62.

———. 1953. Studies on the pathogenesis of a hitherto undescribed virus (hepatoencephalomyelitis) producing unusual symptoms in suckling mice. Aust. J. Exp. Biol. 31:147–59.

Tyler, K.L., and Fields, B.N. 1986. Reovirus infection in laboratory rodents. In *Viral and Mycoplasmal Infections of Laboratory Rodents: Effects on Biomedical Research,* ed. P.N. Bhatt et al., pp. 277–303. New York: Academic.

Walters, M.N.-I., et al. 1963. Murine infection with reovirus. I. Pathology of the acute phase. Br. J. Exp. Pathol. 44:427–36.

Rotaviral Infection

Barthold, S.W. 1997. Murine rotavirus infection, mouse. In *Monographs on Pathology of Laboratory Animals: Digestive System,* ed. T.C. Jones et al., pp. 384–89. New York: Springer-Verlag.

Coelho, K.I.R., et al. 1981. Pathology of rotavirus infection in suckling mice: A study by conventional histology, immunofluorescence, and scanning electron microscopy. Ultrastructural Pathol. 2:59–80.

McNeal, M.M., et al. 1995. Effector functions of antibody and CD8+ cells in resolution of infection and protection against reinfection in mice. Virology 214:387–97.

Riepenhoff-Talty, M., et al. 1987a. Persistent rotavirus infection in mice with severe combined immunodeficiency. J. Virol. 61:3345–48.

———. 1987b. Rotavirus infection in mice: Pathogenesis and immunity. Adv. Exp. Med. Biol. 216:1015–23.

Sheridan, J.F., and Vonderfecht, S. 1986. Mouse rotavirus. In *Viral and Mycoplasmal Infections of Laboratory Rodents: Effects on Biomedical Research,* ed. P.N. Bhatt et al., pp. 217–43. New York: Academic.

Retroviral Infection

Bentvelzen, P., and Hilgers, J. 1980. Murine mammary tumor virus. In *Viral Oncology,* ed. G. Klein, pp. 311–55. New York: Raven.

Kozak, C., et al. 1987. A standardized nomenclature for endogenous mouse mammary tumor viruses. J. Virol. 61:1651–54.

Lilly, F., and Mayer, A. 1980. Genetic aspects of murine type-C viruses and their hosts in oncogenesis. In *Viral Oncology,* ed. G. Klein, pp. 89–108. New York: Raven.

Morse, H.C., III, and Hartley, J.W. 1986. Murine leukemia viruses. In *Viral and Mycoplasmal Infections of Laboratory Rodents: Effects on Biomedical Research,* ed. P.N. Bhatt et al., pp. 349–88. New York: Academic.

Shih, T.Y., and Scolnick, E.M. 1980. Molecular biology of mammalian sarcoma viruses. In *Viral Oncology,* ed. G. Klein, pp. 135–60. New York: Raven.

Zhang, D.J., et al. 1996. Control of endogenous mouse mammary tumor virus superantigen expression in SJL lymphomas by a promoter within the env region. J. Immunol. 157:3510–17.

General Bibliography

Collins, M.J., and Parker, J.C. 1972. Murine virus contaminants of leukemia viruses and transplantable tumors. J. Natl. Cancer Inst. 49:1139–43.

Nicklas, W., et al. 1993. Contamination of transplantable tumors, cell lines, and monoclonal antibodies with rodent viruses. Lab. Anim. Sci. 43:296–300.

BACTERIAL INFECTIONS

BACTERIAL ENTERIC INFECTION

***Citrobacter rodentium* Infection.** *Citrobacter rodentium* causes a syndrome in mice called transmissible murine colonic hyperplasia (TMCH). It has also been termed hyperplastic colitis, catarrhal enterocolitis, and colitis cystica. Unlike most *Citrobacter* spp., pathogenic mouse isolates are nonflagellated and nonmotile. Isolates from different outbreaks possess similar sugar fermentation and other biochemical profiles, but minor differences exist. The causative agent was formerly classified as *C. freundii* but has been reclassified as *C. rodentium.*

EPIZOOTIOLOGY AND PATHOGENESIS. TMCH has been reported in the United States and Europe. Under normal circumstances, *C. rodentium* is not found in mice; its source of introduction into mouse colonies is presumably through contaminated food or bedding. The organism spreads slowly among mice, requiring direct contact or fecal contamination. Following oral inoculation, *C. rodentium* transiently colonizes the small intestine, then selectively colonizes the cecum and colon within 4 d. The bacteria intimately attach in large number to surface mucosa of the descending colon, displacing other aerobic bacteria. Bacterial attachment is mediated by a bacterially derived epithelial transmembrane protein called the translocated intimin receptor, similar to enteropathogenic *Escherichia coli*. Through undefined mechanisms, bacterial colonization elicits an intense mucosal epithelial hyperplasia. A partial explanation is that *C. rodentium*, like murine *Helicobacter*, induces a highly Th1-polarized immune response, with production of IL-12, gamma interferon, and tumor necrosis factor alpha in the lamina propria, resulting in a large increase in the epithelial mitogen, keratinocyte growth factor. As hyperplastic cells migrate to the surface, they displace infected cells, which are exfoliated from the surface. Peak hyperplastic response occurs within 2–3 wk, at which point the causative agent can no longer be isolated from the colon. Clinical signs are most prominent at this interval. Young mice and certain genotypes tend to develop secondary inflammatory and ulcerative lesions in the hyperplastic mucosa. In the ensuing weeks, lesions regress. During regression, excessive goblet cell differentiation and cryptal cysts can develop. By 2 mo, the mucosa appears normal. There is no known carrier state, and recovered mice are refractory to reinfection.

PATHOLOGY. Affected mice can be runted, lose weight, and have sticky, unformed feces that smear the cage walls. Rectal prolapse often occurs. Careful examination of the bowel will reveal a contracted, thickened, opaque, descending colon devoid of feces. Lesions can extend into the transverse colon. The cecum is also frequently but variably involved. During the early stages of infection, the brush border of surface mucosa of affected bowel is heavily colonized by a carpet of intimately attached cocco-bacillary bacteria. As the lesion progresses, these infected cells are pushed aside by uninfected, hyperplastic epithelium, with retention of cells at the extrusion zones. Crypts are elongated and lined by immature basophilic, mitotically active cells (Fig. 1.38). Inflammation and erosion can also occur, especially in infant mice or mice of certain genotypes. As the hyperplasia regresses, cells can undergo differentiation into excessive numbers of goblet cells, and crypts can become distended

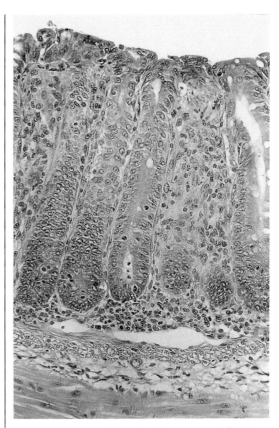

FIG. 1.38—Descending colon from mouse infected with *Citrobacter rodentium.* Note the marked hyperplasia of crypt epithelium with retention of cells on the surface.

with mucin and cellular debris. Once regression is complete, the mucosa returns to normal.

DIAGNOSIS. The causative agent is often absent when clinical signs are most apparent. Infection can be localized to the descending colon, and only a small percentage of mice in the population may be infected because of its low contagiousness. Isolation is enhanced by culturing feces or descending colon from multiple mice in the early stages of infection. *Citrobacter* can be readily isolated on MacConkey agar. Most *Citrobacter* spp. do not utilize lactose, but pathogenic mouse isolates readily ferment lactose and thus resemble *Escherichia coli* on MacConkey agar. An effective way of screening *C. rodentium* from *E. coli* isolates is plating colonies on Malonate agar containing 0.5% lactose. *Citrobacter* will form blue colonies, since it utilizes Malonate and *E. coli* does not. Other differences include nonmotility and lack of indole production. *Differential diagnoses* include other agents that cause enteritis in the mouse, including rotavirus, coronavirus, adenovirus, and reovirus in young mice and *Salmonella* and *Clostridium piliforme* in older mice. Rectal prolapse is frequently associated with TMCH but can also occur spontaneously or in association with enteritis of other causes, particularly *Helicobacter* infections in immunodeficient mice. Hyperplastic colitis has been observed in nude mice chronically infected with enterotropic MHV.

SIGNIFICANCE. *C. rodentium* infections are rare, and infection is transient but can cause low mortality, permanent rectal prolapse, and runting. TMCH represents a possible complication in certain types of research, such as carcinogenesis studies.

Escherichia coli Infection: Coliform Typhlocolitis.
E. coli is a common gut organism in mice that has rarely been considered to be a primary pathogen in this species. A syndrome resembling *Citrobacter rodentium* and *Helicobacter*–associated colonic hyperplasia in immunodeficient mice has been associated with an atypical, non–lactose-fermenting *E. coli.*

EPIZOOTIOLOGY AND PATHOGENESIS. In published reports, large intestinal hyperplastic lesions were observed primarily in young adult triple-deficient N:NIH(s)(homozygous for *nu, xid, bg*) and to a lesser extent double-deficient mice. Other immunocompetent and partially deficient mice were infected without significant hyperplastic lesions. Bacteria were located in the gut lumen and intracellularly within enterocytes. This syndrome has also been observed in SCID mice. The presence of *Helicobacter* in these mice was not determined, as *Helicobacter* was an unrecognized pathogen at the time. Nevertheless, these outbreaks are associated with this unusual, invasive, and non–lactose-fermenting *E. coli,* but its primary role as a pathogen remains to be determined.

PATHOLOGY. Mice are depressed, with perianal fecal staining. Gross necropsy findings are lim-

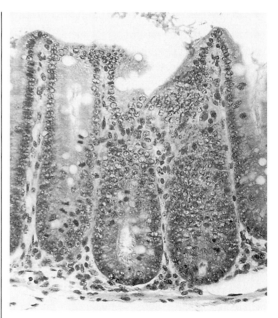

FIG. 1.39—Hyperplastic typhlitis due to *Escherichia coli* infection in SCID mouse. There is marked hyperplasia of enterocytes lining crypts.

ited to mild to moderate thickening of segments of colon or cecum and occasional blood-tinged feces. Microscopic findings consist of mucosal hyperplasia in one or all segments of colon, with variable inflammation and erosion (Fig. 1.39). *E. coli* are present in the gut lumen, attached to the surface and within enterocytes of superficial mucosa of both small and large intestine.

DIAGNOSIS. Segmental hyperplastic lesions in the colon and cecum of immunodeficient mice and isolation of atypical *E. coli* are required in order to confirm the diagnosis. The causative agent is non–lactose-fermenting, an unusual feature of *E. coli. Differential diagnoses* must include hyperplastic typhlocolitis caused by *C. rodentium* (which ferments lactose and is pathogenic in immunocompetent mice), *Helicobacter,* and enterotropic MHV in immunodeficient mice. Unlike *C. rodentium,* which invariably affects descending colon, *E. coli* lesions are segmental and usually affect other portions of the colon.

SIGNIFICANCE. This organism can potentially cause significant illness in immunodeficient mice but is nonpathogenic in other mice.

***Clostridium perfringens* Infection: Necrotizing Enteritis.** Sporadic cases of necrotizing enteritis have been observed in SPF mice that died during the postweaning period. The small intestines of affected animals were dilated and contained blood-stained fluid contents. In affected regions of the small and large intestine, there were fibrinous exudation and effacement of the normal architecture. Large numbers of gram-positive bacilli were present in the exudates, and *C. perfringens* was isolated consistently from the intestinal contents. In one outbreak of diarrhea with mortality in adult germ-free BALB/c mice associated with *C. perfringens* infections, the intestines were distended with dark fluid contents and gas, and inflammatory lesions were present in intestine, lung, and uterus. Lesions also occur in the cecum, and the mucosa of recovering mice may be hyperplastic. It appears that under certain circumstances *C. perfringens* can produce disease with mortality in laboratory mice. The organism is a relatively common inhabitant of the murine intestinal tract and a strict anaerobe. When *C. perfringens* is isolated from filtering organs at necropsy, care must be taken to ensure that it is the primary pathogen and not a contaminant or postmortem invader. Differential diagnosis must include Tyzzer's disease and (in the recovery phase) causes of hyperplastic enteritides (*Citrobacter, Helicobacter, E. coli,* etc.).

***Clostridium piliforme* Infection: Tyzzer's Disease.** Tyzzer's disease was first recognized and characterized by Ernest Tyzzer in 1917 (see the discussion of Tyzzer's disease in Chap. 6). He described an epizootic that decimated a colony of Japanese waltzing mice. The organism is now recognized to produce disease in wide variety of other species, including rats, gerbils, hamsters, guinea pigs, and rabbits. *C. piliforme* infects a wide range of species, but some isolates may have a more limited host range. For decades, the causative agent was called *Bacillus piliformis*. However, based on 16S rRNA sequence analysis, it is now recognized to be a member of the genus *Clostridium* and classified as *C. piliforme*. The organism is a spore-forming, gram-negative, filamentous bacterium that propagates only in living cells. In the laboratory, *C. piliforme* can be grown in the yolk sac of embryonated eggs or in cell culture.

EPIZOOTIOLOGY AND PATHOGENESIS. Shed in the feces, the organism can survive in the sporulated state in contaminated bedding for at least 1 yr. Exposure is considered to be primarily by ingestion, although intrauterine transmission has been produced experimentally in mice inoculated intravenously with *C. piliforme*. Based on serological assessment, up to 80% or more of clinically normal mice from known infected colonies may have detectable antibodies to the organism. Outbreaks of Tyzzer's disease in mice are usually characterized by low morbidity and high mortality in affected animals. Mouse strain, age, and immune status are factors in susceptibility to the disease. For example, DBA/2 mice are susceptible, and B6 mice are resistant to Tyzzer's disease. Depletion of NK cells in resistant adult B6 mice, but not DBA mice, rendered them more susceptible, and neutrophil depletion rendered both juvenile DBA and B6 mice more susceptible to disease. Macrophage depletion did not appear to influence susceptibility to disease. Infected DBA and B6 mice develop elevations in IL-12, and neutralization of IL-12 renders infected mice more susceptible to disease. Disease resistance also appears to be due, at least in part, to B-lymphocyte function. T-cell–deficient nude mice were shown to be as resistant to the disease as immunocompetent mice. However, in a more recent report of a spontaneous outbreak of Tyzzer's disease in a colony of nude mice, homozygous *nu/nu* mice were particularly susceptible with high mortality compared with heterozygous *nu/+* mice. The isolate proved to be the first toxigenic isolate recovered from mice. The cytotoxin may have contributed to the severity of disease in this outbreak. In outbreaks of Tyzzer's disease, predisposing factors include overcrowding, poor sanitation, and experimental procedures that may compromise the immune response. Sudden death and diarrhea may occur. Typically, the organism invades intestinal mucosal epithelium and disseminates to other organs, particularly liver and heart.

PATHOLOGY. Miliary pale foci up to 5 mm in diameter are usually visible throughout the parenchyma of the liver, but foci can be large and umbilicated in immunodeficient mice. The intestine can be moderately congested. Lesions are

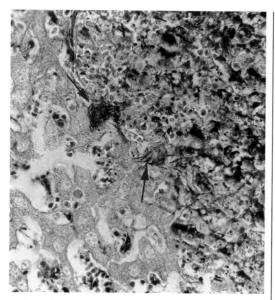

FIG. 1.40—Focus of hepatitis in spontaneous case of Tyzzer's disease stained with the silver impregnation method. Bacilli (*arrows*) are present in the cytoplasm of hepatocytes at the periphery of the lesion.

characterized by multifocal coagulation to caseation hepatic necrosis, with polymorphonuclear leukocyte infiltration. Segmental necrotizing lesions can be present in the terminal ileum and cecum. Foci of necrosis are frequently evident in the mesenteric lymph nodes, and focal myocardial lesions have been observed in experimentally inoculated animals. In tissue sections stained with the Warthin-Starry, Giemsa, or PAS, typical intracytoplasmic bundles of bacilli are usually readily seen in enterocytes and hepatocytes adjacent to necrotic foci (Fig. 1.40).

DIAGNOSIS. The diagnosis of Tyzzer's disease can be confirmed by demonstration of the intracellular bacilli in tissue sections, using the appropriate stains. The typical bacilli may also be visualized in impression smears prepared from liver lesions and stained using the Giemsa method. Serologic assays are available and utilize whole bacterial lysates, prepared from cell-cultured bacteria, as antigen. *C. piliforme* can be isolated in vitro by inoculation of mouse or rat liver cell line cultures. PCR amplification of *C. piliforme*–specific sequences of ribosomal DNA can also be used. *Differential diagnoses* include diseases such as MHV infection, mousepox, salmonellosis, pseudomoniasis, corynebacteriosis, and infections with *Helicobacter* spp.

SIGNIFICANCE. In confirmed outbreaks of Tyzzer's disease, investigations should include a review of husbandry and sanitation practices and possible sources of the infection, including wild mice or other subclinically infected species in the facility. The wide species range of this pathogen, including nonhuman primates and, recently, an HIV-1–infected human, suggest that *C. piliforme* should be considered a zoonotic agent for immunocompromised individuals.

***Helicobacter* spp. Infections.** *Helicobacter* spp. have emerged as a major new group of gastrointestinal pathogens in a number of species, which now inconvertibly include mice. *Helicobacter* spp. are microaerobic, curved to spiral rods with variable numbers of flagella. Each species has a somewhat distinctive electron microscopic appearance. *Helicobacter* spp. are not new to mice, but they have been validated as true pathogens since the early 1990s, due not only to the otherwise pathogen-free status of many colonies but also largely to the rapid growth of genetically engineered immunodeficient mice. Mice are host to *H. hepaticus, H. bilis, H. muridarum, H. rodentium, H. typhlonicus,* and *Flexispira rappini,* which is probably a *Helicobacter* sp. Other species are likely to be added to this list as they are isolated and characterized. *H. hepaticus* and *H. bilis* have received the most attention, because they appear to be most frequently associated with disease in mice.

EPIZOOTIOLOGY AND PATHOGENESIS. In 1992, a bacterium was found by silver staining of livers from mice with hepatitis and from older mice with an increased prevalence of hepatocellular tumors. The agent was shortly thereafter isolated, characterized, and named *H. hepaticus*. Additional studies demonstrated that mouse genotype was pivotal in expression of disease during infection. A, SCID, and C3H/He mice were found to be susceptible to hepatitis and neoplasia, whereas B6 and B6C3F1 mice were disease-resistant. Studies indicate that multiple genes are involved in genetic susceptibility/resistance to the disease. Hepatic lesions are more common in males than females, and the incidence of identifiable disease is increased in mice 6 mo of age or older. Because of awareness of *H. hepaticus, H. bilis* was discovered from bile, livers, and intestines of aged mice with chronic hepatitis. Although original descriptions of *H. hepaticus* included intestinal lesions in SCID mice, the association of *H. hepaticus* with proliferative colitis and rectal prolapse was not confirmed until 2 yr later in SCID and nude mice. Large bowel inflammation has also been reported in some immunocompetent genotypes of mice infected with *H. hepaticus,* including A and C3H/He mice. Natural outbreaks of bowel disease in immunodeficient mice have been associated with *H. hepaticus, H. bilis, H. rodentium, H. typhlonicus,* or (often) mixed infections. Based upon limited surveys, these agents appear to be widespread in academic mouse colonies but are rapidly being eliminated in commercial colonies.

Mice are likely exposed to the organism through ingestion of contaminated feces, and *Helicobacter* spp. are readily transmitted by contaminated bedding. In the liver, *H. hepaticus* and *H. bilis* localize in the biliary system and will persist indefinitely within the bile canaliculi. The pathogenesis of hepatitis and hepatocellular tumors is unknown, but hepatotoxins or autoimmunity to heat shock protein 70 are suspected. Pathogenesis of typhlocolitis, which has marked inflammatory and hyperplastic features, has been extensively studied in mice with selective immune deficiencies. It has been proposed that *Helicobacter* infection induces a highly Th1-polarized mucosal immune response, with production of IL-12, gamma interferon, and tumor necrosis factor alpha in the lamina propria, resulting in expression of the epithelial mitogen, keratinocyte growth factor. This hypothesis does not explain the florid mucosal inflammation and hyperplasia that are seen in SCID and Rag1 knockout mice, which lack T cells.

PATHOLOGY. Hepatic lesions are quite variable. If present, they consist of randomly scattered white foci up to 4 mm in diameter. Early lesions may be confined to one or more lobes of the liver, with focal necrosis and mixed leukocytic infil-

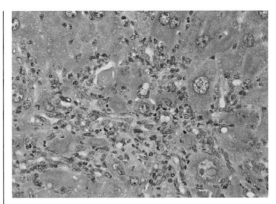

FIG. 1.41—Liver from mouse infected with *Helicobacter hepaticus* with focal necrotizing hepatitis.

trates (Fig. 1.41). As disease progresses, more lobes of the liver become involved. Within a few months, there is marked hypertrophy and hyperplasia of cells lining bile ductules (oval cells) and increased mitotic activity among hepatocytes. There may be prominent ductule formation extending from the portal regions with piecemeal necrosis of hepatocytes. Cellular infiltrates around the biliary system consist primarily of lymphocytes and plasma cells. Changes progress to a different pattern in mice infected for several months. Hepatocytomegaly, postnecrotic fibrosis, lipofuscinlike pigment in Kupffer cells, extensive hyperplasia of bile ductules, peribiliary lymphoid nodule formation, and cholangitis can be prominent at this stage of the disease (Fig. 1.42). In the typical cases of chronic hepatitis, the elongated, helical microorganisms are best demonstrated

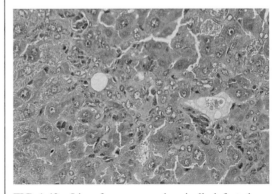

FIG. 1.42—Liver from mouse chronically infected with *Helicobacter hepaticus*. Note the hepatocytomegaly with hyperplasia of bile ductules.

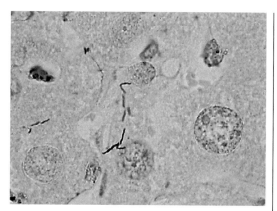

FIG. 1.43—Liver from mouse infected with *Helicobacter hepaticus* stained with the Steiner stain depicting characteristic *Helicobacter* organisms within bile canaliculi.

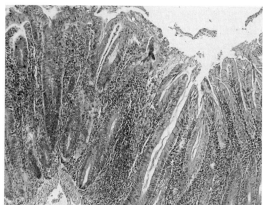

FIG. 1.44—Section of colon from MRL lpr (immunodeficient) mouse chronically infected with *Helicobacter hepaticus*. There is marked mucosal hyperplasia, with mononuclear cell infiltration in the lamina propria.

within biliary canaliculi using the Steiner silver impregnation staining method (Fig. 1.43). Selected strains of mice, such as A mice, develop chronic hepatitis that gives rise to an increased incidence and earlier onset of hepatocellular tumors with similar morphologic features to those occurring spontaneously.

Typhlitis, colitis, and rectal prolapse are typical clinical and pathologic findings observed in a variety of immunodeficient mice. Clinical signs include wasting (often accompanied by pneumocystosis or other forms of pneumonia in immunodeficient mice) and mortality. Feces can be unformed, sticky, mucoid, or hemorrhagic. Rectal prolapse is a frequent, but nonspecific, sign of colitis in mice (it can occur in uninfected mice without bowel inflammation). The prolapsed mucosa is usually eroded and markedly inflamed and hyperplastic. These changes are nonspecific and due to the trauma of prolapse and may not be directly associated with *Helicobacter* spp. Thus, other areas of bowel should be examined to confirm the diagnosis. Segmental areas of cecum and colon are grossly thickened and opaque. Affected mucosa is thickened due to varying degrees of crypt hyperplasia, with markedly immature and mitotically active enterocytes occupying the entire crypt column. Depending upon the mouse genotype and stage of infection, there are varying degrees of mixed leukocytic infiltration in the lamina propria. In some strains, there is marked lymphocytic infiltration (Fig. 1.44). Although there may be extensive lesions in the large intestine, hepatic lesions may be uncommon. Typical *Helicobacter* organisms can be readily demonstrated within crypt lumina of the affected sections of gut, using Steiner or other silver staining methods (Fig. 1.45).

DIAGNOSIS. Diagnosis is based upon the typical liver or intestinal lesions, but other etiologic agents must be considered. Definitive diagnosis requires demonstration of typical organisms within bile canaliculi or crypts using silver stains, PCR, or culture and confirmed by demonstration of *Helicobacter* antibody (in mice capable of producing antibody). Relatively insensitive serologic assays are available that utilize membrane antigen extracts for detecting serum IgG and fecal IgA, but PCR is extensively used to screen feces. PCR amplification of a segment of 16S rDNA can be embellished with restriction enzyme analysis to readily speciate *Helicobacter*. Differential diagnosis of liver lesions includes infections with *Salmonella*, *Proteus*, *Clostridium piliforme*, MHV, ectromelia virus, or nonspecific foci of hepatic necrosis and inflammation. Intestinal lesions must be differentiated from those induced by infection with *Escherichia coli*, *Citrobacter rodentium*, enterotropic MHV, or the nonspecific lesions of rectal prolapse.

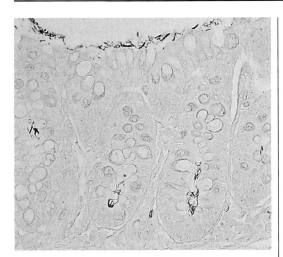

FIG. 1.45—Section of colon from immunodeficient transgenic mouse, stained with the Steiner stain depicting *Helicobacter* organisms on the surface and within crypts. (Courtesy J.M. Ward)

SIGNIFICANCE. *Helicobacter* has growing significance on mouse health and biomedical research. Aside from its direct pathogenic potential, particularly in immunodeficient mice, *Helicobacter* infection can significantly alter research results. *H. hepaticus* (and probably other *Helicobacter* spp.) causes an increase in hepatocellular tumors in certain strains of infected mice, but it has also been shown to promote experimental chemical hepatic carcinogenesis. More importantly, there continues to be widescale misinterpretation of colonic lesions by the scientific community. *Helicobacter* typhlocolitis has been extensively touted as a model for human "inflammatory bowel disease," which is a term reserved for ulcerative colitis and Crohn's disease, neither of which remotely resembles the mouse condition. The role of *Helicobacter* in these "models" continues to be ignored (the disease is often referred to as "spontaneous colitis"), with the widely held belief that lesions are associated with induction of autoreactive thymocytes capable of inducing colitis or are a consequence of dysfunctional T cells responding inappropriately to the normal constituents of the gut. "Inflammatory bowel disease" has been described in a variety of interleukin (IL-2, IL-10), T-cell receptor (alpha, beta, delta), and MHC class II knockout mice, and it occurs in Rag knockout, SCID, nude, and some immunocompetent mice as well.

***Salmonella* Infection: Salmonellosis.** *Salmonella,* gram-negative member of the Enterobacteriaceae, is currently classified into three species: *S. cholerasuis, S. typhi,* and *S. enteritidis.* Mice are infected with *S. enteritidis.* They are non–lactose fermenters and consist of over 1600 recognized serotypes. During the first half of this century, sporadic outbreaks of salmonellosis were a relatively common occurrence in conventional colonies of mice. With improved quality control and health assurance programs and good housing, husbandry, and feeding practices, recognized outbreaks now rarely occur. Nevertheless, *Salmonella* is an extensively utilized experimental model system in mice, allowing increasing opportunity for iatrogenic infections of mouse colonies.

EPIZOOTIOLOGY AND PATHOGENESIS. Exposure is considered to occur primarily by ingestion of contaminated feed or bedding, although conjunctival inoculation requires fewer organisms to establish an infection. Susceptibility/resistance depends on a variety of factors, including age (weanlings are more susceptible than adult mice), gut microflora, strain of mice (CBA and A/J mice are frequently studied resistant strains, and BALB/c and B6 mice are susceptible), virulence and dose of organism, route of inoculation, intercurrent infections, and manipulations that impair the immune response. *S. enteritidis,* serotype *enteritidis* or *typhimurium,* are the most commonly identified natural isolates in mice, and *typhimurium* is a commonly used experimental serovar.

Following exposure by ingestion, the incubation period is usually 3–6 d. Organisms gain entry to mucosa via fimbrial attachment to M cells, followed by multiplication in gut-associated lymphoid tissue. Colonization of the mesenteric lymph nodes precedes spread to the systemic circulation. In a small percentage of animals, there may be intermittent shedding of the organism in the feces for several months. The organism may be also harbored in the upper respiratory tract. *Salmonella* is readily killed by neutrophils, and neutrophil function is an important factor in resistance, but the bacterium has adapted to grow within macrophages, effectively evading clearance. In the liver, bacteria replicate intracellularly within macrophages, producing focal granulomata as the hallmark lesion. Genetically susceptible mice die from massive bacterial proliferation and tissue destruction related to endotoxin.

PATHOLOGY. Clinical signs can include diarrhea, anorexia, weight loss, conjunctivitis, and variable mortality. Gross findings can include splenomegaly, with multifocal pale miliary foci present on the liver. The alimentary tract is frequently essentially normal. In other cases, scanty fluid contents are present in the small and large intestine. Mesenteric lymph nodes can be enlarged and reddened. Microscopic changes include multifocal necrosis and venous thrombosis with leukocytic infiltration in the liver, spleen, Peyer's patches, and mesenteric lymph nodes. The hepatic lesions are typically granulomatous in nature (Fig.1.46). In the terminal small intestine and cecum, there may be edema in the lamina propria and submucosa, with sloughing of enterocytes and leukocytic infiltration.

DIAGNOSIS. Isolation and identification of the organism from sites such as liver, spleen, mesenteric lymph nodes, and intestine are essential and must accompany the standard macroscopic and histopathologic findings. Selenite F broth plus cystine, followed by streaking on brilliant green agar, are recommended for recovery of the organism. When screening a colony for possible *Salmonella* carriers, culturing of individual fecal samples is more sensitive than using pooled samples, and the highest rate of detection among carriers is achieved by culturing mesenteric lymph node, since fecal shedding is intermittent. *Differential diagnoses* include Tyzzer's disease, coronaviral hepatitis, mousepox, *Helicobacter* hepatitis, and pseudomoniasis. Spontaneous mesenteric lymphadenopathy (mesenteric disease) can also occur in aging mice.

SIGNIFICANCE. Murine salmonellosis is relatively rare today in mice. The danger of interspecies transmission is an important consideration; human infections are possible. Investigations into the possible source of the organism should include wild rodents, feed, fomites, human contacts, and iatrogenic introduction of experimental material. The dangers of inapparent shedders in this species should be emphasized

OTHER GRAM-NEGATIVE BACTERIAL INFECTIONS

***Chlamydia* Infection.** Mice can be naturally and/or experimentally infected with both species of *Chlamydia: C. psittaci* and *C. trachomatis.* Both agents are used in laboratory mice as contemporary models for respiratory and genital chlamydiosis and thus can serve as potential iatrogenic sources of infection in mouse colonies. In the early 1940s, a "latent virus" of mice, which caused pneumonitis upon serial intranasal passage, was named the Nigg agent after Clara Nigg, who discovered it during attempts to isolate influenza virus from human throat washings by intranasal inoculation of mice. It is currently called the mouse pneumonitis (MoPn) agent, or *C. trachomatis* MoPn biovar (based upon DNA typing).

EPIZOOTIOLOGY AND PATHOGENESIS. The MoPn biovar does not share type-specific antigens with two human strains of *C. trachomatis* (bivars tra-

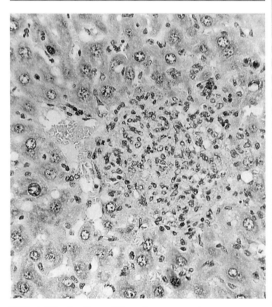

FIG. 1.46—Section of liver from a spontaneous case of murine salmonellosis. The circumscribed lesion consists of aggregations of histiocytic cells.

choma and lymphogranuloma venereum). The agent is believed to be transmitted by respiratory aerosols and/or by venereal transmission. Immunocompetent animals develop transient infections, and infections are typically silent in naturally infected mice. Immunodeficient strains of mice, including B-cell–deficient, T-cell–deficient, or combined deficient (SCID or Rag-1 knockout) strains, have increased susceptibility to infection and disease, as do mice treated with cyclophosphamide.

In addition, *C. psittaci* infects a wide range of mammals (and birds) and can experimentally cause respiratory and septicemic disease in mice. Documentation of natural infections of laboratory mice with *C. psittaci* is largely presumptive. In one case, intraperitoneal passage of mouse tissues resulted in splenomegaly, hepatomegaly, and serofibrinous peritonitis, and intranasal inoculation resulted in pneumonia following mouse passage. In another, an agent was isolated following intranasal inoculation with lung tissue from enzootically infected mice, resulting in pulmonary disease. Speciation of the agents in these cases was presumed to be *C. psittaci,* based upon inaccurate methods (sulfadiazine resistance and glycogen staining).

PATHOLOGY. *Chlamydia* grows intracellularly, forming discernable elementary and reticulate bodies in the cytoplasm of infected cells (bronchiolar epithelium and macrophages). Experimental intranasal inoculation results in pulmonary perivascular and peribronchiolar lymphocyte infiltration and nonsuppurative interstitial pneumonia with atelectasis, which can have significant neutrophilic leukocyte infiltration with passage or high dose. Pulmonary lesions are manifest grossly as pinpoint, elevated gray foci on the pleural surfaces. Organisms grow within bronchiolar epithelium and macrophages, which can possess intracytoplasmic vesicles containing inclusions. The MoPn agent readily disseminates hematogenously and by lymphatics to multiple organs, regardless of route of inoculation, due to its tropism for macrophages. It frequently infects peritoneal macrophages.

DIAGNOSIS. Diagnosis can be made with impression smears, growth in cell culture, or embry-onated chicken eggs. Accurate speciation can now be accomplished by DNA sequencing.

SIGNIFICANCE. *C. pneumoniae* is common in human populations, which may serve as a potential source of infection of mice. The likelihood of this scenario may increase with immunodeficient strains of mice. Furthermore, the role of *C. pneumoniae* in atherosclerosis in humans and experimental mice has expanded use of this agent in mouse colonies, increasing the chances for iatrogenic infections.

Cilia-Associated Respiratory (CAR) Bacillus Infection. CAR bacillus is a widespread and significant respiratory pathogen in the rat, commonly infects rabbits, and probably infects mice at a higher rate than is currently recognized. The CAR bacillus is an unclassified, gram-negative, motile, non–spore-forming bacterium that is closely related genetically to *Flexibacter* spp. and *Flavobacterium* spp., members of the gliding bacteria group. The organism has been associated with chronic respiratory disease in conventional and obese mutant mice dying with the disease. Chronic suppurative cranioventral bronchopneumonia and marked peribronchiolar infiltration with lymphocytes and plasma cells were evident on microscopic examination. Filamentous bacteria were demonstrated in association with the ciliated respiratory epithelium of bronchioles. In one study, representative animals were seropositive for Sendai virus and pneumonia virus of mice, and negative for *Mycoplasma pulmonis.* Thus, it is possible that more than one organism was involved in the evolution of lesions in the respiratory tract. Chronic respiratory disease and seroconversion have been produced in BALB/c mice inoculated intranasally with the CAR bacillus. The infection may be transmitted by direct contact, but airborne transmission to adjacent cages does not appear to occur in mice. Mice appear to be one of the most susceptible species. CAR bacilli possess considerable antigenic diversity among isolates from different host species. Diagnosis is typically achieved by silver staining of respiratory tissue to reveal characteristic organisms among cilia of the respiratory epithelium. Organisms can be isolated and cultured in mouse fibroblast cell lines. Serologic assays utilize bacterial lysates as antigen but are not optimal. PCR is being increasingly utilized to detect mild or subclinical infections in rodents and can be applied to nasal, oral, and tracheal swabs, with the oral cavity the most suitable noninvasive site for detecting early infection.

***Eperythrozoon coccoides* Infection.** *Eperythrozoon* is naturally transmitted by the louse *Polypax serrata;* both the infection and the vector are now nonexistent in laboratory mice. The organism is not transmitted transovarially and is not transmitted by other mouse arthropods (*Myobia, Myocoptes,* and *Radfordia*). Heretofore, *Eperythrozoon* was classified under Rickettsiales: Anaplasmataceae, but recent genetic analysis of *Eperythrozoon* and *Hemobartonella* has revealed that these organisms are more closely related to mycoplasma than to rickettsia, thereby placing them in the class Mollicutes, order Mycoplasmatales. With Giemsa and Romanowsky stains, the organism can be found attached to erythrocytes as well as free in the plasma of peripheral blood. In the early infection, a high level of parasitemia occurs within a few days, with clinical signs ranging from inapparent to severe anemia and death. Splenomegaly is a prominent feature of this infection, and this organ plays a central role in clearance of the parasite from the blood.

***Klebsiella oxytoca* Infection.** An unusually high prevalence of suppurative female reproductive tract lesions has been reported in a large population of aging B6C3F mice. *K. oxytoca* was the most frequently isolated organism from these lesions, but disease could not be experimentally reproduced, suggesting that other factors were involved. Other organisms isolated from affected mice included *K. pneumoniae, Escherichia coli, Enterobacter,* and others. Aged female mice had suppurative endometritis, salpingitis, and perioophoritis and/or peritonitis, often resulting in the formation of abscesses and adhesions. Lesions were severe enough to be life-limiting in some mice. Diagnosis is based on recognition of lesions and isolation of the agent and is not necessarily specific for *K. oxytoca.* Utero-ovarian infection can be life-limiting in aging studies.

***Leptospira* Infection: Leptospirosis.** *Leptospira* are represented by a large number of species or serotypes with a wide host range. Individual serotypes tend to prefer a single primary host but can infect many different host species. Mice can be infected with a number of leptospira serotypes, but *L. ballum* is common. Infection of laboratory mice now appears to be quite rare. Rodents do not become clinically ill when naturally infected and can shed organisms in their urine throughout life. Lesions are absent in naturally acquired infections, but mice are susceptible to disease. Experimental inoculation of C3H/He mice with *L. interrogans* serovar *icterohaemorrhagiae* results in pulmonary fibrinoid vasculitis, thrombosis, and hemorrhage, as well as renal tubular necrosis and interstitial nephritis. T-cell deficiency (CD4 and CD8) increased host susceptibility to disease. The most accurate means of diagnosis is kidney culture, which should be performed on serial 10-fold dilutions of tissue homogenates because growth inhibition can occur in undiluted samples. Serology is also possible; however, mice infected as neonates may become persistently infected but never seroconvert. Under natural conditions, this phenomenon is common. Leptospirosis is a zoonotic disease. Humans can become infected and develop clinical illness when handling asymptomatic mice.

***Mycobacterium avium-intracellularis* Infection.** Although laboratory mice are susceptible to experimental infections with *Mycobacterium,* naturally occurring infections are rare. A single outbreak of infection in laboratory mice with *M. avium-intracellulare* has been documented. *M.avium-intracellulare* complex organisms can be isolated from soil, water, and sawdust, which was the presumed origin of the infection in mice. Infected mice were asymptomatic. At necropsy, there were a few subpleural 1- to 5-mm-diameter tan-colored masses in lung. Microscopic findings consisted of focal accumulations of epithelioid cells, foamy macrophages and lymphocytes in alveolar spaces and septa, with variable amounts of necrosis and neutrophilic leukocyte infiltration. Many of the mice had microgranulomas with occasional Langhans-type giant cells in liver parenchyma and mesenteric lymph nodes. Small numbers of acid-fast bacilli were visualized in some lesions.

Definitive diagnosis can be made by demonstrating acid-fast organisms in granulomas and isolation of *Mycobacterium. Differential diagnoses* for pulmonary granulomas should include *M. pulmonis* and *Corynebacterium kutscheri* infections, as well as lesions associated with the administration of Freund's adjuvant.

Mycoplasma spp. Infection: Mycoplasmosis.

Mycoplasma is a bacterium of the family Mycoplasmataceae. These pleomorphic organisms lack a cell wall and are enclosed by a single limiting membrane. Laboratory mice are host to several *Mycoplasma* species including *M. pulmonis, M. arthritidis, M. neurolyticum,* and *M. collis. M. pulmonis, M. arthritidis,* and *M. neurolyticum* inhabit the upper respiratory tract, and *M. collis* inhabits the genital tract. Only *M. pulmonis* is a significant natural pathogen.

EPIZOOTIOLOGY AND PATHOGENESIS. Prior to and during the 1960s, infections with *M. pulmonis* were widespread in many colonies of mice. With marked improvements in health quality assessment and improved management practices, there has been a marked reduction in the incidence of clinically affected colonies of mice. However, based on some serological surveys, a relatively high percentage of laboratory mice may have detectable antibody to *M. pulmonis,* or to *M. arthritidis,* which cross-reacts with *M. pulmonis* antigenically. Exposure occurs by aerosol transmission. Newborn animals frequently become infected during the first few weeks of life from contact with affected mothers. Compared with the laboratory rat, mice are relatively resistant to the disease. In one study, intranasal inoculation with 10^4 colony-forming units or less of *M. pulmonis* resulted in disease confined to the upper respiratory tract and tympanic bullae. Higher doses resulted in lower respiratory tract disease, with mortality in some animals. Chronic suppurative arthritis has been produced in immunocompetent mice inoculated intravenously with *M. pulmonis.* SCID mice inoculated intranasally with *M. pulmonis* developed extensive polyarthritis with weight loss. However, it appears that spontaneous cases of *M. pulmonis*–associated arthritis rarely occur. In natural outbreaks of disease due to *M. pulmonis,* affected animals may exhibit weight loss, dyspnea, and a characteristic "chattering" sound on clinical examination. *M. pulmonis* colo-

nizes the apical cell membranes of respiratory epithelium and interferes with mucociliary clearance. Mycoplasmosis is exacerbated by viral infections, such as Sendai virus and MHV, by other bacteria, and by environmental ammonia levels. These cofactors probably play a significant role in driving subclinical mycoplasmal infections into overt disease. In outbreaks of chronic respiratory disease and/or otitis media, other contributing factors such as concurrent infections with Sendai virus are important considerations. Sendai virus infection has been shown to have a synergistic effect in *M. pulmonis*-infected mice. Environmental factors, such as high cage-ammonia levels, may aggravate disease. (For additional information on mycoplasmal infections, consult *M. pulmonis* infections in the rat in Chap. 2.)

PATHOLOGY. Infection is often subclinical or mild. Mucopurulent exudate may be present in the nasal passages, with variable involvement of the trachea and major airways. In advanced cases, cranioventral consolidation, bronchiectasis, and abscessation may be evident on gross examination (Fig. 1.47). Otitis media is another frequent manifestation of murine mycoplasmosis (Fig. 1.48). On microscopic examination, suppurative rhinitis,

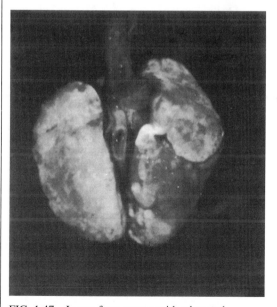

FIG. 1.47—Lungs from mouse with advanced mycoplasmal infection. There is marked mottling and discoloration, particularly in the right lung.

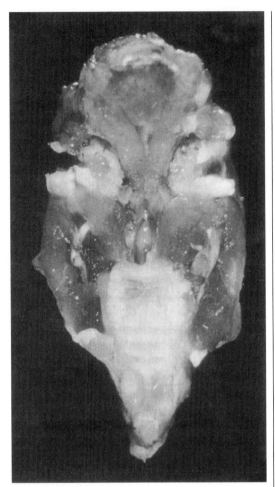

FIG. 1.48—Chronic suppurative otitis media associated with chronic mycoplasmosis. Note the marked thickening of the tympanic membranes and the presence of exudate in the opened tympanic bullae.

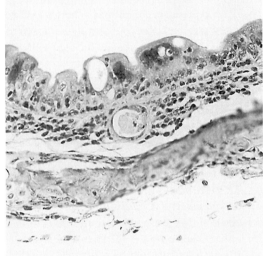

FIG. 1.49—Section of larynx from laboratory mouse with chronic mycoplasmal infection. Multinucleated giant cells are present in the respiratory epithelium. This is a common feature of the disease in this species.

with polymorphonuclear and lymphocytic infiltration and hyperplasia of submucosal glands, are characteristic findings. In the respiratory epithelium of the nasal passages and major airways, there may be loss of cilia and flattening of epithelial lining cells. In association with the chronic suppurative process, syncytia may be present in affected nasal mucosa and larynx (Fig. 1.49). In the lower respiratory tract, lesions vary from discrete peribronchial and perivascular lymphocytic and plasma cell infiltration to chronic suppurative bronchiolitis and alveolitis, with mobilization of alveolar macrophages. In advanced cases, there may be squamous metaplasia of respiratory epithelium, bronchiectasis and bronchiolectasis, and abscessation, with obliteration of the normal architecture. Purulent otitis media is a frequent finding in chronic mycoplasmosis. Mice do not develop the intense peribronchial lymphocytic infiltrates and severe bronchiectasis and bronchiolectasis that are common in mycoplasmosis in the rat.

DIAGNOSIS. Confirmation of *Mycoplasma* infection is achieved by culture. Immunohistochemistry on tissue sections has been utilized, and serology, based upon whole bacterial lysate antigen, is widely used for detecting infection in mouse colonies. For culture, nasopharyngeal flushing and tracheobronchial lavages with *Mycoplasma* broth or phosphate-buffered saline are recommended procedures. Cultures are often negative for *Mycoplasma* in affected animals. Thus additional tests are required. In serological testing, infected mice may have relatively low antibody titers to *M. pulmonis*. In the interpretation of seropositive cases, it is important to be aware of the serological cross-reactivity of *M. pulmonis* and *M. arthritidis*. In view of the recognized role of secondary bacterial infections in the disease, the respiratory tract should also be cultured for bacteria such as *Pasteurella pneumotropica*. Histological assessment should include a search for syncytia in the upper respiratory tract, a characteristic of the disease. Staining procedures such as the Warthin-Starry method should be performed on tissue sections of major airways to determine if there is infection with cilia-associated respiratory (CAR) bacillus, an organism associated with some outbreaks of murine respiratory disease in mice, and often a co-infecting pathogen in mycoplasmosis. *Differential diagnoses* include bronchopneumonia associated with infections with the CAR bacillus, as well as primary infections with Sendai virus with secondary bacterial infections. Otitis media can be caused by a variety of other opportunistic bacteria.

SIGNIFICANCE. Although mice are relatively resistant to clinical disease following infection with *M. pulmonis,* lesions of chronic respiratory disease occasionally occur, particularly in older mice. Outbreaks of lower respiratory disease and otitis can occur in previously asymptomatic, but infected, mouse colonies following introduction of respiratory viruses, such as Sendai virus and MHV. There is evidence that *M. pulmonis* infections may complicate certain types of research, such as tumor metastases studies, and infections may depress humoral and cell-mediated responses.

SIGNIFICANCE OF OTHER MURINE MYCOPLASMAL INFECTIONS. *M. neurolyticum* is the causative agent of "rolling disease," a term used to denote the neurologic signs associated with the exotoxin that follows experimental inoculation of the organism in mice. Spontaneous outbreaks of conjunctivitis have been associated with *M. neurolyticum* infection in young mice, but the organism appears to be relatively nonpathogenic under most conditions and is exceedingly rare or nonexistent anymore. *M. arthritidis* is antigenically related to *M. pulmonis* and causes arthritis when inoculated intravenously into mice but is nonpathogenic under natural conditions. *M. collis* has been isolated from the genital tract, without known adverse effect in mice.

Mice can be naturally infected with "gray lung virus," a nonculturable agent that can be transmitted by intranasal inoculation. Based upon 16S rDNA homology, the agent is now considered to be a mycoplasma. It appears to be distantly related to *M. pulmonis* (84% homology) and more closely related to *M. hominis* (94% homology). Furthermore, electron microscopy revealed *Mycoplasma*-like organisms in lung tissue. The name *M. ravipulmonis* (ravi'gray; pulmonis'lung) has been proposed.

***Pasteurella pneumotropica* Infection.** *P. pneumotropica* is a gram-negative coccobacillus that frequently infects rodents, without clinical evidence of disease; it can be associated with a number of lesions in mice. It should be considered an opportunist, since its true nature as a primary pathogen is questionable. However, with the increased use of genetically engineered and immunocompromised mice, the incidence of clinical disease is on the increase.

EPIZOOTIOLOGY AND PATHOGENESIS. *P. pneumotropica* frequently exists as an inapparent infection and may be recovered from the respiratory or enteric tracts in a significant percentage of clinically normal animals in infected premises. Severe pneumonia has been documented in B-cell–deficient mice co-infected with *Pneumcystis carinii.* Seroconversion normally occurs only in mice with overt disease. Clinical signs associated with *P. pneumotropica* infections include conjunctivitis, periorbital abscessation, panophthalmitis, rhinitis, cervical lymphadenitis, and subcutaneous abscessation. Immunocompromised and some genetically altered mice are especially susceptible to disease. Severe pneumonia has been documented in B-cell–deficient mice co-infected with *Pneumocystis carinii. P. pneumotropica* has also been associated with respiratory disease in mice, primarily as a secondary invader in mycoplasmal infections. Reproductive disorders attributed to *P. pneumotropica* have included abortions, infertility, and infections of the male accessory sex glands. In one report, abortions with necrotizing metritis were associated with *P. pneumotropica* infection. However, the organism has been recovered from the reproductive tracts of clinically normal male and female mice; thus the role of this organism in genital tract disease requires further study. Based on biochemical profiles, a bacterium classified as *Haemophilus influenzaemurium* has been isolated repeatedly from mice in one facility in Europe. Based on 16S rDNA sequences, the organism has been grouped with the Pasteurellaceae.

PATHOLOGY. In animals with suppurative lesions, patterns may vary. Purulent conjunctivitis, periorbital abscessation, subcutaneous abscesses, abscessation of the cervical lymph nodes, rhinitis, and bronchopneumonia are possible manifestations of infection. The suppurative nature of the inflammatory process is confirmed on histological examination (Fig. 1.50). Suppurative metritis has also been associated with infection.

DIAGNOSIS. Culture of the organism from lesions, with subsequent identification, is required. In screening colonies for the organism, serology is not particularly helpful, since subclinically infected mice are normally seronegative. *Differential diagnoses* include infections from other pyogenic organisms, such as staphylococci, corynebacteria, or streptococci; fighting injuries; and respiratory tract disease due to *M. pulmonis*. *Klebsiella oxytoca* has also been associated with suppurative endometritis and salpingitis.

SIGNIFICANCE. *P. pneumotropica* infections represent a potential complicating disease in research facilities, particularly as an opportunistic infection. The organism has been isolated from organs such as reproductive tract in clinically normal animals; therefore the significance of positive isolations must be interpreted with care. A careful search for other possible pathogens or predisposing factors should be an essential step in the investigation.

***Proteus mirabilis* Infection.** *Proteus* infection has been observed in both immunocompetent and immunodeficient laboratory mice. In immunocompetent C3H/HeJ mice, infection was observed most frequently in females. *P. mirabilis* has been isolated from the intestinal tract of both clinically affected and asymptomatic animals, but the nasopharynx may be another important portal of entry. In spontaneous cases in SCID mice, clinical signs were characterized by weight loss, hunched posture, and dehydration.

PATHOLOGY. Suppurative pyelonephritis and septicemia may occur, and there is some evidence that the renal lesions are hematogenous in origin. In immunodeficient mice, splenomegaly and multifocal hepatic lesions are typical macroscopic findings. In some cases, fibrinopurulent exudate is present in the peritoneal cavity (Fig. 1.51). On

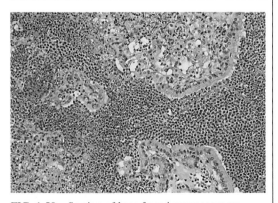

FIG. 1.50—Section of lung from immunocompromised mouse with concomitant pneumocystosis and *Pasteurella pneumotropica* infection. The suppurative bronchopneumonia is consistent with a pasteurella infection.

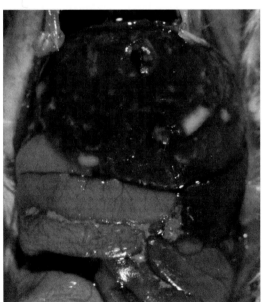

FIG. 1.51—Viscera of SCID mouse naturally infected with *Proteus mirabilis*. Note the irregular focal to coalescing hepatic lesions and the fibrinous exudate in peritoneal cavity.

microscopic examination, there are multifocal areas of coagulation necrosis present in the subcapsular regions of the liver and around central veins and minimal to moderate infiltration with neutrophils (Fig. 1.52). Septic thrombi may be present in vessels of tissues such as liver, intestinal serosa, and pancreas. Pulmonary lesions, when present, are characterized by alveolar flooding and mobilization of alveolar macrophages.

DIAGNOSIS. In addition to the presence of histological lesions consistent with bacterial sepsis, the recovery of large numbers of *P. mirabilis* from sites such as liver, peritoneal cavity, and intestine will serve to confirm the diagnosis.

SIGNIFICANCE. Infections with *P. mirabilis* may cause significant mortality in colonies of SCID mice, and infections have also been observed in immunocompetent mice. Meticulous sanitation practices and reduced population densities should alleviate the problem.

***Pseudomonas aeruginosa* Infection: Pseudomoniasis.** *Pseudomonas aeruginosa* is a gram-negative, non–spore-forming rod that is widespread in warm, moist environments. It is frequently isolated from soil, water, and normal human skin.

EPIZOOTIOLOGY AND PATHOGENESIS. The organism is not part of the normal microflora. Following procedures that impair granulocyte production and/or immune function, bacteremia is initiated when ingested organisms penetrate nasal and oral mucous membranes. Following treatment with cyclophosphamide, bacterial antigen is detectable at the nasal squamocolumnar junction and gingival epithelium, followed by invasion of regional lymph nodes and subsequent systemic disease. Invasion of *P. aeruginosa* from the intestinal tract, particularly the cecum and colon, is another likely source of the organism in systemic infections. In one study, coinvasion with group B streptococci from the oral cavity may have facilitated the invasion of *Pseudomonas* into the systemic circulation. Similarly, disease with mortality in a colony of SCID mice was attributed to concurrent infections with enterococci and *Pseudomonas aeruginosa*. Clinical signs may include weight loss, conjunctivitis, nasal discharge, and subcutaneous edema around the head. There is a strain-related variation in susceptibility to experimental *P. aeruginosa* infections of the respiratory tract. The increased susceptibility of some strains of mice was attributed to their inability to recruit large numbers of neutrophils and to a defect in tumor necrosis alpha production.

PATHOLOGY. Microscopic changes include necrosis of epithelium at sites of invasion in the upper respiratory tract and gingival tissues, with ulceration, and necrosis of the regional lymph nodes. Vasculitis, thrombosis, necrosis, and hemorrhage may occur in other organs, such as spleen and liver. *Pseudomonas* is also associated with otitis media.

DIAGNOSIS. A history of experimental procedures that could impair the immune response and/or leukocyte function usually precedes the onset of systemic disease. The presence of typical lesions and the recovery of the organism confirm the diagnosis. In the septicemic form of the disease, *P. aeruginosa* may be recovered from sites such as the blood, spleen, and oral cavity. *Differential diagnoses* include postimmunosuppression deaths due to other opportunistic bacteria such as

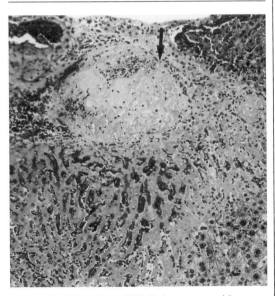

FIG. 1.52—Liver from SCID/beige mouse with systemic *Proteus mirabilis* infection. There is thrombophlebitis with coagulation necrosis of hepatic parenchyma and thrombosis of a hepatic vein (*arrow*).

Corynebacterium kutscheri. Other possible causes are bacterial septicemias due to other gram-negative organisms.

SIGNIFICANCE. *Pseudomonas* is relatively ubiquitous, even in commercial barrier facilities. The diagnosis of pseudomoniasis requires a thorough investigation of management and sanitation practices. The drinking water is the usual source of the organism. Predisposing factors, including procedures that impair granulocyte function or the immune response, should be evaluated. *Pseudomonas* infections may result in high mortality under these conditions and represent an important potential complication in certain types of research. Mice have been studied as an animal model for persistent pulmonary infections with *P. aeruginosa,* a condition commonly seen in patients with cystic fibrosis.

Streptobacillus moniliformis Infection: Streptobacillosis

EPIZOOTIOLOGY AND PATHOGENESIS. Streptobacillosis is a septicemic disease of mice caused by *S. moniliformis.* The organism is normally carried in the nasopharynx of wild rats and occasionally laboratory rats. It is no longer common in laboratory rats, and the disease in mice has likewise become rare. In documented outbreaks of streptobacillosis in mice, carrier rats were maintained in the same room, but mouse-to-mouse transmission can also occur. Following oral inoculation, *S. moniliformis* can be isolated from submaxillary and cervical lymph nodes within 48 hr, with subsequent septicemia. A large number of organisms can be isolated from the blood during this stage.

PATHOLOGY. Clinical signs include diarrhea, hemoglobinuria, and conjunctivitis. There are disseminated foci of necrosis and inflammation in liver, spleen, and lymph nodes, with petechial and ecchymotic hemorrhages on serosal surfaces. Suppurative embolic interstitial nephritis, dermatitis, and mastitis were associated with one outbreak of *S. moniliformis* infection in breeding female mice. Some mice, particularly those that survive the acute phase, can develop suppurative polyarthritis.

DIAGNOSIS Definitive diagnosis of streptobacillosis is made by isolation from infected tissues, using blood agar. Organisms are nonmotile, gram-negative rods that are highly pleomorphic, with long filamentous forms under ideal growth conditions. *Differential diagnoses* must include other forms of septicemic disease that cause disseminated lesions, such as pseudomoniasis, corynebacterial, staphylococcal, and streptococcal infections.

SIGNIFICANCE. Streptobacillosis is an unlikely pathogen in contemporary laboratory mouse colonies but is a major reason for not cohabitating mice and rats in the same room. *S. moniliformis* causes rat-bite fever (Haverhill fever) in humans, and human infections have been acquired through contact with laboratory animals.

INFECTIONS WITH GRAM-POSITIVE BACTERIA

Corynebacterium kutscheri Infection: Pseudotuberculosis.

Corynebacterium kutscheri is a gram-positive diphtheroid bacillus that causes a syndrome in mice and rats termed pseudotuberculosis. This was one of the first infectious disease syndromes to be recognized in laboratory mice and rats in 1894 by D. Kutscher. Once quite common in these species, it is now rare. However, it remains a significant pathogen that occasionally infects colonies of mice and rats.

EPIZOOTIOLOGY AND PATHOGENESIS. Infection is believed to enter through oral or enteric mucosa, from which the organisms spread to regional lymph nodes and to other internal organs by bacteremia. The organism may persist as a subclinical infection for long periods with no detectable circulating antibodies. The usual sites for the colonization of *C. kutscheri* in mice are the oral cavity, cecum, and colon. Clinical manifestations of the disease usually occur in conjunction with predisposing factors that compromise the immune response. A variation in susceptibility to *C. kutscheri* among strains of mice has been attributed to the efficacy of the mononuclear phagocyte system.

PATHOLOGY. Cervical lymph nodes may be enlarged. At necropsy, raised, gray-white nodules up to 1 cm in diameter may be present in liver and kidney and, to a lesser extent, in other tissues. Lesions may contain material that varies from friable caseous exudate to liquefied pus. Suppurative arthritis is occasionally present in affected mice. The carpometacarpal and tarsometatarsal joints are most frequently affected and may be markedly swollen on gross examination. Microscopically the nodules, when present in viscera, consist of an area of coagulation to caseation necrosis, with peripheral aggregations of leukocytes, neutrophils predominating. Thrombosis and embolization involving the mesenteric and portal vessels may be evident, with leukocytic infiltration. Suppurative lesions may be present in the joints.

DIAGNOSIS. Bacterial colonies are usually readily evident within suppurative lesions and are best visualized in tissue sections stained with preparations such as Brown and Brenn. The distribution and nature of the lesions consistent with pseudotuberculosis require recovery and identification of *C. kutscheri.*

SIGNIFICANCE. Pseudotuberculosis represents an important potentially complicating disease in mice, particularly when subjected to immunosuppression. Sanitation procedures and the likelihood of carrier animals should be important considerations.

***Corynebacterium bovis* Infection: Coryneform Hyperkeratosis.** An organism initially categorized as *Corynebacterium pseudodiphtheriticum* was associated with scaling dermatitis in nude mice. The agent has subsequently been classified as *C. bovis.* The disease is characterized by weight loss and diffuse hyperkeratotic dermatitis.

EPIDEMIOLOGY AND PATHOGENESIS. The organism may be transmitted by topical application to the skin, by direct contact with infected mice, and by fomites. The organism has been isolated from asymptomatic immunocompetent haired mice, and these mice are one possible source of the organism in infected colonies. However, infections are usually transient in immunocompetent animals, and nude mice are the most likely source of the infection when outbreaks do occur. Local-

ized skin lesions have been observed in SCID mice, but not in immunocompetent mice infected with *C. bovis.* In infected colonies of nude mice, the morbidity is frequently high, but mortality usually occurs only in suckling mice. Skin lesions are usually transient in older animals. The bacterium can be isolated from the oral cavity and skin of infected mice.

PATHOLOGY. On gross examination, there is a diffuse, scaling dermatitis (Fig. 1.53). Microscopically, there is marked epidermal hyperplasia, orthokeratotic hyperkeratosis, and a sparse mononuclear and polymorphonuclear cell infiltrate in the underlying dermis (Fig. 1.54). In gram-stained sections, small gram-positive coryneform rods can be demonstrated in the keratin layers. In SCID mice, lesions, when present,

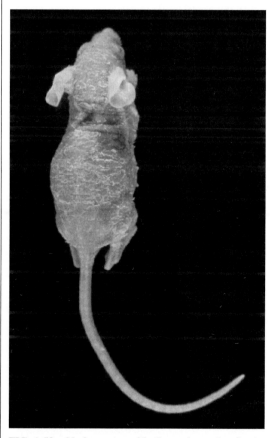

FIG. 1.53—Nude mouse with *Corynebacterium bovis* hyperkeratosis. (Courtesy C. Richter and R.J. Rahija)

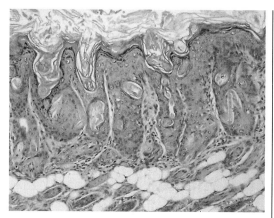

FIG. 1.54—Skin from athymic mouse with chronic *Corynebacterium bovis* infection. There is a marked epidermal hyperplasia and hyperkeratosis associated with the disease. (Courtesy C. Richter and R.J. Rahija)

consist of areas of alopecia with scaling dermatitis on the back, flanks, neck, and cheeks. *Differential Diagnoses:* The disease must be differentiated from hyperkeratosis associated with low ambient humidity.

SIGNIFICANCE. Complications reported include increased toxicity of chemotherapeutic agents and decreased tumor growth in affected nude mice.

***Corynebacterium* spp.-Associated Keratoconjunctivitis.** Keratoconjunctivitis with ulcerative keratitis has been reported in aged B6 mice. A *Corynebacterium* spp. was the most consistent isolate and was deemed the primary pathogen. Older mice inoculated in the conjunctival sac with the organism developed the typical lesions, but younger mice were resistant to the disease. *C. hoffmani* is a frequent isolate from BALB/c mice with conjunctivitis. Other causes of conjunctivitis include infections with *Pasteurella pneumotropica,* foreign bodies, and genetic factors in some mouse strains, such as entropion or microophthalmia and other ocular anomalies in B6 mice.

Staphylococcal Infections. Staphylococci, grampositive bacteria that are common inhabitants of the skin and mucous membranes, include potentially pathogenic strains of *Staphylococcus aureus* and the relatively nonpathogenic strains *S. epidermidis* and *S. xylosus.*

EPIZOOTIOLOGY AND PATHOGENESIS. Staphylococci are often carried asymptomatically on the skin, in the nasopharynx, and intestine. There are several factors identified that may have an influence on the appearance of clinical disease, including strain of mouse. For example, nude mice, with sparse protective pelage, distorted vibrissal shaft growth, and impaired T-cell function, may develop periorbital abscesses and nasal furunculosis due to *S. aureus* infections. In one outbreak involving male nude mice, multifocal full thickness necrotizing skin lesions were associated with *S. xylosus* infections. Various strains of mice, particularly B6 mice, are prone to ulcerative dermatitis that is associated with *Staphylococcus aureus.* Staphylococcal botryomycosis with abscessation and visceral lesions occurs in normal mice, but also urokinase plasminogen activator-deficient mice. In addition to immune status, lack of competing bacteria, nutritional deficiencies, breaks in the integument associated with trichotillomania (as in B6 mice), mite hypersensitivity (see Ectoparasitic Infestations), fighting injuries, and the prevalence of staphylococci in the environment are recognized to be contributing factors.

PATHOLOGY. Clinical signs include abscessation of cervical lymph nodes, inflammation and abscessation of preputial and lacrimal glands, conjunctivitis, superficial pyoderma, and severe ulcerative dermatitis, particularly around the muzzle, head, and shoulders. Skin infections are frequently accompanied by pruritus with self-excoriation. Ulcerative skin lesions are reminiscent of burns due to production of epidermolytic toxins by prominent colonies of gram-positive cocci within the overlying exudate, with underlying coagulation necrosis of epidermis and dermis to varying depths. Full thickness necrosis of the epidermis has occurred in *S. xylosus* infections in immunocompromised mice. Varying degrees of necrosis, leukocytic infiltration, and granulation are found in ulcerative skin lesions. In nude mice, severe folliculitis and furunculosis occur on the muzzle, with a marked neutrophilic leukocyte infiltration. Regional lymph nodes may also be

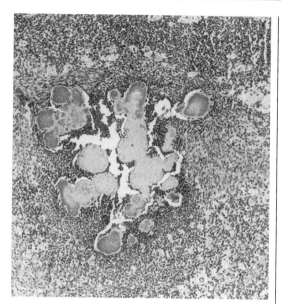

FIG. 1.55—Cervical lymph node, illustrating the typical inflammatory reaction in a case of botryomycosis due to localized staphylococcal infection. There are bacterial colonies and central aggregates of eosinophilic material interpreted to be antigen-antibody complexes.

involved. In chronic suppurative lesions, particularly involving lymph nodes, botryomycotic granules (Splendore-Hoeppli material) are prominent (Fig. 1.55).

DIAGNOSIS. Gram-positive coccoid bacteria are readily identified on the surface of skin lesions and within abscesses. Confirmation requires isolation of a coagulase-positive staphylococcus that may produce beta hemolysis on blood agar and grow well on mannitol-salt agar. Some strains of coagulase-negative staphylococci are potentially pathogenic in immunocompromised mice. *Differential diagnoses* include abscessation due to other bacterial infections, mite infestation, and fighting injuries.

SIGNIFICANCE. The isolation of a coagulase-positive staphylococcus must be correlated with the presence of lesions attributable to the organism, since potentially pathogenic staphylococci may be recovered from the skin of clinically normal animals. Staphylococcal infections are particularly troublesome to nude mice, which tend to develop furunculosis around their muzzles,

lacrimal gland abscesses, and preputial gland infections. In the event of disease, investigations into the problem should include a study of possible contributing factors, such as immune status, genetic predisposition, self-trauma associated with mite infestation, or fighting injuries.

Streptococcal Infections: Dermatitis. Outbreaks of dermatitis have been associated with Lancefield type G streptococcal infections. Affected animals had a progressive necrotizing dermatitis. Posterior paralysis and mortality were also observed. Beta-hemolytic streptococci can be recovered from skin lesions, the pharynges, and spleen of affected mice. The disease has been reproduced in some animals inoculated with the bacterial isolate.

PATHOLOGY. Lesions in this disease appear to occur most frequently in the lumbar, shoulder, and hip regions. They consist of dry, brown, gangrenous areas on gross examination. Microscopic examination reveals a necrotizing dermatitis, with ulceration and polymorphonuclear cell infiltration, sometimes with concurrent phlebitis and lymphangitis of adjacent vessels. In sections stained with the appropriate procedure, gram-positive cocci are usually evident in the dermis underlying ulcerated areas. *Differential diagnoses* include mite infestation with secondary bacterial invaders, staphylococcal infections, and fighting injuries.

Streptococcal Infections: Systemic. Generalized streptococcal infections can occasionally occur in both immunocompetent and immunocompromised mice. One outbreak in recently shipped conventional mice was attributed to a beta-hemolytic streptococcal infection. Lesions were characterized by septicemia and endocarditis with mural thrombus formation. Bacterial colonies were present within thrombi and within vessels of the myocardium. Endogenous streptococcal infections can become systemic in experimentally immunosuppressed mice. Multifocal suppurative streptococcal myocarditis was observed in weanling mice recently shipped to a research facility. Lesions were confined to the myocardium. Systemic infections with other strains have been identified. Group B *S. agalactiae* was associated with

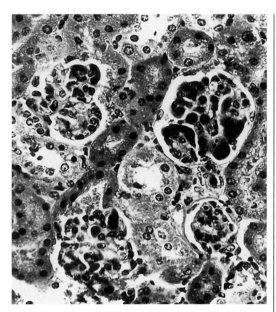

FIG. 1.56—Kidney from C.B-17 mouse (SCID/beige mouse) with a generalized alpha-hemolytic streptococcal infection. Numerous bacterial colonies are present in glomerular vessels.

an epizootic in DBA/2 mice. The pathogenesis of the infection was attributed to ascending pyelonephritis with subsequent septicemia resulting in suppurative lesions in a variety of organs including heart, liver, and lung. Human carriers are one possible source of *S. agalactiae*. Hepatic abscesses have been associated with *S. equisimilis* infections in SPF mice. Systemic disease due to alpha-hemolytic streptococci may occur in colonies of SCID mice. Bacterial colonies were observed within glomerular tufts and vessels within the medulla of the kidney (Fig. 1.56) and myocardium. Septicemia with mortality has been associated with concurrent enterococcal and pseudomonas infections in SCID mice. Confirmation of streptococcal infections requires the consistent isolation of the organism in pure culture from affected tissues.

BIBLIOGRAPHY
FOR BACTERIAL INFECTIONS

Citrobacter rodentium Infection
Barthold, S.W. 1980. The microbiology of transmissible murine colonic hyperplasia. Lab. Anim. Sci. 30:167–73.

Barthold, S.W., and Adams, R.L. 1986. *Citrobacter freundii.* In *Manual of Microbiologic Monitoring of Laboratory Animals,* ed. A.M. Allen and T. Nomura. Natl. Inst. Health Pub. No. 86-2498. Washington, D.C.: Government Printing Office.

Barthold, S.W., et al. 1978. Transmissible murine colonic hyperplasia. Vet. Pathol. 15:223–36.

———. 1977. Dietary, bacterial, and host genetic interactions in the pathogenesis of transmissible murine colonic hyperplasia. Lab. Anim. Sci. 27:938–45.

———. 1976. The etiology of transmissible murine colonic hyperplasia. Lab. Anim. Sci. 26:889–94.

Bienick, H., and Tober-Meyer, B. 1976. Zur Atiologie der Colitis und des Prolapses recti bei der Maus. Z. Versuch. 18:337–48.

Brennan, P.C., et al. 1965. *Citrobacter freundii* associated with diarrhea in laboratory mice. Lab. Anim. Care 15:266–75.

Ediger, R.D., et al. 1974. Colitis in mice with a high incidence of rectal prolapse. Lab. Anim. Sci. 24:488–94.

Higgins, L.M., et al. 1999a. Role of bacterial intimin in colonic hyperplasia and inflammation. Science 285:588–91.

———. 1999b. *Citrobacter rodentium* infection in mice elicits a mucosal Th1 cytokine response and lesions similar to those in murine inflammatory bowel disease. Infect. Immun. 67:3031–39.

Schnaur, D.B., et al. 1995. Genetic and biochemical characterization of *Citrobacter rodentium* sp.nov. J. Clin. Microbiol. 33: 2064–68.

Silverman, J., et al. 1979. A natural outbreak of transmissible murine colonic hyperplasia in A/J mice. Lab. Anim. Sci. 29:209–13.

Clostridium perfringens Infection
Matsushita, S., and Matsumoto, T. 1986. Spontaneous necrotic enteritis in young RFM/Ms mice. Lab. Anim. 20:114–17.

Sanchez, S., and Rozengurt, N. 1994. Lesions caused by *Clostridium perfringens* in germ-free mice. Lab. Anim. Sci. 44:397.

Clostridium piliforme Infection
Duncan, A.J. 1993. Assignment of the agent of Tyzzer's disease *Clostridium piliforme* comb.nov. On the basis of 16S r RNA sequence analysis. J. Syst. Bacteriol. 43:314–18.

Franklin, C.L., et al. 1994. Tyzzer's infection: Host specificity of *Clostridium piliforme* isolates. Lab. Anim. Sci. 44:568–72.

Fries, A.S. 1977. Studies on Tyzzer's disease: Application of immunofluorescence for detection of *Bacillus piliformis* and for the demonstration and determination of antibodies to it in sera from mice and rabbits. Lab. Anim. 11:69–73.

Ganaway, J.R., et al. 1971. Tyzzer's disease. Am. J. Pathol. 64:711–32.

Livingston, R.S., et al. 1996. A novel presentation of *Clostridium piliforme* infection (Tyzzer's disease) in nude mice. Lab. Anim. Sci. 46:21–25.

Motzel, S.L., et al. 1991. Detection of serum antibodies to *Bacillus piliformis* in mice and rats using an enzyme-linked immunoabsorbent assay. Lab. Anim. Sci. 41:26–30.

Smith, K.J., et al. 1996. *Bacillus piliformis* infection (Tyzzer's disease) in a patient with HIV-1: Confirmation with 16S ribosomal RNA sequence analysis. J. Am. Acad. Dermatol. 34:343–48.

Tyzzer, E.E. 1917. A fatal disease of the Japanese waltzing mouse caused by a spore-bearing bacillus (*Bacillus piliformis* N.sp.). J. Med. Res. 37:307–38.

Van Andel, R.A., et al. 1998. Interleukin-12 has a role in mediating resistance of murine strains to Tyzzer's disease. Infect. Immun. 66:4942–46.

———. 1997. Effects of neutrophil, natural killer cell, and macrophage depletion on murine *Clostridium piliforme* infection. Infect. Immun. 65: 2725–31.

Waggie, K.S., et al. 1981. A study of mouse strain susceptibility to *Bacillus piliformis* (Tyzzer's disease): The association of B-cell function and resistance. Lab. Anim. Sci. 31:139–42.

Escherichia coli Infection

Waggie, K.S., et al. 1988. Cecocolitis in immunodeficient mice associated with an enteroinvasive lactose negative *E. coli*. Lab. Anim. Sci. 38:389–93.

Helicobacter spp. Infections

Cahill, R.J., et al. 1996. Inflammatory bowel disease: An immunity-mediated condition triggered by bacterial infection with *Helicobacter hepaticus*. Infect. Immun. 65:3126–31.

Foltz, C.J., et al. 1996. Evaluation of various oral antimicrobial formulations for eradication of *Helicobacter hepaticus*. Lab. Anim. Sci. 46:193–97.

Fox, J.G., and Lee, A. 1997. The role of *Helicobacter* species in newly recognized gastrointestinal tract disease of animals. Lab. Anim. Sci. 47:222–55.

Fox, J.G., et al. 1996a. Persistent hepatitis and enterocolitis in germ-free mice infected with *Helicobacter hepaticus*. Infect. Immun. 64:3673–81.

———. 1996b. Chronic proliferative hepatitis in A/JCr mice associated with persistent *Helicobacter hepaticus* infection: A model of *Helicobacter*-induced carcinogenesis. Infect. Immun. 64:1548–58.

———. 1995. *Helicobacter bilis* sp. nov., a novel *Helicobacter* species isolated from bile, livers, and intestines of inbred mice. J. Clin. Microbiol. 33:445–54.

———. 1994. *Helicobacter hepaticus* sp. nov., a microaerophilic bacterium isolated from livers and intestinal mucosal scrapings from mice. J. Clin. Microbiol. 32:1238–45.

Franklin, C.L., et al. 1999. Enteric lesions in SCID mice infected with "*Helicobacter typhlonicus*," a novel urease-negative *Helicobacter* species. Lab. Anim. Sci. 49:496–505.

———. 1998. Enterohepatic lesions in SCID mice infected with *Helicobacter bilis*. Lab. Anim. Sci. 48:334–39.

Hailey, J.R., et al. 1998. Impact of *Helicobacter hepaticus* infection in B6C3F1 mice from twelve national toxicology program two-year carcinogenesis studies. Toxicol. Pathol.: 26:602–11.

Higgins, L.M., et al. 1999. Regulation of T cell activation in vitro and in vivo by targeting the OX40-OX40 ligand interaction: Amelioration of ongoing inflammatory bowel disease with an OX40-IgG fusion protein, but not with an OX40 ligand-IgG fusion protein. J. Immunol. 162:486–93.

Ihrig, M., et al. 1998. Characterization of the response to *Helicobacter hepaticus* infection in recombinant inbred strains of mice. Contemp. Top. 37(4):90–91.

Livingston, R.S., et al. 1998. Transmission of *Helicobacter hepaticus* infection to sentinel mice by contaminated bedding. Lab. Anim. Sci. 48:291–93.

Riley, L.K., et al. 1996. Identification of murine helicobacters by PCR and restriction enzyme analysis. J. Clin. Microbiol. 34:942–46.

Schauer, D.B., et al. 1993. Isolation and characterization of "*Flexispira rappini*" from laboratory mice. J. Clin. Microbiol. 31:2709–14.

Shames, B., et al. 1995. Identification of widespread *Helicobacter hepaticus* infection in feces in commercial mouse colonies by culture and PCR assay. J. Clin. Microbiol. 33:2968–72.

Shen Z., et al. 1997. *Helicobacter rodentium* sp. nov., a urease negative *Helicobacter* species isolated from laboratory mice. Int. J. Syst. Bacteriol. 47:627–34.

Shomer, N.H., et al. 1998. A novel urease-negative intestinal *Helicobacter* species causes a severe proliferative typhlocolitis in *scid* mice with defined flora. Contemp. Top. 37(4):90.

Strober, W., and Ehrhardt, R.O. 1993. Chronic intestinal inflammation: An unexpected outcome in cytokine or T cell receptor mutant mice. Cell 75:253–61.

Taylor, N.S., et al. 1995. *In vitro* hepatotoxic factor in *Helicobacter hepaticus, H. pylori*, and other *Helicobacter* species. J. Med. Microbiol. 42:48–52.

Ward, J.M., et al. 1996a. Autoimmunity in chronic active *Helicobacter* hepatitis of mice. Am. J. Pathol. 148:509–17.

———. 1996b. Inflammatory large bowel disease associated in immunodeficient mice naturally infected with *Helicobacter hepaticus*. Lab. Anim. Sci. 46:15–20.

———. 1994a. Chronic active hepatitis in mice caused by *Helicobacter hepaticus*. Am. J. Pathol. 145:959–68.

———. 1994b. Chronic active hepatitis and associated liver tumors in mice caused by a persistent bacterial infection with a novel *Helicobacter* species. J. Natl. Cancer Inst. 86:1222–27.

Whary, M.T., et al. 1999. Serologic monitoring of sentinel mice and the epidemiology of naturally acquired infection of rodent colonies with *Helicobacter hepaticus, H. bilis,* and *H. rodentium*. Lab. Anim. Sci. 49:433–34.

Salmonella Infection

Bassiloyanakopoulos, A.P., et al. 1998. The crucial role of polymorphonuclear leukocytes in resistance to

Salmonella dublin infections in genetically susceptible and resistant mice. Proc. Natl. Acad. Sci. USA 95:7676–81.

Caseboldt, D.B., and Schoeb, T.R. 1988. An outbreak in mice of salmonellosis caused by *Salmonella enteritidis* serotype *enteritidis*. Lab. Anim. Sci. 38:190–92.

Clark, M.A., et al. 1998. Inoculum composition and *Salmonella* pathogenicity island 1 regulate M-cell invasion and epithelial destruction by *Salmonella typhimurium*. Infect. Immun. 66:724–31.

Khan, S.A., et al. 1998. A lethal role for lipid A in *Salmonella* infections. Mol. Microbiol. 29:571–79.

Margard, W.L., et al. 1963. Salmonellosis in mice-diagnostic procedures. Lab. Anim. Care 13:144–65.

Moncure, C.W., et al. 1998. Comparative histopathology in mouse typhoid among genetically diverse mice. Int. J. Exp. Pathol. 79:183–92.

Richter-Dahlfors, A., et al. 1997. Murine salmonellosis studied by confocal microscopy: *Salmonella typhimurium* resides intracellularly inside macrophages and exerts a cytotoxic effect on phagocytes in vivo. J. Exp. Med. 186:569–80.

Stott, J.A., et al. 1975. Incidence of salmonellae in animal feed and the effect of pelleting on content of Enterobacteriaceae. J. Appl. Bacteriol. 39:41–46.

Tannock, G.W., and Smith, J.M.B. 1971. A *Salmonella* carrier state involving the upper respiratory tract of mice. J. Infect. Dis. 123:502–6.

Chlamydia Infection

Ata, F.A., et al. 1971. Inapparent respiratory infection of inbred Swiss mice with sulfadiazine-resistant, iodine-negative chlamydia. Infect. Immun. 4:506–7.

Gogalak, F.M. 1953. The histopathology of murine pneumonitis infection and the growth of the virus in mouse lung. J. Gen. Microbiol. 15:292–304.

Karr, H.V. 1943. Study of a latent pneumotropic virus of mice. J. Infect. Dis. 72:108–16.

Kaukoranta-Tolvanen, S.S.E., et al. 1993. Experimental infection of *Chlamydia pneumoniae* in mice. Microb. Pathog. 15:293–302.

Masson, N.D., et al. 1995. Relevance of *Chlamydia pneumoniae* murine pneumonitis model to evaluation of antimicrobial agents. Antimicrob. Agents Chemother. 39:1959–64.

Moazed, T.C., et al. 1998. Evidence of systemic dissemination of *Chlamydia pneumoniae* via macrophages in the mouse. J. Infect. Dis. 177:1322–25.

Nigg, C. 1942. Unidentified virus which produces pneumonia and systemic infection in mice. Science 95:49–50.

Nigg, C., and Eaton, M.D. Isolation from normal mice of a pneumotropic virus which forms elementary bodies. J. Exp. Med. 79:496–510.

Yang, X., and Brunham, R.C. 1998. Gene knockout B cell–deficient mice demonstrate that B cells play an important role in the initiation of T cell responses to *Chlamydia trachomatis* (mouse pneumonitis) lung infection. J. Immunol. 161:1439–46.

Yang, X., et al. 1998. Different roles are played by alpha beta and gamma delta T cells in acquired immunity to *Chlamydia trachomatis* pulmonary infection. Immunology 94:469–75.

Yang, Z.P., et al. 1995. Systemic dissemination of *Chlamydia pneumoniae* following intranasal inoculation in mice. J. Infect. Dis. 171:736–38.

Cilia-Associated Respiratory (CAR) Bacillus Infection

Cundiff, D.D., et al. 1994. Characterization of cilia-associated respiratory bacillus isolates from rats and rabbits. Lab. Anim. Sci. 44:305–12.

Goto, K., et al. 1995. Detection of cilia-associated respiratory bacillus in experimentally and naturally infected mice and rats by the polymerase chain reaction. Exp. Anim. 44:333–36.

Griffith, J.W., et al. 1988. Cilia-associated respiratory (CAR) bacillus infection in obese mice. Vet. Pathol. 25:72–76.

Hook, R.R. Jr., et al. 1998. Antigenic analyses of cilia-associated respiratory (CAR) bacillus isolates by use of monoclonal antibodies. Lab. Anim. Sci. 48:234–39.

Matsushita, S., et al. 1989. Transmission experiments of cilia-associated respiratory bacillus in mice, rabbits and guinea pigs. Lab. Anim. 23:96–102.

Shoji-Darkye, Y., et al. 1992. Pathogenesis of CAR bacillus in rabbits, guinea pigs, Syrian hamsters, and mice. Lab. Anim. Sci. 41:567–71.

Eperythrozoon Infection

Baker, H.J., et al. 1971. Research complications due to *Hemobartonella* and *Eperythrozoon* infections in experimental animals. Am. J. Pathol. 64:625–56.

Berkenkamp, S.D., and Wescott, R.B. 1988. Arthropod transmission of *Eperythrozoon coccoides* in mice. Lab. Anim. Sci. 38:398–401.

Rikihisa, Y., et al. 1997. Western immunoblot analysis of *Haemobartonella muris* and comparison of 16S rRNA gene sequence of *H. muris, H. felis,* and *Eperythrozoon suis.* J. Clin. Microbiol. 35:823–29.

Klebsiella oxytoca and *Klebsiella pneumoniae* Infections

Bolister, N.J., et al. 1992. The ability of airborne *Klebsiella pneumoniae* to colonize mouse lungs. Epidemiol. Infect. 109:121–31.

Davis, J.K., et al. 1987. The role of *Klebsiella oxytoca* in utero-ovarian infection of B6C3F1 mice. Lab. Anim. Sci. 37:159–66.

Rao, G.N., et al. 1987. Utero-ovarian infection in aged B6C3F1 mice. Lab. Anim. Sci. 37:153–58.

Schneemilch, H.D. 1976. A naturally acquired infection of laboratory mice with *Klebsiella* capsule type 6. Lab. Anim. 10:305–10.

Leptospira Infection

Birnbaum, S., et al. 1972. The influence of maternal antibodies on the epidemiology of leptospiral carrier state in mice. Am. J. Epidemiol. 96:313–17.

Friedman, C.T.H., et al. 1973. *Leptospirosis ballum* contracted from pet mice. Calif. Med. 118:51–52.

Pereira, M.M., et al. 1998. Morphological characterization of lung and kidney lesions in C3H/HeJ mice infected with *Leptospira interrogans* serovar *icterohaemorrhagiae:* Defect of CD4+ and CD8+ T-cells are prognosticators of the disease progression. Exp. Toxicol. Pathol. 50:191–98.

Stoenner, H.G. 1957. The laboratory diagnosis of leptospirosis. Vet. Med. 52:540–42.

Stoenner, H.G., and Maclean, D. 1958. *Leptospirosis (ballum)* contracted from Swiss albino mice. Arch. Intern. Med. 101:706–10.

Mycoplasma spp. Infection

Andrewes, C.H., and Glover, R.E. 1946. Grey lung virus: An agent pathogenic for mice and other rodents. Br. J. Exp. Path. 26:379–87.

Evengard, B.K., et al. 1994. Intranasal inoculation of M*ycoplasma pulmonis* in mice with severe combined immunodeficiency (SCID) causes a wasting disease with grave arthritis. Clin. Exp. Immunol. 98:388–94.

Kishima, M., et al. 1989. Cell-mediated and humoral immune responses in mice during experimental infection with *Mycoplasma pulmonis.* Lab. Anim. 23:138–42.

Lai, W.C., et al. 1989. *Mycoplasma pulmonis* depresses humoral and cell-mediated responses in mice. Lab. Anim. Sci. 39:11–15.

———. 1986. *Mycoplasma pulmonis* infection of mice influences tumor metastasis research. Lab. Anim. Sci. 36:568.

Neimark, H., et al. 1998. An approach to characterizing uncultivated prokaryotes: The grey lung agent and proposal of a candidatus taxon for the organism, "Candidatus Mycoplasma ravipulmonis." Int. J. Syst. Bacteriol. 48:389–94.

Niven, J.S.F. 1950. The histology of "grey lung virus" lesions in mice and cotton rats. Br. J. Exp. Pathol. 31:759–78.

Saito, M., et al. 1981. Synergistic effect of Sendai virus on *Mycoplasma pulmonis* infection in mice. Jap. J. Vet. Res. 43:43–50.

Temenetsky, J., and De Luca, R.R. 1998. Detection of *Mycoplasma pulmonis* from rats and mice of Sao Paulo/SP, Brazil. Lab. Anim. Sci. 48:210–13.

Pasteurella pneumotropica Infection

Arwohl, J.E., et al. 2000. Outbreak of *Pasteurella pneumotropica* in a closed colony of STOCK-Cd[tm1Mak] mice. Contemp. Top. 39(1):39–41.

Boot, R., et al. 1993. Colonization and antibody response in mice and rats experimentally infected with *Pasteurellaceae* from different rodent species. Lab. Anim. 28:130–37.

Brennan, P.C., et al. 1969. Role of *Pasteurella pneumotropica* and *Mycoplasma pulmonis* in murine pneumonia. J. Bacteriol. 97:337–49.

Davis, J.K., et al. 1987. The role of *Klebsiella oxytoca* in utero-ovarian infection of B6C3F1 mice. Lab. Anim. Sci. 37:159–66.

Erdman, S.E., et al. 1999. *P. pneumotropica* infection in E2F-4 deficient transgenic mice impedes phenotypic characterization. Lab. Anim. Sci. 49:440.

Goelz, M.F., et al. 1996. Efficacy of various therapeutic regimens in eliminating *Pasteurella pneumotropica* from the mouse. Lab. Anim. Sci. 46:280–85.

Macy, J.D., et al. 2000. Dual infection with *Pneumcystis carinii* and *Pasteurella pneumotropica* in B cell–deficient mice: Diagnosis and therapy. Comp. Med. 50:49–55.

Needham, J.R., and Cooper, J.E. 1975. An eye infection in laboratory mice associated with *Pasteurella pneumotropica.* Lab. Anim. 9:197–200.

Nicklas, W., et al. 1998. Phenotypic and molecular characterization of *Haemophilus influenzaemurium* isolated from laboratory mice. Contemp. Top. 37(4):93–94.

Wagner, J.E., et al. 1969. Spontaneous conjunctivitis and dacryoadenitis of mice. J. Am. Vet. Med. Assoc. 155:1211–17.

Ward, G.E.R., et al. 1978. Abortion in mice associated with *Pasteurella pneumotropica.* J. Clin. Microbiol. 8:177–80.

Weisbroth, S.H., et al. 1969. *Pasteurella pneumotropica* abscess syndrome in a mouse colony. J. Am. Vet. Med. Assoc. 155:1206–10.

Proteus mirabilis Infection

Jones, J.B., et al. 1972. *Proteus mirabilis* infection in a mouse colony. J. Am. Vet. Med. Assoc. 161:661–64.

Scott, R.A.W. 1989. Fatal *Proteus mirabilis* infection in a colony of SCID/bg immunodeficient mice. Lab. Anim. Sci. 39:470–71.

Scott, R.A.W., et al. 1991. Diagnostic exercise: Hepatitis in SCID-beige mice. Lab. Anim. Sci. 41:166–68.

Wensinck, F. 1961. The origin of endogenous *Proteus mirabilis* bacteremia in irradiated mice. J. Pathol. Bacteriol. 81:395–401.

Pseudomonas aeruginosa Infection

Brownstein, D.G. 1978. Pathogenesis of bacteremia due to *Pseudomonas aeruginosa* in cyclophosphamide-treated mice and potentiation of virulence of endogenous streptococci. J. Infect. Dis. 137:795–801.

Dietrich, H.M., et al. 1996. Isolation of *Enterococcus durans* and *Pseudomonas aeruginosa* in a scid mouse colony. Lab. Anim. 30:102–7.

Furuya, N., et al. 1993. Mortality rates amongst mice with endogenous septicemia caused by *Pseudomonas aeruginosa* isolates from various clinical sources. J. Med. Microbiol. 39:141–46.

Lindsey, J.R. 1986. Prevalence of viral and mycoplasmal infections in laboratory rodents. In *Viral and Mycoplasmal Infections of Laboratory Rodents: Effects on Biomedical Research,* ed. P.N. Bhatt et al., pp. 801–8. New York: Academic.

Morisset, C., et al. 1996. Lung phagocyte bacterial function in strains of mice resistant and susceptible to *Pseudomonas aeruginosa.* Infect. Immun. 64:4984–92.

Pier, G.B., et al. 1992. A murine model of chronic mucosal colonization by *Pseudomonas aeruginosa.* Infect. Immun. 60:4768–76.

Streptobacillus moniliformis Infection

Anderson, L.C., et al. 1983. Rat-bite fever in animal research laboratory personnel. Lab. Anim. Sci. 33:292–94.

Feundt, E.A. 1959. Arthritis caused by *Streptobacillus moniliformis* and pleuropneumonia-like organisms in small rodents. Lab. Invest. 8:1358–75.

Glastonbury, J.R.W., et al. 1996. *Streptobacillus moniliformis* infection in Swiss white mice. J. Vet. Diagn. Invest. 8:202–9.

Wullenweber, M., et al. 1990. *Streptobacillus moniliformis* epizootic in barrier-maintained C57BL/6J mice and susceptibility to infection of different strains of mice. Lab. Anim. Sci. 90:608–12.

Wullenweber, M. 1994. *Streptobacillus moniliformis*–a zoonotic pathogen. Taxonomic considerations, host species, diagnosis, therapy, geographical distribution. Lab. Anim. 29:1–15.

Corynebacterium kutscheri Infection

Amao, H., et al. 1995. Natural habitats of *Corynebacterium kutscheri* in subclinically infected ICGN and DBA/2 strains of mice. Lab. Anim. Sci. 45:6–10.

McWilliams, T.S., et al. 1993. Corynebacterium species–associated keratoconjunctivitis in aged male C57BL/6J mice. Lab. Anim. Sci. 43:509–12.

Corynebacterium bovis Infection

Clifford, C.B., et al. 1995. Hyperkeratosis in athymic nude mice caused by a coryneform bacterium: Microbiology, transmission, clinical signs, and pathology. Lab. Anim. Sci. 45:131–39.

Gobbi, A., et al. 1999. *Corynebacterium bovis* infection in immunocompetent hirsute mice. Lab. Anim. Sci. 39:209–11.

Richter, C.B., et al. 1991. D2 coryneforms as a cause of severe hyperkeratotic dermatitis in athymic nude mice. Lab. Anim. Sci. 40:545.

Russell, S., et al. 1998. Identification of *Corynebacterium bovis* as the etiologic agent of hyperkeratosis in nude mice and development of a diagnostic polymerase chain reaction assay. Contemp. Top. 37(4):93.

Scanziani, E., et al. 1998. Hyperkeratosis-associated coryneform infection in severe combined immunodeficient mice. Lab. Anim. 32: 330–36.

———. 1997. Outbreaks of hyperkeratotic dermatitis of athymic mice in northern Italy. Lab. Anim. 31:206–11.

Staphylococcal Infections

Bradfield, J.F., et al. 1993. Epizootic of fatal dermatitis in athymic nude mice due to *Stapylococcus xylosus.* Lab. Anim. Sci. 43:111–13.

McBride, D.F., et al. 1981. An outbreak of staphylococcal furunculosis in nude mice. Lab. Anim. Sci. 31:270–72

Shapiro, R.L., et al. 1997. Urokinase-type plasminogen activator-deficient mice are predisposed to staphylococcal botryomycosis, pleuritis, and effacement of lymphoid follicles. Am. J. Pathol. 150:359–69.

Wardrip, C.L., et al. 1994. Diagnostic exercise: Head and neck swelling in A/JCr mice. Lab. Anim. Sci. 44:280–82.

Streptococcal Infections

Dietrich, H.M., et al. 1996. Isolation of *Enterococcus durans* and *Pseudomonas aeruginosa* in a scid mouse colony. Lab. Anim. Sci. 30:102–7.

Duignan, P.J., and Percy, D.H. 1992. Diagnostic exercise: Unexplained deaths in recently acquired C3H3 mice. Lab. Anim. Sci. 42:610–11.

Geistfield, J.G., and Weisbroth, S.H. 1993. An epizootic of beta hemolytic group B type V streptococcus in DBA and DBA hybrid mice. Lab. Anim. Sci. 43:387–88.

Geistfield, J.G., et al. 1998. Epizootic of group B *Streptococcus agalactiae* serotype V in DBA/2 mice. Lab. Anim. Sci. 48:29–33.

Greenstein, G., et al. 1994. Isolation of *Streptococcus equisimilis* from abscesses detected in specific-pathogen-free mice. Lab. Anim. Sci. 44:374–76.

Morris, T.H. 1992. Sudden death in young mice. Lab. Anim. 21(9):15–17.

Percy, D.H., and Barta, J.R. 1993. Spontaneous and experimental infections in SCID and SCID/beige mice. Lab. Anim. Sci. 43:127–32.

Schenkman, D.I., et al. 1994. Outbreak of group B streptococcal meningoencephalitis in athymic mice. Lab. Anim. Sci. 44:639–41.

Stewart, D.D., et al. 1975. An epizootic of necrotic dermatitis in laboratory mice caused by Lancefield group G streptococci. Lab. Anim. Sci. 25:296–302.

Mycobacterium Infection

Waggie, K.S., et al. 1983a. A naturally occurring outbreak of *Mycobacterium avium-intracellulare* infections in C57BL/6N mice. Lab. Anim. Sci. 33:249–53.

———. 1983b. Experimental murine infections with a *Mycobacterium avium-intracellulare* complex organism isolated from mice. Lab. Anim. Sci. 33:254–57.

Spontaneous Diseases Associated with Immunocompromised and Genetically Engineered Mice

Brownstein, D.G. 1998. Genetically engineered mice: The holes in the sum of their parts. Lab. Anim. Sci. 48:121–22.

Smith, A.L. 1998. International conference on emerging infectious diseases. Lab. Anim. Sci. 48:225–27.

Viguera, C., et al. 1978. Clinical and pathological conditions of female nude (athymic) mice in two conventional maintained colonies. J. Am. Vet. Med. Assoc. 173:1198–1201.

General Bibliography

Caseboldt, D.B., et al. 1988. Prevalence rates of infectious agents among commercial breeding populations of rats and mice. Lab. Anim. Sci. 38:327–29.

Ganaway, J.R. 1982. Bacterial and mycotic diseases of the digestive system. In *The Mouse in Biomedical Research. II. Diseases,* ed. H.L. Foster, pp. 1–20. New York: Academic.

Nicklas, W., et al. 1999. Implications of infectious agents on results of animal experiments. Bact.: Lab. Anim. 33:S1.67–76.

Shultz, L.D., and Sidman, C.L. 1987. Genetically determined murine models of immunodeficiency. Annu. Rev. Immunol. 5:367–403.

Sparrow, S. 1976. The microbiological and parasitological status of laboratory animals from accredited breeders in the United Kingdom. Lab. Anim. 10:365–73.

Williford, C.B., and Wagner, J.E. 1982. Bacterial and mycotic diseases of the integumentary system. In *The Mouse in Biomedical Research. II. Diseases,* ed. H.L. Foster, pp. 55–75. New York: Academic.

MYCOTIC INFECTIONS

Dermatomycosis

EPIZOOTIOLOGY AND PATHOGENESIS. *Trichophyton mentagrophytes* is the predominant dermatophyte among mice, although other dermatophytes, including *Microsporum canis,* have been isolated. Two varieties of *T. mentagrophytes* have been recovered from mice: *T. mentagrophytes* var. *quinckeanum* and *T. mentagrophytes* var. *mentagrophytes. T. mentagrophytes* occurs worldwide. Its true prevalence in laboratory mouse colonies is unclear, since the great majority of infections are subclinical, especially among adult mice. The most severe manifestation, favus, is usually associated with *T. mentagrophytes* var. *quinckeanum.* Other predisposing factors probably play a role in the manifestation of this disease.

PATHOLOGY. Favus is characterized by dull yellow, cuplike crusts on the muzzle, head, ears, face, tail, and extremities. These crusts are composed of epithelial debris, exudate, mycelia, and masses of arthrospores, with underlying dermatitis. Hair invasion has not been observed in mouse favus. Other lesions attributed to *T. mentagrophytes* include alopecia and focal crusts, particularly on the head, but the majority of infections are subclinical.

DIAGNOSIS. Lesions of dermatomycosis are characteristic. Arthrospores and mycelia can be visualized with fungal strains and are Schiff-positive. *Differential diagnoses* include other forms of dermatitis and alopecia. *Trichophyton* can be readily grown on Sabaroud's agar.

SIGNIFICANCE. *Trichophyton* appears to be relatively nonpathogenic in mice. Subclinical carriers are the norm among mice and have been shown to occur in high prevalence in some mouse populations. *Trichophyton* is nonselective in its host range and can infect other laboratory animals and human contacts.

Pneumocystis carinii Infection: Pneumocystosis.

P. carinii is a microorganism that is widespread in the rodent population. Based on current information, *P. carinii* should be classified as a fungus and not a protozoon. Pneumocystis pneumonia is a major complication in immunosuppressed humans and has emerged as a significant natural pathogen in immunodeficient mice.

EPIZOOTIOLOGY AND PATHOGENESIS. *P. carinii* can exist as a saprophytic infection in the lungs of several species, including mice, rats, and humans. Significant antigenic differences have been observed among *Pneumocystis* recovered from different species. Based on current information, it is unlikely that interspecies infections occur. Normally, infected animals are asymptomatic, and detection of infection in such mice is difficult, even by PCR. Nevertheless, these carrier mice can inefficiently transmit infection to other mice by direct contact. Immunosuppression of carrier mice will result in pneumocystis pneumonia and more efficient transmission to contact animals. Spontaneous enzootics of pneumocystis pneumonia are now common in a variety of immunodeficient strains of mice. Superimposed viral infection can exacerbate disease, and superimposed bacterial infections, such as *Pasteurella pneumotropica,* may result in suppurative bronchopneumonia. Immunocompromised mice subclinically infected with *P. carinii* inoculated with

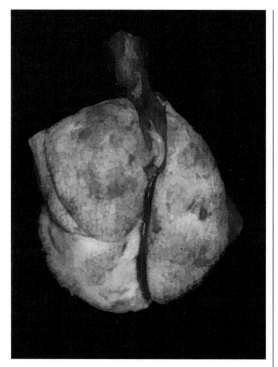

FIG. 1.57—Lungs from immunodeficient mouse with pneumocystosis. The lungs are pale and fleshy and collapse poorly, typical gross findings with this disease.

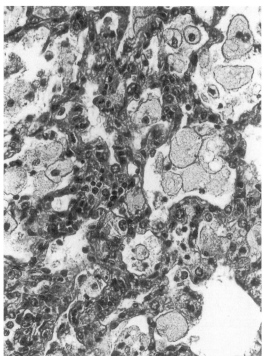

FIG. 1.58—Section of lung from athymic mouse with spontaneous pneumocystis pneumonitis. Alveolar septa are hypercellular, with mononuclear cell infiltration. Foamy proteinaceous exudate and alveolar macrophages are present in many alveoli.

PVM developed severe respiratory tract lesions attributed to the dual infection.

PATHOLOGY. Clinical signs of pneumocystis pneumonia in immunodeficient mice include dyspnea, wasting, hunched posture, and dry, scaly skin. Lungs collapse poorly and have a rubbery consistency, with pale, patchy areas of consolidation (Fig.1.57). Microscopic examination reveals an interstitial alveolitis, with proteinaceous exudation into the alveolar lumina. There is marked thickening of alveolar septa and infiltration with mononuclear leukocytes (Fig. 1.58). Finely vacuolated, eosinophilic material and alveolar macrophages are scattered in affected alveoli. In tissue sections from affected lung stained with the PAS or methenamine silver procedures, numerous rounded and irregularly flattened cyst forms 3-5 μm in diameter are present in reactive areas (Fig. 1.59). Electron microscopy reveals numerous trophozoites (vegetative forms) with long filapodia (involved in cell attachment) intermixed

with thicker-walled cysts. The quality of the pneumonia associated with pneumocystis in immunodeficient mice can be quite variable, depending upon the immune deficiency. Some types of mice may have very few visible cysts or alveolar exudation, with principally an interstitial pneumonia.

DIAGNOSIS. The history of experimental procedures leading to immunosuppression or the presence of disease in genetically immunodeficient mice are critical predisposing factors. Organisms should be demonstrated in the typical foamy alveolar exudate, using the methenamine silver or PAS staining procedure. The organisms are best visualized with the methenamine silver staining method. *Differential diagnoses* include viral pneumonitis, particularly Sendai virus and pneumonia virus of mice, and pulmonary edema secondary to congestive heart failure.

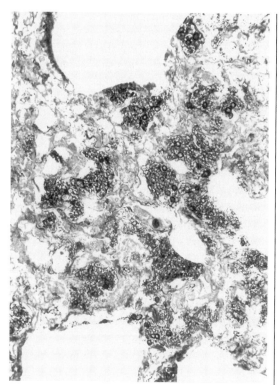

FIG. 1.59—Lung from mouse in FIGure 1.57, stained with methenamine silver method. Large numbers of cyst forms are present in alveoli.

SIGNIFICANCE. *Pneumocystis* infections pose a major threat in colonies of immunodeficient mice, with high mortality. There currently is no evidence of interspecies transmission.

Other Mycotic Infections. The yeast *Candida albicans* is frequently present as a member of the normal flora of the alimentary tract in laboratory rodents. When microscopic examination of the murine stomach reveals scattered pseudohyphae in the keratinized epithelium of the forestomach, it is usually regarded as an incidental finding. However, there have been reports of extensive gastric candidiasis with mortality in immunocompromised mice. These mice have thickening of the squamous portion of the stomach with necrotic debris adherent to the surface forming a pseudomembrane. There is marked epithelial hyperplasia with hyperkeratosis and leukocytic infiltration. The typical filamentous structures with pseudohyphae formation are readily visualized with PAS or silver stains. T-cell–deficient mice are particularly at risk. Fungal hyphae can be found incidentally in microscopic sections of the nasal passages of mice, associated with chronic inflammation. Contaminated bedding is a possible source for a variety of fungal agents, including *C. albicans, Aspergillus fumigatus,* and *Cryptococcus* spp.

BIBLIOGRAPHY
FOR MYCOTIC INFECTIONS

Dermatomycosis

Dolan, M.M., et al., 1958. Ringworm epizootics in laboratory mice and rats: Experimental and accidental transmission of infection. J. Invest. Dermatol. 30:23–25.

Mackenzie, D.W.R. 1961. *Trichophyton mentagrophytes* in mice: Infections of humans and incidence amongst laboratory animals. Sabouradia 1:178–82.

Papini, R., et al. 1997. Survey of dermatophytes isolated from the coats of laboratory animals in Italy. Lab. Anim. Sci. 47:75–77.

Pneumocystis carinii Infection

Barthold, S.W. 1991. A review of common infectious disease agents of laboratory mice and rats: Potential influence on *Pneumocystis carinii*. J. Protozool. 38:131S–33S.

Bauer, N.L., et al. 1993. *Pneumocystis carinii* organisms obtained from rats, ferrets, and mice are antigenically different. Infect. Immun. 61:1315–19.

Beck, J.M., et al. 1996. Role of CD8+ lymphocytes in host defense against *Pneumocystis carinii* in mice. J. Lab. Clin. Med. 128:477–87.

Bray, M.V., et al. 1993. Exacerbation of *Pneumocystis carinii* pneumonia in immunodeficient (*scid*) mice by concurrent infection with a pneumovirus. Infect. Immun. 61:1586–88.

Macy, J.D., et al. 2000. Dual infection with *Pneumocystis carinii* and *Pasteurella pneumotropica* in B cell-deficient mice: Diagnosis and therapy. Comp. Med. 50:49–55.

Powles, M.A., et al. 1992. Mouse model for *Pneumocystis carinii* pneumonia that uses natural transmission to initiate infection. Infect. Immun. 60:1397–1400.

Serikawa, T., et al. 1991. A survey of *Pneumocystis carinii* infection in research colonies in Japan. Lab. Anim. Sci. 41:411–14.

Shultz, L.D., and Sidman, C.L. 1987. Genetically determined murine models of immunodeficiency. Annu. Rev. Immunol. 5:367–403.

Soulez, B., et al. 1991. Introduction of *Pneumocystis carinii* in a colony of SCID mice. J. Protozool. 38:123S–25S.

Stringer, J.R. 1993. The identity of *Pneumocystis carinii:* Not a single protozoan, but a diverse group of exotic fungi. Infect. Agents Dis. 2:109–17.

Walzer, P.D., et al. 1989. Outbreaks of *Pneumocystis carinii* pneumonia in colonies of immunodeficient mice. Infect. Immun. 57:62–70.

———. 1979. Experimental *Pneumocystis carinii* pneumonia in different strains of cortisonized mice. Infect. Immun. 24:939–47.

Weir, E.C., et al. 1986. Spontaneous wasting disease in nude mice associated with *Pneumocystis carinii* infection. Lab. Anim. Sci. 36:140-44.

Other Mycotic Infections

Dixon, D., et al. 1993. Diagnostic exercise: Gastritis in athymic nude mice. Lab. Anim. Sci. 43:497–99.

Mayeux, P., et al. 1995. Massive fungal contamination in animal care facilities traced to bedding supply. Appl. Environ. Microbiol. 61:2297–2301.

PARASITIC DISEASES

ECTOPARASITIC INFESTATIONS

Fur Mite Infestations: Acariasis. Laboratory mice are commonly infested with mixed populations of fur mites, including *Myobia musculi, Radfordia affinis,* and *Myocoptes musculinis. Myobia musculi* is the most clinically significant mouse mite. *Trichoecius romboutsi* closely resembles *Myocoptes,* and its actual prevalence is therefore unknown.

EPIZOOTIOLOGY, LIFE CYCLES, AND PATHOGENESIS. *Myobia* infestations are widespread in mouse populations. Eggs are laid on hair shafts adjacent to the epidermis. Larvae hatch in 7–8 d, and egg-laying adults may evolve as early as 16 d after the eggs are laid. *Myobia* mites feed on skin secretions and interstitial fluid but apparently not on blood. This intimate feeding pattern is unique to *Myobia,* resulting in immune sensitization of the host, resulting in a high frequency of immune-mediated paraphenomena in some strains of mice. Transmission is by direct transfer of adult mites. Adults may migrate to sucklings from infested mothers at around 1 wk. Infestation corresponds with the appearance of pelage on the young mice. The presence of hair shafts is critical for successful colonization. Newborn mice are not susceptible until pelage erupts, and nude mice are resistant to experimental infection. In newly infested mice, the mite numbers increase for the first 8-10 wk, but host immunity diminishes the populations to a point of equilibrium. This state of equilibrium persists for months to years, with cyclic variations corresponding to waves of egg hatches. Factors recognized to influence parasite load include strain of mouse, age, self-grooming, and mutual grooming. Impairment of grooming function by procedures such as hind toe amputation or Elizabethan collars result in increased parasite load.

Adverse effects of *Myobia* infestation are highly varied and often difficult to prove with certainty. *Myobia* can sensitize the host, resulting in severe pruritis, with self-inflicted ulcerative lesions that often have secondary bacterial components. Sensitivity is genetically associated, and strains such as B6 are highly prone to hypersensitivity dermatitis. Lesion susceptibility is affected by a non-H-2-linked gene or gene combination shared by all B6 background strains. Cutaneous allergy due to mite infestation may also occur in other strains, including BALB/c mice. The hypersensitivity component was confirmed by the histopathologic findings and the markedly elevated serum IgE levels present in affected mice. Manifestations of acariasis range from ruffled fur and alopecia on the head, eyelids, neck, or shoulder regions to severe ulcerative dermatitis with marked pruritis, occasionally resulting in traumatic amputation of the ear pinnae. Self-trauma is an important factor in the development of these lesions (Fig. 1.60). Other adverse effects include reduced life span, weight loss, and infertility.

Radfordia affinis is also common among mice, but its life cycle is not well studied. Its close resemblance to *Myobia* has led to confusion to its actual prevalence and effects. It does not induce overt disease like *Myobia* and often exists in mixed infestations.

Myocoptes musculinis is the most common of the mouse fur mites and usually exists as a mixed infestation with *Myobia. Myocoptes* is a surface dweller and feeds upon material in the superficial epidermis. Transmission occurs by close contact, and mites can be transferred within 1 wk of birth to newborns. *Myocoptes* tends to be peripatetic, spreading all over the body. In mixed infestations, *Myobia* tends to dominate the head and shoulder pelage, and *Myocoptes* can be found primarily in the inguinal, ventral abdomen, and back. Clinical

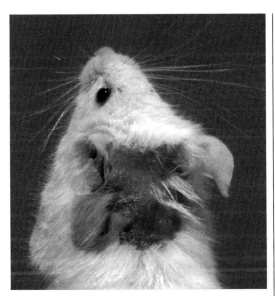

FIG. 1.60—Ulcerative dermatitis with denuding of hair associated with acariasis and secondary staphylococcal infection. Pruritis associated with the infestation may lead to self-inflicted skin abrasions with superimposed bacterial infection.

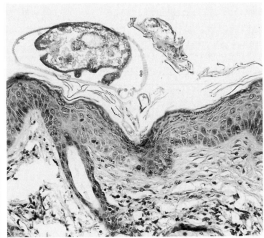

FIG. 1.61—Histological section of skin from a case of acariasis in C57BL mouse. There is epidermal hyperplasia, with mononuclear cell infiltration in the dermis. A mite is present on the surface of the lesion.

signs are usually mild, including patchy hair loss, erythema, and mild pruritis. However, severe pruritis with ulcerative dermatitis has been observed in BALB/c mice infected with *Myocoptes musculinus* only (with the caveat that mixed infestations are common and often overlooked).

Microscopic examination of fur mite–induced skin lesions will reveal mild epidermal hyperplasia and hyperkeratosis, with variable dermal infiltrates of mononuclear leukocytes and mast cells. In ulcerated lesions, exudation and secondary bacterial colonization (see Staphylococcal Infections) are often present, with underlying fibrovascular proliferation, mixed leukocyte infiltration, and hyperplasia of the adjacent intact epidermis. Mites may be present on the surface of the lesions, particularly in early, mild lesions (Fig. 1.61).

DIAGNOSIS. Fur mites can be demonstrated by placing the mouse or a portion of the skinned pelt (head and shoulder regions) in a Petri dish for 1 or more hours. The mites will climb up the hair

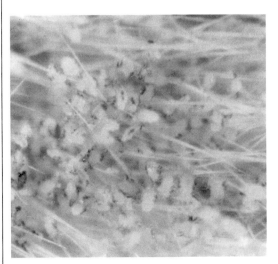

FIG. 1.62—*Mycoptes musculinus* infestation. Large numbers of mites are present on the pellage (dissecting microscope preparation). (Courtesy J.P. Lautenslager)

shafts and can then be visualized under a dissecting microscope (Fig. 1.62), collected, and identified under a light or stereoscopic microscope. Skin scrapings or cellophane tape applied to the hair can then be placed on a glass slide for microscopic evaluation. A number of points are important to consider in the diagnosis of acariasis. The number of mites will be greatest in young mice, before immune-mediated equilibrium has occurred. For this reason, the number of mites on mice with severe hypersensitivity-induced lesions may be exceedingly few. Infestations are usually mixed, so identification of a single mite will not reflect the true population. Finally, *Myobia* is the most clinically significant, but clinical signs are variable, depending on host factors. One does not have to be a sophisticated acarologist to identify mouse fur mites. A few distinguishing features allow simple speciation. *Myobia* and *Radfordia* are remarkably similar in morphology, with slightly elongated bodies possessing bulges between their legs. If the second pair of legs is carefully examined, *Myobia* has a single terminal tarsal claw, while *Radfordia* has two of unequal length. *Myocoptes* is oval, with heavily chitinized, pigmented third and fourth legs and suckers on its tarsi. *Differential diagnoses* for fur mite infestation includes pediculosis, trauma, bacterial dermatitis, dermatophytosis, hair chewing, and mechanically induced muzzle alopecia.

SIGNIFICANCE. Complications include reduced life span, infertility, weight loss, modified immune responsiveness, and secondary amyloidosis. The association with amyloidosis is not absolute but is suspected. Mice of the B6 background are particularly at risk and may develop a severe hypersensitivity reaction to mite infestations. Cutaneous allergy with wasting has also been observed in BALB/c mice.

Follicle Mite Infestations. *Mus musculus* is susceptible to infestation with *Demodex musculi,* but this parasite has not been noted in contemporary laboratory mouse colonies for decades. Considering this fact, and the high degree of host specificity of *Demodex* species, it is remarkable that *D. musculi* infestation has been recently reported in a colony of transgenic mice lacking mature T cells and NK cells. Mites were located in the superficial dermis of the dorsal thorax, at the opening of hair follicles, with no inflammatory reaction. Infection of immunocompetent mice was documented, but they harbored very few

mites. Contact transmission of the mites to SCID mice was readily accomplished. Diagnosis can be achieved by examination of plucked hair or skin sections. Older accounts of demodex infestations in *Mus musculus* include observations of mites in the tongue (unknown species)and preputial and clitoral glands (*D. flagellarus*).

Psorergates simplex was once common among laboratory mice but is now rare. It remains common in wild and pet mice. This small mite inhabits hair follicles, inciting the formation of comedones in the skin of the head, shoulders, and lumbar areas, and, less commonly, elsewhere. The life cycle of this mite is not known, but all of its life stages can be found within a single hair follicle.

PATHOLOGY. Mice infested with fur mites display varying degrees of pruritis, with hyperactive, agitated behavior. Skin lesions include scruffiness, varying degrees of alopecia and dermatitis. Mice highly sensitized to *Myobia* develop self-inflicted ulcerative dermatitis, with secondary pyoderma. Pruritis may be intense in these mice, resulting in self-mutilation. Regional lymph nodes are often enlarged. *Psorergates* infection results in the formation of follicular cysts, which can be seen as white nodules on the subcutaneous side of the dermis. These are most common around the head and neck. *Psorergates* infestation can be diagnosed by microscopic examination of cystic hair follicles or their contents. Follicles are filled with keratin squames, and mites are present along the epidermis.

***Ornithonyssus bacoti* Infestation.** *O. bacoti,* or tropical rat mite, is a blood-sucking mesostigmate mite that infests wild rats, as well as other species. It is nonselective in its host range. It inhabits its host only to feed and then hides in nearby niches. It causes intense pruritis, and its presence in a rodent population is often first manifest on human handlers. Its complete life cycle can occur within 2 wk, allowing massive infestation to occur within a short period of time. Because of its nonselective nature, *Ornithonyssus* has been found in laboratory mouse colonies.

Louse Infestation: Pediculosis. *Polyplax serrata* is a relatively common louse of wild mice, and at one time it infested laboratory mice throughout the world. It is now essentially nonexistent in laboratory mouse colonies. Eggs attach to the base of hair shafts and hatch through an operculum at their top. Stage I nymphs can be found over the entire body, but the later four stages tend to prefer the anterior dorsum of the body. Eggs hatch within 5-6 d, and nymphs develop into adults within 1 wk. Transmission is by direct contact. Host immunity appears to develop, as parasite numbers diminish with time. As sucking lice, heavy infestations can result in anemia and debilitation. Bites are pruritic, resulting in intense scratching and dermatitis. *Polyplax* once played a significant role as a vector of *Eperythrozoon coccoides.*

ENDOPARASITIC INFECTIONS

Protozoal Infections. Coccidia, *Cryptosporidium muris, Giardia muris,* and *Spironucleus muris* are examples of protozoal organisms found in the intestinal tract that are considered to be relatively nonpathogenic. Under some circumstances, they may represent opportunistic infections associated with overt disease. *Eimeria muris* is more overtly pathogenic, but it is rare in laboratory mice. Another coccidian, *Klossiella muris,* is also rare in laboratory mice. *Trichomonas muris* is an intestinal flagellate that can grow to abundance in the large intestine of mice, but it is not a pathogen. It is frequently included in lists of mouse parasites, but it is a commensal organism.

COCCIDIAL INFECTIONS: COCCIDIOSIS. Mice are host to several species of *Eimeria,* with *E. falciformis* being the most significant. Intestinal coccidiosis rarely occurs in well-managed facilities. Intestinal coccidiosis is very common among wild mice, where it causes marked colitis (Fig. 1.63) and runting in juvenile animals. Oocysts can be found in the mucosa of older mice without discernible lesions.

Renal coccidiosis due to *Klossiella muris* is rarely observed in laboratory mice but is quite common in wild mice. Infection probably occurs by the ingestion of sporocysts, with hematogenous spread to glomerular capillaries and schizogony. Gametogeny and sporogony occur in epithelial cells lining convoluted tubules. On microscopic examination, lesions are usually con-

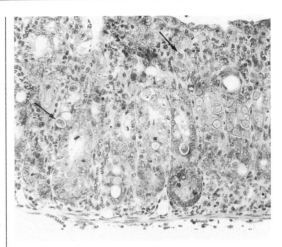

FIG. 1.63—Section of colon from case of intestinal coccidiosis in laboratory mouse. There is a marked hyperplastic colitis. Sloughed cells, leukocytes, and a few developing oocysts (*arrows*) are present on the surface of the gut. Macrogametocytes are evident in some enterocytes.

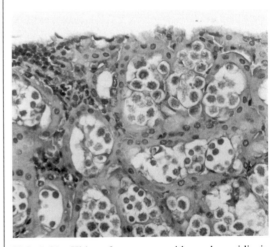

FIG. 1.64—Kidney from mouse with renal coccidiosis due to *Klossiella muris.* Large numbers of sporocysts are present in epithelial cells of renal tubules.

fined to the convoluted tubules. Organisms appear as eosinophilic spherical structures within the cytoplasm of epithelial cells, with minimal inflammatory response (Fig. 1.64).

SIGNIFICANCE. *Klossiella* infections are rarely detected in laboratory mice. They are considered to be an incidental finding, but if present, they indicate the need for improved sanitation practices. There have been anecdotal reports of transmission of *K. muris* to guinea pigs, but this species has its own *Klossiella* (*K. cobayae*).

CRYPTOSPORIDIUM INFECTION: CRYPTOSPORIDIOSIS. *Cryptosporidium muris* occurs primarily on the surface of the gastric mucosa of mice. It is relatively nonpathogenic in this species. Similarly, *C. parvum* is a marginally pathogenic inhabitant of the small intestine. The prevalence of infection is not known, but it can be associated with enteritis, probably secondary to viral infections in young mice. Suckling mice are particularly at risk. It may also ascend the biliary tract in nude and SCID mice, resulting in chronic cholangiohepatitis with focal hepatic coagulative necrosis (Fig. 1.65). Intestinal microflora may play a role in susceptibility/resistance to clinical disease. The presence of cryptosporidia in a colony of mice suggests that improved sanitation practices are warranted. Possible sources of the organism include a contaminated water supply. The possibility of transmission to human contacts, and the potential danger posed by *Cryptosporida* spp. to immunocompromised mice, should be emphasized.

GIARDIA MURIS INFECTION: GIARDIASIS

EPIZOOTIOLOGY AND PATHOGENESIS. *Giardia muris* is a flagellate that normally resides primarily in the lumen of the duodenum. Mice, hamsters, rats, and other rodents are natural hosts. In the naturally occurring disease, trophozoites proliferate in the small intestine and adhere to the microvilli of enterocytes near the base of villi by means of concave sucking disks. Organisms also wedge in furrows on the epithelial surface and lodge in mucus overlying intestinal epithelium. Clearance of the parasite has been associated with intraluminal lymphocyte migration and attachment to the organism. *Giardia* infects both young and adult mice. In heavy infestations, animals have a rough hair coat and distended abdomen, usually with no evidence of diarrhea. Based on some surveys, the incidence of positive colonies may be up to 60%.

PATHOLOGY. At necropsy, the small intestine is usually distended, with yellow to white watery contents. Microscopic examination of tissue sections of the small intestine reveals trophozoites that are pear-shaped, with a broadly rounded anterior sucking disk. There may be a reduction in crypt:villus ratio, with increased numbers of inflammatory cells in the lamina propria. Intestinal invasion may occur in immunocompromised mice.

DIAGNOSIS. The demonstration of typical trophozoites and cysts on wet mount preparations of feces is the basis for the diagnosis of giardiasis.

SIGNIFICANCE. Infections are frequently subclinical in the absence of other predisposing factors. Complications may include significant morbidity and mortality in nude or thymectomized mice. Cytokinetic studies have demonstrated a marked increase in cryptal enterocyte turnover in the small intestine of infected mice. Suppression of the immune response to sheep erythrocytes has been observed in infected mice.

SPIRONUCLEUS (HEXAMITA) MURIS INFECTION: SPIRONUCLEOSIS

EPIZOOTIOLOGY AND PATHOGENESIS. This flagellated protozoan parasite is frequently present in the alimentary tract of clinically normal mice. In surveys of commercial suppliers, over 60% of colonies studied were positive for *Spironucleus*. Other species commonly infected include rats and hamsters. Both *Spironucleus* and *Giardia* are

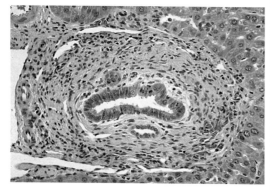

FIG. 1.65—Section of liver from athymic mouse with chronic cryptosporidiosis. There is a chronic cholangitis with peribiliary fibrosis. Organisms are present on the surface of the biliary epithelium.

transmissible from hamsters to mice. The organism is usually associated with clinical disease (spironucleosis, previously termed hexamitiasis) only in young mice, and often there are identifiable predisposing factors. The organism colonizes the small intestine, primarily in the crypts in the duodenum. *Spironucleus* divides by longitudinal fission. Animals become infected by the ingestion of trophozoites or cysts. Clinical manifestations are usually associated with immunosuppression or environmental stress, and there may be a concomitant infection with other pathogens, such as enterotropic mouse hepatitis virus. Animals 3-6 wk of age are particularly at risk. Clinical signs include depression, weight loss, dehydration, hunched posture, diarrhea, and mortality rates of up to 50% in young animals.

PATHOLOGY. The small intestine is distended with dark red to brown watery contents and gas. In tissue sections of small intestine examined microscopically from animals with the acute form of the disease, there may be edema of the lamina propria, with mild leukocytic infiltration, neutrophils predominating. Crypts and intervillous spaces are distended with elongated, pear-shaped trophozoites (Fig. 1.66). Organisms may also be present between enterocytes and within the lamina propria. Other intestinal microflora may play a role in the development of these lesions. In the chronic form of the disease, the cellular infiltrate consists primarily of lymphocytes and plasma cells. Scattered duodenal crypts may be markedly dilated and contain leukocytes and cellular debris. The trophozoites stain well with the PAS staining technique, while the organism is poorly delineated in H & E–stained preparations.

DIAGNOSIS. Trophozoites with fast straight or zigzag movements can be visualized microscopically on direct wet mount smears prepared from small intestine. Typical banded "Easter egg" cysts are present in the intestinal contents.

SIGNIFICANCE. It is frequently difficult to determine the significance of *Spironucleus* infections, since infected animals are normally asymptomatic. Investigations should include a search for underlying disease or other predisposing factors.

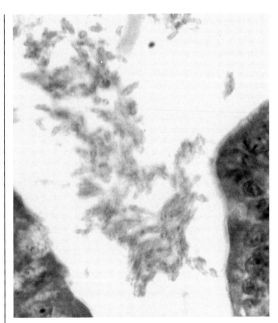

FIG. 1.66—Spironucleosis (*Spironucleus muris* infection) in young laboratory mouse with diarrhea. In this section of duodenum, large numbers of trophozoites are present on the mucosal surface.

Copathogens may include concurrent viral infections, such as enterotropic murine coronavirus. Complications in research associated with heavy infestations with *Spironucleus* include impaired immune response and macrophage function in euthymic mice, chronic doubling of enterocyte turnover in the small intestine, and shortened life span in nude mice. Interspecies transmission has been demonstrated between hamsters and mice, but not to rats.

Helminth Infections: Pinworms (Oxyuriasis). *Syphacia obvelata* and *Aspicularis tetraptera* are extremely common pinworms in the laboratory mouse.

EPIZOOTIOLOGY AND LIFE CYCLE. Pinworm infestations remain a relatively common problem. This is in part due to the high degree of environmental resistance of eggs, and their propensity to drift in air and dust. Pinworms are often the first break in rederived mouse colonies. The life cycle of *Syphacia* is direct and is completed in approximately 12–15 d. Following the ingestion of eggs, larvae emerge and migrate to the cecum. They develop into adults and mate, and females then migrate to the perianal region for egg deposition. Eggs become infective within a few hours. Young mice are particularly susceptible to pinworm infestation. Dual infections with *Aspicularis* and *Syphacia* also occur. The life cycle of *A. tetraptera* is direct and takes approximately 23–25 d. Mature females lay eggs in the terminal colon, which are then passed in the feces. Eggs require incubation at room temperature for 6–7 d in order to become infective and can survive for weeks outside the host. Most mice with pinworm infections are asymptomatic. Clinical signs associated with heavy infestations include rectal prolapse, intussusception, fecal impaction, and diarrhea.

DIAGNOSIS. Visualization and identification of adult worms present in the cecum or colon at necropsy is a standard procedure. These nematodes are frequently found in tissue sections of cecum and colon (Fig. 1.67). Identification of worm eggs will require fecal flotation for *Aspicu-laris* spp., but cellophane tape applied to the perianal region is the recommended method of collection of *Syphacia* eggs for microscopic identification. Ova can be readily differentiated. *Aspicularis* ova are bilaterally symmetrical, while *Syphacia* ova are banana-shaped.

SIGNIFICANCE. Complications attributed to pinworm infestations include decreased weight gains, behavioral changes, and altered immune responses. Nude (and presumably other immunodefient) mice are especially susceptible to heavy infestations. In immunodeficient mice, mucosal invasion with colitis can be noted on occasion. These ascarids are readily treated with drugs such as ivermectin, but treatment seldom completely cures the colony of infection, and maintaining colonies free from the parasite is a difficult matter.

Helminth Infections: Tapeworms

HYMENOLEPIS INFECTIONS. Wild and laboratory rodents can be infected with three separate species of *Hymenolepis,* including *H. nana* (dwarf tapeworm), *H. diminuta,* and *H. microstoma.* The latter two species are no longer found in laboratory mice, since husbandry conditions preclude the necessary intermediate arthropod host.

EPIZOOTIOLOGY, LIFE CYCLE, AND PATHOGENESIS. A variety of species of laboratory animals are susceptible to infection with the dwarf tapeworm, including mice, rats, and hamsters. Its wide host range also includes humans. Husbandry conditions have essentially eliminated *H. diminuta* and *H. microstoma* and have greatly reduced the prevalence of *H. nana* in laboratory mouse populations. These tapeworms all utilize arthropods as intermediate hosts, but *H. nana* can also have a direct life cycle in which onchospheres penetrate the mucosa and develop into the cercocystis stage, subsequently emerging into the lumen as adults. The entire life cycle can occur in the intestine within 20–30 d. Thus, superinfections can occur in the absence of an intermediate host. Immunity develops to these worms, with reduction of parasite numbers over time. Clinical signs associated with heavy infestations include poor weight gains and diarrhea.

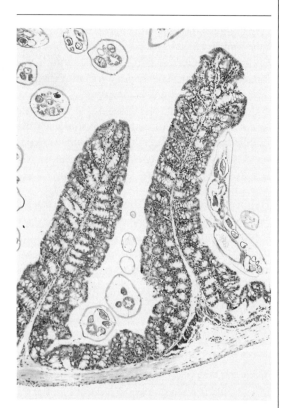

FIG. 1.67—Adult pinworms *(Syphacia obvelata)* present in the cecum of adult athymic mouse.

PATHOLOGY. *H. nana* adults are threadlike worms in the small intestine. Microscopic findings include the presence of cysticeri within the lamina propria and adults (approximately the size of villi) with prominent serrated edges in the lumen. Occasionally, cysticeri can be found in the mesenteric lymph nodes. *H. diminuta* adults are much larger, and intermediate forms do not appear in the mucosa. *H. microstoma* adults are the size of *H. diminuta* and often lodge in the bile or pancreatic ducts, inciting inflammatory and atrophic changes in the pancreas and cholangitis.

DIAGNOSIS. The worms can be identified grossly. Only *H. nana* and *H. diminuta* are likely to be encountered in laboratory animals. *H. nana* is typically threadlike (1 mm wide), while the other species are much larger (4 mm wide). The *H. nana* scolex possesses hooks, and the ova have polar filaments while those of *H. diminuta* do not.

SIGNIFICANCE. In addition to transient damage to the intestinal mucosa and weight loss, there is danger of interspecies spread, including human infections.

TAENIA TAENIAFORMIS INFECTION. Mice can serve as the intermediate host for this cat tapeworm. The larval form, *Cysticercus fasciolaris,* consists of a scolex and segments within a cyst and thus resembles an adult tapeworm (Fig. 1.68).

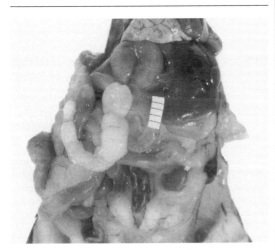

FIG. 1.68—Laboratory mouse with *Cysticercus fasciolaris* infestation of the liver. The lesion has been opened. Note the scolex and identifiable segments of the parasite.

The liver is the most frequent location for cysticerci. The source of the parasite is usually via feed contaminated with cat feces. While cysticercosis should be nonexistent in laboratory mice, the authors have seen infected laboratory mice on multiple occasions.

BIBLIOGRAPHY FOR PARASITIC DISEASES

Ectoparasitic Infestations

Bukva V. 1985. *Demodex flagellarus* sp. n. (Acari: Demodicidae) from the preputial and clitoral glands of the house mouse, *Mus musculus*. Folia Parasitol. 32:73–81.

Burdett, E.C., et al. 1997. Evaluation of five treatment regimens and five diagnostic methods for murine mite (*Myocoptes musculinus* and *Myobia musculi*). Contemp. Top. 36(2):73–76.

Csiza, C.K., and McMartin, D.N. 1976. Apparent acaridal dermatitis in a C57BL/6Nya mouse colony. Lab. Anim. Sci. 26:781–87.

Dawson, D.D., et al. 1986. Genetic control of susceptibility to mite-associated ulcerative dermatitis. Lab. Anim. Sci. 36:262–67.

French, A.W. 1987. Elimination of *Ornithonyssus bacoti* in a colony of aging mice. Lab. Anim. Sci. 37:670–72.

Friedman, S., and Weisbroth, S.H. 1975. The parasitic ecology of the rodent mite, *Myobia musculi*. II. Genetic factors. Lab. Anim. Sci. 25:440–45.

Hill, L.R., et al. 1999. *Demodex musculi* in the skin of transgenic mice. Contemp. Top. 38(6):13–18.

Hirst, S. 1917. Remarks on certain species of the genus *Demodex,* Owen (the *Demodex* of man, the horse, dog, rat and mouse). Ann. Mag. Nat. Hist. 20:233–35.

Jungmann, P., et al. 1996. Murine acariasis. 1. Pathological and clinical evidence suggesting cutaneous allergy and wasting syndrome in BALB/c mouse. Res. Immunol. 147:27–38.

Tuzdil, N. 1957. Das vorkommen von Demodex in der zunge einer maus. Z. Tropenmedez. Parasitol. 8:274–78.

Weisbroth, S.H. 1982. Arthropods. In *The Mouse in Biomedical Research. II. Diseases,* ed. H.L. Foster et al., pp. 388–90. New York: Academic.

Weisbroth, S.H., et al. 1976. The parasitic ecology of the rodent mite *Myobia musculi*. III. Lesions in certain host strains. Lab. Anim. Sci. 26:725–35.

———. 1974. The parasitic ecology of the rodent mite *Myobia musculi*. I. Grooming factors. Lab. Anim. Sci. 24:510–16.

Wharton, G.W. 1940. Life cycle and feeding habits of *Myobia musculi*. J. Parasitol. 40:29.

Coccidial Infections

Haberkorn, A., et al. 1983. Control of an outbreak of coccidiosis in a closed colony. Lab. Anim. 17:59–64.

Taylor, J.L., et al. 1979. *Klossiella* parasites of animals: A literature review. Vet. Parasitol. 5:137–44.

Cryptosporidium Infection
Fernandez, P.E., et al. 1996. Cryptosporidiosis in mice in Argentina. Lab. Anim. Sci. 46:685–86.

Harp, J.A.W., et al. 1992. Resistance of combined immunodeficient mice to infection with *Cryptosporidium parvum:* The importance of intestinal microflora. Infect. Immun. 60:3509–12.

Kuhls, T.L., et al. 1992. Cryptosporidiosis in adult and neonatal mice with severe combined immunodeficiency. J. Comp. Pathol. 113:399–410.

Mead, J.R., et al. 1991. Chronic *Cryptosporidium parvum* infections in congenitally immunodeficient SCID and nude mice. J. Infect. Dis. 163:1297–1304.

Giardia muris Infection
Belosevic, M., et al. 1985. Suppression of primary antibody response to sheep erythrocytes in susceptible and resistant mice infected with *Giardia muris.* Infect. Immun. 47:21–25.

Hsu, C-K. 1982. Protozoa. In *The Mouse in Biomedical Research. II. Diseases,* ed. H.L. Foster et al., pp. 359–72. New York: Academic.

Kunstyr, I., et al. 1992. Host specificity of *Giardia muris* isolates from mouse and golden hamster. Parasit. Res. 78:621–22.

Lindsey, J.R. 1986. Prevalence of viral and mycoplasmal infections in laboratory rodents. In *Viral and Mycoplasmal Infections of Laboratory Rodents: Effects on Biomedical Research,* ed. P. N. Bhatt et al., pp. 801–8. New York: Academic.

MacDonald, T.T., and Ferguson, A. 1978. Small intestinal epithelial cell kinetics and protozoal infection in mice. Gastroenterology 74:496–500.

Owen, R.L., et al. 1979. Ultrastructural observations on giardiasis in a murine model. I. Intestinal distribution, attachment, and relationship to the immune system of *Giardia muris.* Gastroenterology 76:757–69.

Sparrow, S. 1976. The microbiological and parasitological status of laboratory animals from accredited breeders in the United Kingdom. Lab. Anim. 10:365–73.

Venkatesan, P., et al. 1997. A comparison of mucosal inflammatory responses to *Giardia muris* in resistant B10 and susceptible BALB/c mice. Parasite Immunol. 19:137–43.

Spironucleus (Hexamita) muris Infection
Boorman, G.A., et al. 1973. *Hexamita* and *Giardia* as a cause of mortality in congenitally thymus-less (nude) mice. Clin. Exp. Immunol. 15:623–27.

Flatt, R.E., et al. 1978. Hexamitiasis in a laboratory mouse colony. Lab. Anim. Sci. 28:62–65.

Meshorer, A. 1969. Hexamitiasis in laboratory mice. Lab. Anim. Care 19:33–37.

Ruitenberg, E.J., and Kruyt, B.C. 1975. Effect of intestinal flagellates on immune response in mice. Abstr. Parasitol. 71:xxx.

Sebesteny, A. 1979. Transmission of *Spironucleus* and *Giardia* spp. and some non-pathogenic intestinal protozoa from infested hamsters to mice. Lab. Anim. 13:189–91.

Shagemann, G., et al. 1990. Host specificity of cloned *Spironucleus muris* in laboratory rodents. Lab. Anim. 24:234–39.

Van Kruinigen, H.J., et al. 1978. Hexamitiasis in laboratory mice. J. Am. Vet. Med. Assoc. 173:1202–4.

Whitehouse, A., et al. 1993. *Spironucleus muris* in laboratory mice. Aust. Vet. J. 70:193.

Helminth Infections
Balk, M.W., and Jones, S.R. 1970. Hepatic cysticercosis in a mouse colony. J. Am. Vet. Med. Assoc. 157:678–79.

Flynn, R.J. 1973. *Parasites of Laboratory Animals.* Ames: Iowa State University Press.

Jacobson, R.H., et al. 1974. The thymus dependency of resistance to pinworm infections in mice. J. Parasitol. 60:976–79.

Kelment, P., et al. 1996. An oral ivermectin regimen that eradicates pinworms (*Syphacia* spp.) in mice. Lab. Anim. Sci. 46:286–90.

Lindsey, J.R. 1986. Prevalence of viral and mycoplasmal infections in laboratory rodents. In *Viral and Mycoplasmal Infections of Laboratory Rodents: Effects on Biomedical Research,* ed. P.N. Bhatt et al., pp. 801–8. New York: Academic.

Skopets, B., et al. 1996. Ivermectin toxicity in young mice. Lab. Anim. Sci. 46:111–12.

Sparrow, S. 1976. The microbiological and parasitological status of laboratory animals from accredited breeders in the United Kingdom. Lab. Anim. 10:365–73.

Taffs, L.F. 1976. Pinworm infections in laboratory rodents: A review. Lab. Anim. 10:1–13.

Wescott, R.B. 1982. Helminths. In *The Mouse in Biomedical Research. II. Diseases,* ed. H.L. Foster et al., pp. 373–84. New York: Academic.

General Bibliography for Protozoal Infections
Hsu, C-K. 1982. Protozoa. In *The Mouse in Biomedical Research. II. Diseases,* ed. H.L. Foster et al., pp. 359–72. New York: Academic.

Lindsey, J.R. 1986. Prevalence of viral and mycoplasmal infections in laboratory rodents. In *Viral and Mycoplasmal Infections of Laboratory Rodents: Effects on Biomedical Research,* ed. P.N. Bhatt et al., pp. 801–8. New York: Academic.

MacDonald, T.T., and Ferguson, A. 1978. Small intestinal epithelial cell kinetics and protozoal infection in mice. Gastroenterology 74:496–500.

Owen, D.G. 1992. Parasites of Laboratory Animals. London: Royal Society of Medicine Services Ltd.

Sparrow, S. 1976. The microbiological and parasitological status of laboratory animals from accredited breeders in the United Kingdom. Lab. Anim. 10:365–73.

NUTRITIONAL AND METABOLIC DISORDERS

Amyloidosis. Amyloid (from the Greek *amylon*, "starch") was so named by Virchow because it stained with iodine similar to that seen with cellulose. Amyloidosis is an important disease of laboratory mice, both as a spontaneously occurring, life-limiting disease and as an experimentally induced disease.

EPIZOOTIOLOGY AND PATHOGENESIS. Amyloid is a chemically diverse family of insoluble proteins that are deposited in tissues but have in common a biophysical polymerized conformation known as the beta-pleated sheet. It is now known that there are three systemic forms of amyloid. Primary and myeloma-associated amyloid contains immunoglobulin light chains or fragments (called amyloid AL, for amyloid, light chain). Secondary amyloid contains byproducts of the acute phase response and occurs in secondary inflammatory processes. Local tissue injury elicits a complex of events in which macrophages release monokines, including interleukin 1 and tumor necrosis factor, which in turn stimulate serum amyloid A (SAA) synthesis in liver. SAAs are polymorphic apoproteins isolated with serum high-density lipoproteins known as acute phase reactants and are a precursor to amyloid A (AA), which is deposited extracellularly in tissues. A third type of systemic amyloid, found in humans as a hereditary trait, is composed of prealbumin. In addition, a number of localized forms of amyloidosis occur, such as in endocrine tumors, ovaries, and the brain (in Alzheimer's disease), each with differing composition. All amyloids possess amyloid P (protein) component, which is a plasma glycoprotein with homology to the acute phase protein, C-reactive protein. It is not known why these native biological products are not catabolized.

Spontaneous amyloidosis is a common event in certain strains of aging laboratory and wild mice. Primary amyloidosis occurs with high prevalence and at a relatively young age in some strains of mice such as A and SJL and with high prevalence but later onset in strains such as B6 mice; it can be extraordinarily rare in other strains, such as BALB/c and C3H mice. Unlike Syrian hamsters, there does not appear to be a sex-related predisposition in most strains of mice. The patterns of tissue deposition also vary somewhat, depending upon mouse genotype. Secondary amyloidosis can also occur spontaneously in laboratory mice and is related to chronic inflammatory diseases and acariasis. The line of distinction between spontaneous primary and secondary amyloidosis is vague on a morphological basis, but the spleen and liver are only mildly affected in primary amyloidosis and are usually the most severely affected in secondary amyloidosis. The prevalence of spontaneous amyloidosis can be affected by stress (fighting) and ectoparasitism. In one study, mice singly caged in an SPF facility had the lowest incidence of amyloidosis compared with their counterparts. Experimental secondary amyloidosis can be readily induced in a variety of laboratory mouse strains with casein injections. The order of susceptibility (in decreasing order) among common mouse strains is CBA, B6, outbred Swiss, C3H/He, BALB/c, and SWR. Localized forms of amyloidosis can also be found in mice. Tumor-associated amyloid can be found, even in the low-amyloid BALB/c strain, and ovarian corpora luteal amyloidosis can be found with frequency in CBA and DBA mice in the absence of systemic disease.

PATHOLOGY. Amyloid has a characteristic hypocellular eosinophilic appearance in H & E-stained sections. When stained with Congo red and subjected to polarized light, amyloid is birefringent. Amyloid deposition occurs in renal glomeruli (Fig. 1.69), renal interstitium, lamina propria of the intestine (Fig. 1.70), myocardium, nasal submucosa (Fig. 1.71), parotid salivary gland, thyroid gland, adrenal cortex, myocardium, perifollicular areas of the spleen, pulmonary alveolar septa, periportal tissue of the liver, tongue, testes, ovary, myometrium, aorta, pancreas, and other tissues. Amyloidosis is often associated with cardiac atrial thrombosis with left- or right-sided congestive heart failure. The mechanism for this association is unknown but probably is related to renal disease. Mice with amyloid deposition in the renal medullary interstitium can develop papillary necrosis. Healed lesions give the illusion of hydronephrosis.

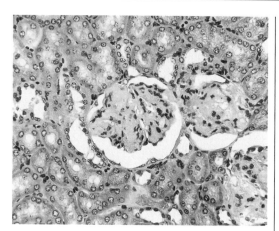

FIG. 1.69—Section of kidney from mouse with renal amyloidosis. There is deposition of amyloid on glomerular basement membranes, with partial obliteration of the normal architecture.

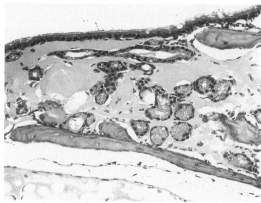

FIG. 1.71—Longitudinal section of turbinates from aged mouse with marked nasal amyloidosis. There is extensive deposition of amyloid around identifiable submucosal glands.

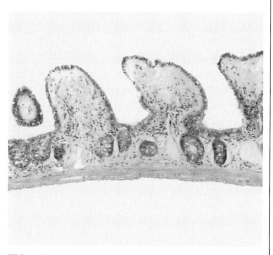

FIG. 1.70—Section of ileum from mouse with intestinal amyloidosis. There is marked deposition of amorphous material in the lamina propria.

Soft-tissue Calcification (Cardiac Calcinosis/ Myocardial Calcification)

EPIZOOTIOLOGY AND PATHOGENESIS. Spontaneous mineralization/calcification of the heart and other soft tissues is a common necropsy finding in strains of mice such as BALB/c, C3H, and DBA, most notably in the DBA strain. Epicardial and corneal mineralization has also been observed in C.B.17/ICR SCID mice. In DBA/2 mice, myocardial lesions may be evident at necropsy in up to 100% of males and females by 10 wk of age. In this strain, calcification may be observed as early as 3 wk of age, with increased incidence in older animals. A variety of factors have been implicated in this condition, including environmental or dietary change, concomitant disease, and elevated levels of corticosteroids. Female mice appear to be particularly at risk. Calcification may occur in a variety of other tissues, particularly in DBA and C3H mice. Focal mineralization most frequently occurs in the myocardium, muscles of the tongue, muscles of the axial skeleton, cornea, and aorta. Calcified lesions at these sites are usually present as an incidental finding at necropsy. The mineralization appears to be dystrophic in nature, since there is no evidence of elevated serum calcium levels in affected mice.

PATHOLOGY. There may be chalky linear streaks evident on the heart, particularly on the epi-

DIAGNOSIS. The diagnosis is confirmed by the typical appearance of amyloid and its staining characteristics. *Differential diagnoses* must include age-related glomerular disease (glomerular hyalinosis), glomerulonephritis, hydronephrosis, and spontaneous cardiac atrial thrombosis.

SIGNIFICANCE. Amyloidosis is a major life-limiting disease in aging mice and can be exacerbated by stress and other disease states.

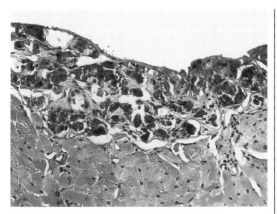

FIG. 1.72—Myocardial calcinosis in DBA mouse, illustrating mineralization and fibrous tissue proliferation in epicardial region.

cardium of the right ventricles. On microscopic examination, myocardial lesions are most frequently present in the right and left ventricles, atria, and epicardium of the right ventricle (Fig. 1.72). Changes vary from single mineralized fibers (grade 1) to grade 3 lesions, which are characterized by extensive linear calcification. In recent lesions, there may be interstitial edema. In lesions interpreted to be of some duration, frequently there is concurrent fibrosis and mononuclear cell infiltration. Foci of calcification in the tongue, when present, are often concentrated in the musculature adjacent to the lamina propria, frequently with concurrent granulomatous inflammatory response in the adjacent regions. Lesions may be distributed anywhere along the area from the apex to the root of the tongue. Ulceration of the epithelium overlying affected areas is an infrequent finding. Foci of calcification, when present in the aorta, are characterized by mineralization of the elastic lamina and smooth muscle of the vessel wall. Corneal lesions are characterized by degeneration of Bowman's membrane, with extension into the adjacent collagen fibers of the corneal stroma.

DIAGNOSIS. The strain of mouse, the demonstration of calcium in lesions by the appropriate staining procedure (e.g., alizarin red), and the nature and distribution of lesions are sufficient to confirm the diagnosis.

SIGNIFICANCE. Soft-tissue calcification commonly occurs in strains such as DBA mice. It is usually an incidental finding at necropsy, although it is likely that there is some impairment of cardiac function, particularly in animals with extensive myocardial lesions.

Reye's-Like Syndrome. Reye's syndrome, an important cause of morbidity and mortality among human infants and children, is characterized as encephalopathy and fatty degeneration of viscera. Antecedent viral infections and aspirin therapy are precipitating factors in this disease. Spontaneous Reye's-like syndrome has also been reported in mice but not in other species.

EPIZOOTIOLOGY AND PATHOGENESIS. Outbreaks of Reye's-like syndrome, although relatively rare, do occur, with high morbidity and mortality. The disease has so far been associated only with BALB/cByJ mice. Precipitating factors have not been defined but may be linked to enterotropic mouse hepatitis virus or other infections. Reye's syndrome in humans is characterized by a rapidly deteriorating encephalopathy secondary to hepatic dysfunction with hyperammonemia. The metabolic defect is unknown, but mitochondrial swelling with dysfunction in hepatocytes is the probable primary lesion. Affected mice become precipitously stuporous and comatose with hyperventilation. Death occurs in most cases within 6–18 hr after onset, but some mice regain consciousness.

PATHOLOGY. Livers are swollen, greasy, and pale, and kidneys are swollen, with pale cortices. Intestines can be fluid- and gas-filled, with empty ceca. Microscopic findings include marked microvesicular fatty change and swelling of hepatocytes, with sinusoidal hypoperfusion (Fig. 1.73). Moderate numbers of fat vacuoles are also present in renal proximal convoluted tubular epithelium. Neurological lesions consist of swelling of protoplasmic astrocyte nuclei (Alzheimer type II astrocytes) in the neocortex, corpus striatum, hippocampus, and thalamus. Intestinal lesions consistent with enterotropic mouse hepatitis virus are variably present.

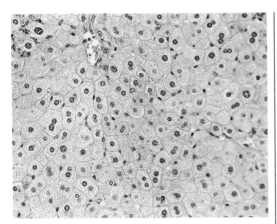

FIG. 1.73—Section of liver from a case of Reye's-like syndrome in BALB/c mouse. Note the increased cytoplasmic volume and the diffuse vacuolation of the hepatocyte cytoplasm.

DIAGNOSIS. Clinical signs and gross liver lesions are distinctive. Microscopic changes in liver and brain, coupled with hyperammonemia, are diagnostic. *Differential diagnoses* must include other causes of hepatocellular fatty change in BALB/c mice, which normally possess a moderate degree of this change.

SIGNIFICANCE. Although rare, outbreaks of the syndrome can be devastating. If the syndrome could be experimentally reproduced, it would serve as a valuable model of Reye's syndrome in humans.

BIBLIOGRAPHY FOR NUTRITIONAL AND METABOLIC DISORDERS

Amyloidosis
Cohen, A.S., and Shirahama, T. 1980. Amyloidosis, model no. 17. In *Handbook: Animal Models of Human Disease,* ed. C.C. Capen et al. Washington, D.C.: Registry of Comparative Pathology, Armed Forces Institute of Pathology.
Cohen, A.S., et al. 1983. Amyloid proteins, precursors, mediators and enhancers. Lab. Invest. 48:1–4.
Conner, M.W., et al. 1983. Spontaneous amyloidosis in outbred CD-1 mice. Surv. Synth. Pathol. Res. 1:67–78.
Lipman, R.D., et al. 1993. Husbandry factors and the prevalence of age-related amyloidosis in mice. Lab. Anim. Sci. 43: 439–44.

Soft-Tissue Calcification
Brownstein, D.G. 1983. Genetics of dystrophic epicardial mineralization in DBA/2 mice. Lab. Anim. Sci. 33:247–48.

Meador, V.P., et al. 1992. Epicardial and corneal mineralization in clinically normal severe combined immunodeficiency (SCID) mice. Vet. Pathol. 29:247–249.
Vargas, K.J., et al. 1996. Dystrophic cardiac calcinosis in C3H/HeN mice. Lab. Anim. Sci. 46:572–75.
Van Vleet, J.F., and Ferrans, V.J. 1991. Inherited dystrophic cardiac calcinosis, mouse. In *Monographs on Pathology of Laboratory Animals: Cardiovascular and Muscular Systems,* ed. T.C. Jones, pp. 9–14. New York: Springer-Verlag.
Yamate, J., et al. 1987. Observations on soft tissue calcification in DBA/2NCrj mice in comparison with CRJ:CD-1 mice. Lab. Anim. 21:289–98.

Reye's-like Syndrome
Brownstein, D.G., et al. 1984. Spontaneous Reye's-like syndrome in BALB/cByJ mice. Lab. Invest. 51:386–95.

BEHAVIORAL DISORDERS

The mouse is highly gregarious and thrives in communal groups. Social harmony requires the establishment of a dominance hierarchy, which can be easily destabilized. The reproductive cycles of mice are significantly influenced by pheromones, which in turn are intimately associated with the dominance hierarchy and presence of foreign members. Infertility, manifested as altered estrous cycles, fetal resorption, and anestrus, as well as maternal cannibalism, can result from pheromone-driven responses. Mouse behavior and pheromones have been well studied and are recommended subjects for further reading (reviewed in Whittingham and Wood 1976). Stereotypy occurs among caged mice but is often overlooked because of their nocturnal activity patterns. Individual mice can display aberrant circling behavior, unrelated to neurological or vestibular disease. Bar chewing and polydypsia are among other behavioral vices in individual mice. Normal behavior patterns are disrupted in specific strains of mice with retinal degeneration (such as C3H mice), deafness (such as B6 mice), hippocampal and corpus callosum defects (such as 129 and BALB mice), hydrocephalus (common in many strains), pituitary adenomas (FVB mice), and numerous other neurologic anomalies.

Barbering and Pugilistic Dermatitis. Adult male mice will fight savagely unless reared as sib-

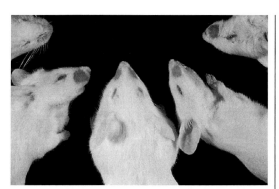

FIG. 1.74—Mice illustrating barbering of vibrissae. Note the culprit with the intact vibrissae (upper left).

lings or peers from infancy. Certain strains, such as BALB and SJL, are notorious in this respect. Fight wounds can be diffuse, but they are often oriented around the tail and genitalia. Barbering is a common dominance-associated vice of both sexes (but particularly females) and can be manifest in different patterns, depending upon genotype or individual idiosyncrasies. A common form is whisker chewing, which is common among Swiss, B6, and C3H mice. Vibrissae chewing often leads to muzzle alopecia, which must be differentiated from mechanical abrasion associated with feeding devices (Fig. 1.74). Barbering of the pelage on other parts of the body is common, and often with a well-defined, clipped edge. Typically, the dominant mouse within a group is unaffected.

ENVIRONMENT-RELATED DISEASE

Mechanical Muzzle Alopecia. Hair loss in the muzzle region occurs occasionally in laboratory mice. *Differential diagnoses* include "barbering" and mechanical denuding due to improperly constructed openings for feeders or watering devices.

"Ringtail". Low ambient humidity can cause skin dryness, which can be a significant problem in infant mice. Dry dermatitis can cause "ringtail," or annular constrictions of the tail and occasionally digits, resulting in edema of the distal extremity and dry gangrene. Hairless strains of mice are also prone to skin problems as adults, which may be manifest as inflammation and gangrene without the classic "ringtail" antecedent

stage. These phenomena are probably exacerbated by environmental temperature extremes, particularly low temperatures, and nutritional factors. However, the nature of the predisposing factors and the precise pathogenesis of the condition are yet to be resolved.

Sloughing of Extremities Due to Cotton Nesting Material. Necrosis and sloughing of limb extremities in suckling mice have been associated with infarction due to the wrapping of absorbent cotton (cotton wool) nesting material around one or more legs or digits.

Hypothermia and Hyperthermia. Although mice are highly adaptable to living in different climates, they are inefficiently homeothermic and cannot tolerate sudden and extreme changes in environmental temperature. In a stabile environment, core body temperature will normally fluctuate several degrees in a day, depending upon activity. Hypothermia and hyperthermia are all too common occurrences during shipping, when crates are moved from one environment to another. Water bottle "accidents" often cause mortality from hypothermia. All of these factors can result in high mortality with few, if any, discernible lesions.

Dehydration. Mice require relatively large volumes of drinking water and easily become dehydrated. Hydration can be evaluated at necropsy by skin plasticity, "stickiness" of tissues, pale and contracted spleens, vascular hypovolemia, or elevated hematocrit. Thorough anamnesis will often reveal failure of watering devices. Even if water bottles are full, sipper tubes can become obstructed, or if new, they can contain metal filings that interfere with water flow. Dehydration can also occur when water bottle sipper tubes are too high for young mice to reach or if newly arrived mice are unaccustomed to automatic watering devices. Dehydration frequently accompanies other diseases that preclude drinking, such as hydrocephalus. A consistent microscopic finding in dehydrated mice is massive thymic apoptosis (stress reaction).

BIBLIOGRAPHY FOR BEHAVIORAL DISORDERS AND ENVIRONMENT-RELATED DISEASE

Litterst, C.L. 1974. Mechanically self-induced muzzle alopecia in mice. Lab. Anim. Sci. 24:806–9.

Long, S.Y., et al. 1972. Hair-nibbling and whisker-trimming as indicators of social hierarchy in mice. Anim. Behav. 20:10–12.

Percy, D.H., et al. 1994. Diagnostic exercise: Sloughing of limb extremities in immunocompromised suckling mice. Contemp. Top. 33(1):66–67.

Rowson, K.E.K., and Michaels, L. 1980. Injury to young mice caused by cottonwool used as nesting material. Lab. Anim. 14:187.

Strozik, E., and Festing, M.F.W. 1981. Whisker trimming in mice. Lab. Anim. 15:309–12.

Svendsen, P. 1994. Environmental impact on animal experiments. In *Handbook of Laboratory Animal Science. Vol.1*, ed. P. Svendson and J. Hau, pp. 191–202. Boca Raton: CRC Press.

Thornburg, L.P., et al. 1973. The pathogenesis of the alopecia due to hair-chewing in mice. Lab. Anim. Sci. 23:843–50.

Whittingham, D.G., and Wood, M.J. 1976. Reproductive physiology. In *The Mouse in Biomedical Research. III. Normative Biology, Immunology, and Husbandry*, ed. H.L. Foster et al., pp. 137–64. New York: Academic.

AGING, DEGENERATIVE, AND MISCELLANEOUS DISORDERS

Alopecia and Dermatitis in B6 (C57BL/6) Mice. B6 (C57BL/6) mice are prone to a number of skin disorders, with frequent overlap of syndromes in the individual mouse, and in the minds of pathologists. First, juvenile B6 mice may manifest transient alopecia, which can be eliminated by delaying weaning or changing the diet. Alopecia also occurs in older mice, due to dominance-associated self- and peer grooming/barbering among females (trichotillomania). Over time, there can be inflammation of the underlying dermis. Ulcerative dermatitis has been recognized to occur in mice of this genetic background for decades, and this can be associated with barbering, as well as hypersensitivity dermatitis due to ectoparasitism. B6 mice that are infested with *Myobia* often develop cutaneous allergy with severe pruritis. The resultant self-trauma may progress to ulcerations and secondary cutaneous bacterial infections. However, in some cases, other factors may be involved. In one report, older mice on the B6NNia background developed spontaneous ulcerative dermatitis with pruritis. Affected animals were negative for primary ectoparasitic, bacterial, or mycotic infections. Histopathologic examination and immunofluo-

rescent microscopy revealed an underlying vasculitis attributed to immune complex deposition on dermal vessels. Dietary factors have also been implicated in the development of the ulcerative dermatitis in B6 mice. These include dietary restriction and varying ingredients in the diet. Weaning of the females at a later date has been another strategy used to alleviate the problem, with variable success.

Alopecia Areata in C3H Mice. Aging C3H mice develop irregular, diffuse alopecia of the ventral and dorsal trunk, which closely mimics human alopecia areata. Hair loss increases with age, particularly after 6 mo of age, in both males and females. Microscopic examination of affected skin reveals densely packed anagen follicles with dystrophic hair formation, "melanin incontinence," interfollicular epidermal thickening, and perifollicular mononuclear leukocyte infiltrates.

Malocclusion. Malocclusion due to improperly aligned upper and lower incisor teeth may result in marked overgrowth, particularly of the lower incisors. This condition has a hereditary basis, and culling is recommended.

Liver Disorders. In mice, a progressive increase in ploidy occurs in hepatocyte nuclei with age. The change in the number of chromosomes (polyploidization) may increase to ploidy values of 16 or 32. Thus karyomegaly and anisokaryosis are normal incidental findings, particularly in older animals. Intranuclear cytoplasmic invaginations occur as clearly delineated eosinophilic structures within the karyoplasm (Fig. 1.75). Eosinophilic cytoplasmic inclusions are also common. They are most frequently observed in hepatocytes of older mice and transgenic mice. Hepatocellular fatty change is a normal finding in BALB mice, and the livers of these mice are typically paler than in other strains.

Ileus in Lactating Mice. A spontaneous disease with relatively high mortality has been recognized in female mice, usually during the second week of their first lactation. Mortality rates may be up 40%, and mice of various genetic back-

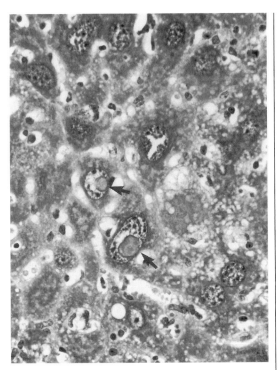

FIG. 1.75—Polyploidy of hepatocytes with cytoplasmic invaginations (*arrows*) into hepatocyte nuclei in aged mouse.

grounds appear to be susceptible to the disease. The condition has been called paralysis/ paresis of peristalsis.

PATHOLOGY. At necropsy, there is frequently abdominal distension. There may be fecal staining in the perineal region. The stomach is usually slightly dilated and filled with watery fluid. The proximal small intestine is distended with fluid contents. Firm, conical fecal plugs are frequently present in the ileum and the tip of the cecum. The ileum caudal to the plug may be empty, or it may contain fecal pellets. The colon and rectum are also usually empty, or they may contain a few fecal pellets or mucous material. Histological findings are usually unremarkable, and pathogenic organisms have not been recovered from the intestine or other tissues.

EPIZOOTIOLOGY AND PATHOGENESIS. Several possible etiologies have been proposed: clostridial enterotoxemia and exogenous toxins are two suggested causes. *Citrobacter*-induced colitis was associated with the problem in one facility. "Exhaustion" with concurrent imbalance of, for example, calcium, sodium and/or other electrolytes, or glucose has been proposed as the underlying cause, with subsequent impaired peristalsis and resultant impaction. *Differential diagnoses* include differentiation from advanced autolysis and postpartum bacterial septicemia.

SIGNIFICANCE. Postpartum ileus has been recognized as a significant cause of mortality in primiparous female mice in Europe, and there is one report from the USA. It is likely that the problem occurs sporadically elsewhere. The etiopathogenesis of the condition is yet to be resolved.

Vestibular Syndrome. Head tilt, circling, and more severe manifestations of vestibular disease are common clinical signs in mice. It is often due to bacterial otitis and, less often, to central nervous system disease. An undescribed but frequent cause of vestibular disease also appears to be necrotizing arteritis of undetermined cause. This lesion occurs in a number of mouse strains in the absence of detectable viral and bacterial pathogens. The internal and middle ear structures are normal, but careful examination of surrounding tissues will reveal active necrotizing and/or inflammatory changes in medium-size arteries (Fig. 1.76). Similar segmental inflammatory changes will be found in arteries of the heart and mesentery.

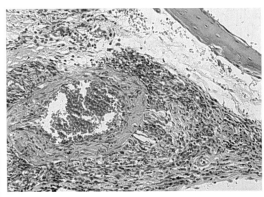

FIG. 1.76—Vasculitis of artery in region of the middle and inner ear of a mouse with vestibular syndrome.

Cardiovascular Disorders. Left- or right-sided heart failure is a frequent, but sporadic manifestation of atrial thrombosis. Atrial thrombosis typically involves organizing thrombi in the auricles. In left atrial thrombosis, the process may extend into the pulmonary veins. This syndrome is typically precipitated by multisystemic amyloidosis. Atrial thrombosis is one cause of spontaneous mortality in older mice, and the findings are similar to those seen in the hamster (see Chap. 3). For discussion of cardiac calcinosis, see under nutritional and metabolic disorders.

Left heart failure is the most common cause of noninfectious dyspnea in mice. *Differential diagnoses* include viral pneumonia, aspiration pneumonia, pneumocystis pneumonia (in immunodeficient mice), bacterial pneumonia, thymic lymphoma, and bronchioloalveolar adenoma. The distribution and nature of the lesions seen with polyarteritis in mice are similar to those seen in rats (see Chap. 2). Immune complexes have been demonstrated within affected vessels.

Perivascular Lymphoid Infiltrates. Mild to severe infiltrates of lymphoid cells can be found in the adventitia of pulmonary vessels, with extension into adjacent alveolar septa. This is invariably in response to antigenic stimuli, such as a prior virus infection. They should not be present in pathogen-free mice. They also appear in lymphoproliferative disorders, accompanied by similar perivascular infiltrates in salivary glands, kidneys, and other organs.

Alveolar Hemorrhage. Regardless of the cause of death, acute extravasation of blood into alveolar spaces is a common agonal finding in mice. It must be differentiated from congestive heart failure and other causes.

Freund's Adjuvant Pulmonary Granulomata. Focal histiocytic granulomata can be found in the lungs of mice that have been immunized with Freund's adjuvant, regardless of the site of immunization (Fig. 1.77).

Aspiration Pneumonia. Accidental inhalation of foreign material can occur under a number of circumstances, but especially when shipping

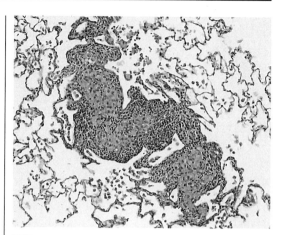

FIG. 1.77—Section of lung from a murine recipient of Freund's adjuvant. Note the typical focal granulomatous inflammatory response and the prominent epithelioid cells.

crates containing wood shavings are handled roughly in transit. Foreign plant material can be readily identified in airways (Fig. 1.78).

Pulmonary Histiocytosis/Lipoproteinosis/ Crystal Pneumonitis. Focal accumulations of lipid-laden macrophages are frequently observed in the peripheral (particularly subplural) regions in the lung of aging mice of all types. Some of the macrophages may contain cholesterol crystalloid material. Alveolar lipoproteinosis is another, more severe condition, in which there is progressive intra-alveolar accumulation of granular pale eosinophilic phospholipid (surfactant), with a relative paucity of macrophages and secondary response. This lesion is rare in pathogen-free mice. A more striking syndrome is the presence of eosinophilic crystals of varying size and shape in terminal airways, alveolar ducts, alveolar spaces, and bronchiolar glands of certain strains of mice, particularly in aging B6 mice. These crystals are usually within the cytoplasm of alveolar macrophages; large crystals, however, can be extracellular (Fig. 1.79). Similar crystals can be found in the gallbladder. The crystalline material is complex, but ultrastructural analysis reveals that crystals are the breakdown product of granulocytes, particularly eosinophils. Crystal pneumonitis can be very extensive, leading to dyspnea in some mice. Crystal pneumonitis is accelerated in mice with immune deficiencies, such as mice

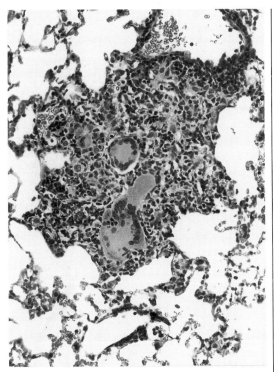

FIG. 1.78—Section of lung from mouse with pneumonia (following aspiration of plant fibers). Note the granulomatous inflammatory response and the multinucleated giant cell formation.

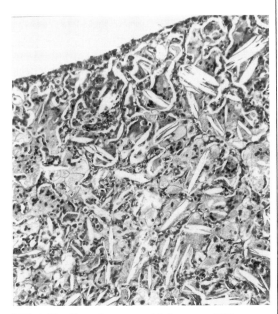

FIG. 1.79—Crystal pneumonitis in an aged B6 mouse. Note prominent cholesterol clefts within alveolar macrophages.

with the "motheaten" mutation (a B6 mutant with a complex and not fully defined immunodeficiency). Crystal pneumonitis is a prominent feature of GM-CSF knockout mice (B6 background) and is touted as a model for human progressive alveolar proteinosis. The condition is associated with immunodeficiency in humans.

Spontaneous Corneal Opacity. Corneal opacities have been observed in a variety of strains of mice. Opacities are characterized by acute to chronic inflammatory changes of the corneal epithelium and anterior corneal stroma, including acute keratitis with corneal erosion to ulceration, vascularization of the corneal stroma, and mineralization of corneal basement membranes. In some cases, the problem can be alleviated by more frequent cage cleaning, and it was concluded that an environmental factor, such as ammonia, may play an important role in the development of the disease.

Suppurative Conjunctivitis/Ulcerative Blepharitis. Suppurative conjunctivitis with ulcerations at the mucocutaneous junction have been observed in 129, BALB, and other strains of mice. Suppuration with abscessation of the meibomian glands also occurred. A variety of bacteria were isolated from affected conjunctivae, including *Corynebacterium,* coagulase-negative *Staphylococcus,* and *Pasteurella pneumotropica.* These are likely to be opportunistic infections, and the specific etiopathogenesis is unknown.

Retinal Degeneration

EPIZOOTIOLOGY AND PATHOGENESIS. Retinal degeneration is a very common lesion that can be considered a normal characteristic of certain inbred strains of mice; it also occurs in outbred stocks and wild mice. It may have different modes of inheritance but appears histologically identical between mouse strains. Commonly affected strains include C3H, CBA, and Swiss mice, while strains A, AKR, BALB/c, B6, and DBA mice have normal retinas. The retinal degeneration of C3H/He mice is the best characterized and is inherited as a recessive trait. Mice are born with normal-appearing retinas, and the disorder involves both arrested development and subsequent degeneration of photoreceptor cells.

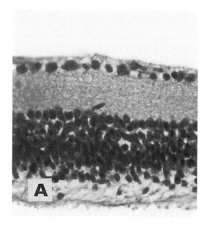

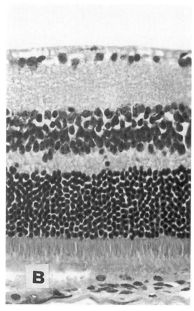

FIG. 1.80—Retinal degeneration in a C3H mouse (**A**) compared with a normal mouse (**B**). Note the marked reduction in the thickness of the retina and the loss of identifiable outer plexiform and bipolar cell layers in the affected mouse.

PATHOLOGY. Microscopic changes include absence or degeneration of the rods, outer nuclear layer, and outer plexiform layer (Fig. 1.80). Active degenerative changes can be encountered in young mice, but the lesion evolves rapidly and is nearly complete by weaning age. *Differential diagnosis* should include light-induced retinal degeneration.

SIGNIFICANCE. Mice do not appear to manifest clinical signs. If ophthalmic or behavioral studies are contemplated, the strain of mouse to be used should be carefully selected.

Mesenteric Disease. In this disorder, mesenteric lymph nodes are enlarged and filled with blood. Lymphoid elements are atrophic. This lesion occurs sporadically in aging mice of various strains, appearing more frequently in C3H mice. Its etiology is unknown. Mesenteric lymph nodes are grossly enlarged and appear bright red. Microscopically, lymphoid tissue is often atrophic, and medullary sinuses are filled with blood. *Differential diagnoses* must include various causes of mesenteric lymphadenomegaly, including *Salmonella.* This is an incidental finding and of no clinical significance.

GENITOURINARY DISORDERS

Chloroform Toxicity. Mice can develop renal tubular necrosis and mineralization when exposed to chloroform fumes. Mature male mice of certain genotypes such as DBA and C3H are exquisitely sensitive, with high mortality. One factor associated with the sex-related susceptibility appears to be the increased renal binding of chloroform in males, compared with females, and castration of males will eliminate their susceptibility to chloroform nephrotoxicity. Severely affected mice develop swollen, pale kidneys. Microscopic changes are characterized by coagulation necrosis of renal tubules, particularly the proximal convoluted tubules. Surviving mice have residual nephrocalcinosis. "Outbreaks" of mortality, with selective deaths among male mice, have been described.

Chronic Glomerulonephritis/Glomerulopathy. Renal lesions are relatively common in certain strains of older mice, such as AKR, BALB/c, and CBA mice. Mice with naturally occurring autoimmune disease, such as the (NZB × NZW) F$_1$ hybrid, usually have developed extensive glomerular lesions by the time they reach 12 or more months of age. However, there are a variety of other factors that may be involved, including viral agents, bacteria or bacterial products, and the deposition of antigen-antibody complexes on glomerular basement membranes. Persistent retroviral infections are an example of a condition that may result in the deposition of antigen-antibody complexes on glomerular tufts.

PATHOLOGY. On gross examination, there may be marked pitting of the cortical surfaces in advanced cases, and small cysts may be evident on the cut surface. Microscopic changes are characterized by thickening of glomerular basement membranes due to the deposition of PAS-positive material that does not stain for amyloid. There may be proliferation of mesangial cells and, in advanced cases, obliteration of the normal architecture of affected glomeruli. Focal to diffuse mononuclear cell infiltration and varying degrees of fibrosis in the interstitial regions are other changes that commonly occur. *Differential diagnoses* include renal amyloidosis and chronic pyelonephritis.

SIGNIFICANCE. In advanced cases of glomerulopathy, there will be manifestations of renal insufficiency, including proteinuria and abnormalities in blood biochemistry. Depending on the strain of mouse affected, investigations into the underlying factors may be warranted.

Interstitial Nephritis. The etiopathogenesis of tubulointerstitial disease in mice is similar to other species and includes sequelae to infections with bacteria such as *Proteus mirabilis, Pseudomonas aeruginosa,* or *Staphylococcus aureus;* sequelae to viruses such as lymphocytic choriomeningitis virus; and sequelae following chemically induced disease. Frequently the etiology cannot be resolved. The nature of the lesions vary, depending on the duration and extent of the disease process. Frequently renal lesions are observed as an incidental finding, although they may be of sufficient magnitude to contribute to the demise of the animal, particularly if there is significant glomerular involvement. In such cases, the carcass is usually pale, with irregular pitting of the renal cortices and often marked ascites. "Metastatic" calcification of target tissues is not a feature of renal failure in the mouse. On microscopic examination, lesions may vary from discrete aggregations of mononuclear cells in perivascular regions in the cortex, to segmental to diffuse involvement with distortion and loss of tubules, and to obliteration of the normal architecture in advanced cases. *Differential diagnoses* include renal amyloidosis, glomerulonephritis, and pyelonephritis.

HYDRONEPHROSIS. Unilateral or bilateral hydronephrosis is a common, usually incidental finding. Hydronephrosis can occur in high prevalence among certain strains or lines of mice or be secondary to urinary obstruction or pyelonephritis. *Differential diagnoses* should include renal papillary necrosis due to amyloidosis, creating an *ex vacuo* pelvic enlargement. Presence of the renal papillus should be verified.

RENAL INFARCTION. Wedge-shaped infarcts of the kidney with scarring is a common finding in aged mice and is presumed to be the aftermath of arteritis of the interlobular arteries.

POLYCYSTIC DISEASE. Certain strains of mice, such as BALB mice, are prone to congenital cysts of varying size in the kidneys. In some cases, these cysts are quite large and impinge on renal function, resulting in mortality.

URINARY OBSTRUCTION/UROLOGIC SYNDROME. This spontaneous disease occurs occasionally in male mice and may be manifest as an acute or chronic condition. Clinical signs may vary from dribbling of urine and wetting of the perineal region to cellulitis with ulceration of the preputial area. In acute cases, animals may be found dead in the cage.

The perineal area may be wet, with varying degrees of swelling and ulceration in the preputial area. Paraphimosis is a variable finding. In acute cases, the urinary bladder is usually markedly distended with urine, and dull white, firm, proteinaceous plugs are often evident in the neck of the urinary bladder and proximal urethra. In chronic cases, the bladder may be distended with cloudy urine and/or calculi. The vesicular glands are sometimes distended with inspissated material, and there may be some evidence of hydronephrosis. On microscopic examination, in acute cases amorphous eosinophilic material containing spermatozoa may be present in the proximal urethra, with minimal to no inflammatory response. In chronic obstruction, there may be varying manifestations of inflammatory response, such as prostatitis, cystitis, urethritis, and balanoposthitis.

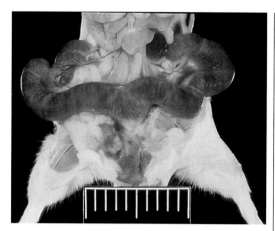

FIG. 1.81—Congenital mucometra in a young adult mouse. The uterine horns are distended with opaque mucoid material.

Differential diagnoses include bacterial cystitis and pyelonephritis, as well as agonal release of secretions from the accessory sex glands at death, which could be confused with a bona fide antemortem urinary obstruction. Urinary obstruction can also occur as a result of fighting injuries to the external genitalia.

Mucometra/Hydrometra. Mucometra is a relatively common phenomenon in laboratory mice. The condition has been identified in a variety of strains including animals with the BALB/c, B6, and DBA backgrounds. It is most commonly encountered among large groups of presumably pregnant mice in which a few never whelp. The abdomen is often distended. One or both uterine horns are dilated (Fig. 1.81). Some mice have congenital imperforate lower reproductive tracts, while, in others, the cause cannot be determined. Mice with an imperforate vagina frequently present with bilobed distention in the perineal region, resembling a scrotum. Imperforate vagina with mucometra or hydrometra appears to be inherited as a complex recessive genetic defect. *Differential diagnoses* must include pyometra (which may occur secondary to mucometra), retained fetuses, and neoplasia. The uterus of mice and rats normally contains small amounts of retained fluid during certain stages of the estrous cycle.

Cystic Endometrial Hyperplasia. Cystic endometrial hyperplasia of endometrial glands is a frequent finding in aged female mice. It may be associated with secondary bacterial pyometras (*Klebsiella oxytoca*).

Preputial Gland Infections. The preputial glands of both male and female mice are prone to bacterial infections, resulting in abscessation. This is particularly common in nude mice. A number of bacteria can be associated with this syndrome, including *Pasteurella pneumotropica*.

Other Disorders. Other nonneoplastic conditions that occur in older mice include gastric mucosal hyperplasia, polyarteritis (see vestibular syndrome and renal infarction), sternal necrosis, and sternal fibro-osseous dysplasia. For additional information on these and other age-related conditions, see Frith and Ward (1988), Maronpot et al. (1999), and Mohr et al. (1996).

BIBLIOGRAPHY FOR AGING, DEGENERATIVE, GENIOURINARY, AND MISCELLLANEOUS DISORDERS

Alopecia and Dermatitis in C57BL (B6) Mice
Andrews, A.G., et al. 1994. Immune complex vasculitis with secondary ulcerative dermatitis in aged C57BL/6NNia mice. Vet. Pathol. 31:293–300.
Stowe, H.D., et al. 1971. A debilitating fatal murine dermatitis. Lab. Anim. Sci. 21:892–97.
Thigpen, J.E. 1998. The role of specific dietary ingredients in reducing the severity of skin lesions in female C57BL/6J mice. Contemp. Top. 37(4):81.
Thornberg, L.P., et al. 1973. The pathogenesis of the alopecia due to hair chewing in mice. Lab. Anim. Sci. 23:843–50.
Witt, W.M. 1989. An idiopathic dermatitis in C57BL/6N mice effectively modulated by dietary restriction. Lab. Anim. Sci. 39:470.

Alopecia Areata in C3H Mice
Sundberg, J.P., et al. 1994. Alopecia areata in aging C3H/HeJ mice. J. Invest. Dermatol. 102:847–57.

Liver Disorders
Hollander, C.F., et al. 1987. Anatomy, function, and aging in the mouse liver. Arch. Toxicol. (Suppl.) 10:244–50.

Ileus in Lactating Mice
Kunstyr, I. 1986. Paresis of peristalsis and ileus lead to death in lactating mice. Lab. Anim. 20:32–35.
Rollman, C., et al. 1998. Abdominal distension in lactating mice: Paresis (paralysis) of peristalsis in lactating mice. Lab. Anim. 27(1):19–20.

Cardiovascular Disorders

Good, M.E., and Whitaker, M.S. 1989. Idiopathic cardiomyopathy in C3H/Bd mice. Lab. Anim. Sci. 39:137–41.

Hewicker, M., and Trautwein, G. 1987. Sequential study of vasculitis in MRL mice. Lab. Anim. 21:335–41.

Maeda, N., et al. 1986. Development of heart and aortic lesions in DBA/2NCrj mice. Lab. Anim. 20:5–8.

Vargas, K.J. 1996. Dystrophic cardiac calcinosis in C3H/HeN mice. Lab. Anim. Sci. 46:572–75.

Pulmonary Histiocytosis/Lipoproteinosis/ Crystal Pneumonitis

Mohr, U., et al. 1996. *Pathobiology of the Aging Mouse.* Volume 1. Washington, D.C.: ILSI Press.

Murray, A.B., and Luz, A. 1990. Acidophil macrophage pneumonia in laboratory mice. Vet. Pathol. 27:274–81.

Reed, J.A., et al. 1999. Aerosolized GM-CSF ameliorates pulmonary alveolar proteinosis in GM-CSF-deficient mice. Am. J. Physiol. Apr., 276(4, pt. 1):L556–63.

Ward, J.M. 1978. Pulmonary pathology of the motheaten mouse. Vet. Pathol. 15:170–78.

Yang, Y.H., and Campbell, J.S. 1964. Crystalline excrements in bronchitis and cholecystitis of mice. Am. J. Pathol. 45:337–45.

Eye Disorders

Keeler, C.E. 1927. Rodless retina, an ophthalmic mutation in the house mouse, *Mus musculus.* J. Exp. Zool. 46:355–407.

Sidman, R.L., and Green, M.C. 1965. Retinal degeneration in the mouse. Location of the rd locus in linkage group XVIII. J. Hered. 56:23–29.

Sundberg, J.P., et al. 1991. Suppurative conjunctivitis and ulcerative blepharitis in 129/J mice. Lab. Anim. Sci. 41:516–18.

Van Winkle, T.J., and Balk, M.W. 1986. Spontaneous corneal opacities in laboratory mice. Lab. Anim. Sci. 36:248–55.

Mesenteric Disease

Dunn, T.B. 1954. Normal and pathologic anatomy of the reticular tissue in laboratory mice. J. Natl. Cancer Inst. 14:1281–1433.

Urinary Disorders

Bendle, A.M., and Carlton, W.W. 1986. Urologic syndrome, mouse. In *Monographs on Pathology of Laboratory Animals: Urinary System,* ed. T.C. Jones et al., pp. 369–75. New York: Springer-Verlag.

Carlton, W.W., and Engelhardt, J.A. 1986. Chloroform nephrosis, male mouse. In *Monographs on Pathology of Laboratory Animals: Urinary System,* ed. T.C. Jones et al., pp. 225–29. New York: Springer-Verlag.

Deringer, M.K., et al. 1953. Results of exposure of strain C3H mice to chloroform. Proc. Soc. Exp. Biol. Med. 83:474–79.

Jacobsen, L., et al. 1964. Accidental chloroform nephrosis in mice. Acta Pathol. Scand. 61:503–13.

Montgomery, C.A. 1986a. Interstitial nephritis, mouse. In *Monographs on Pathology of Laboratory Animals: Urinary System,* ed. T.C. Jones et al., pp. 210–15. New York: Springer-Verlag.

———. 1986b. Suppurative pyelonephritis, mouse. In *Monographs on Pathology of Laboratory Animals: Urinary System,* ed. T.C. Jones et al., pp. 215–19. New York: Springer-Verlag.

Sass, B. 1986. Glomerulonephritis, mouse. In *Monographs on Pathology of Laboratory Animals: Urinary System,* ed. T.C. Jones et al., pp. 192–210. New York: Springer-Verlag.

Reproductive Tract

Sundberg, J.P., and Brown, K.S. 1994. Imperforate vagina and mucometra in inbred laboratory mice. Lab. Anim. Sci. 44:380–82

Musculoskeletal

Albassam, M.A., et al. 1991. Spontaneous fibroosseous proliferative lesions in the sternums and femurs of B6C3F1 mice. Vet. Pathol. 28:381–388.

Yamasaki, K. 1996. Vertebral disk changes in B6C3F$_1$ mice. Lab. Anim. Sci. 46:576–78.

General References

Frith, C.H., and Ward, J.M. 1988. *Color Atlas of Neoplastic and Non-neoplastic Lesions in Aging Mice.* New York: Elsevier.

Maronpot, R.R., et al. 1999. *Pathology of the Mouse.* Vienna, Ill.: Cache River Press

Mohr, U., et al. (ed). 1996. *Pathobiology of the Aging Mouse.* New York: Springer-Verlag.

NEOPLASMS

Neoplasms of the Hematopoietic/ Lymphoreticular System

EPIZOOTIOLOGY AND PATHOGENESIS. In general, the incidence of malignancies of the hematopoietic system are estimated to be 1–2%, but there are marked variations in the incidence of the various tumors, depending on the strain and environmental conditions. For example, AKR mice develop nearly 100% incidence of lymphoma by 1 yr. SCID mice also develop a high incidence of thymic lymphomas (Fig. 1.82). In contrast, BALB/c mice develop a high incidence of multicentric lymphomas (Fig. 1.83).

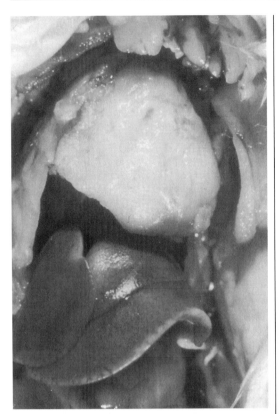

FIG. 1.82—Thymic lymphoma in adult SCID mouse. These neoplasms are relatively common in SCID mice.

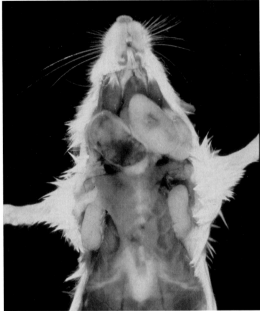

FIG. 1.83—Multicentric lymphoma in a BALB/c mouse. Note the striking lymphadenopathy involving cervical and axillary lymph nodes.

Retroviral infections play a key role in the development of most neoplasms of these systems (see Retroviral Infection).

Lymphoma. The classification of lymphomas continues to be in flux. Recently, mouse lymphomas were reclassified using the Kiel classification for human lymphomas, but this scheme is not likely to survive. As it stands, lymphomas can best be classified in the following manner.

FOLLICULAR LYMPHOMAS. The terminology is more accurate than the follicular center lymphomas and includes the centrocytic/centroblastic/immunocytoma B-cell tumors that were previously termed Dunn's "Type B" (reticulum cell) tumors (Fig. 1.84). These neoplasms commonly occur in B6 mice and involve the spleen, Peyer's patches, and mesenteric lymph nodes. These tumors often arise in germinal centers within the white pulp of the spleen, with a nodular appearance to the white pulp, which is evident at necropsy. There may be marked enlargement of mesenteric lymph nodes and Peyer's patches.

Microscopically, neoplastic cells have large, vesicular, irregularly folded to cleaved nuclei, moderate amounts of cytoplasm, poorly delineated cytoplasmic boundaries, and concurrent lymphocytic infiltration.

LYMPHOCYTIC LYMPHOMAS. Lymphocytic lymphomas are either of B- or T-cell origin, and are composed of uniform solid sheets of small lymphocytes with low mitotic activity. They occur most frequently in the spleen.

LYMPHOBLASTIC LYMPHOMAS. Lymphoblastic lymphomas are of either B- or T-cell origin and consist of solid sheets of cells interspersed with tingible body macrophages ("starry sky effect"). They have a high mitotic index and tend to involve lymph nodes and spleen in a widespread distribution. Thymic lymphomas of AKR and C58 mice are T-cell lymphomas, usually of lymphoblastic type.

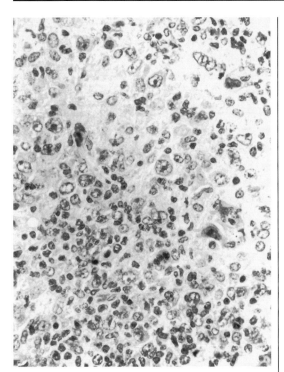

FIG. 1.84—Follicular center lymphoma (previously termed Dunn's type B reticulum cell sarcoma). The tumor consists of neoplastic cells with large cleaved nuclei and a population of well-differentiated lymphocytes.

MARGINAL ZONE LYMPHOMAS. Marginal zone lymphomas arise in the marginal zones of the splenic white pulp and are monocytoid in character. Early lesions are often multicentric in the spleen, with extension from the marginal zone into the red pulp as the disease progresses. They consist of small to medium cells of B-cell origin with plentiful gray cytoplasm when Giemsa-stained. These neoplasms have been traditionally rare in mice but are appearing with increasing frequency in genetically altered mice.

IMMUNOBLASTIC LYMPHOMAS. Immunoblastic lymphomas are composed of large cells with vesicular nuclei and single, large nucleoli that are interspersed with variable numbers of other lymphoid types. These tumors are of B-cell origin.

PLASMACYTOMAS. Plasmacytomas are typically associated with mineral oil, pristane, plastics, and other foreign material injected intraperitoneally in BALB/c mice. They consist of easily discernible plasma cells with moderate mitotic activity. Transplantable hybridomas have this same morphology.

DIAGNOSIS. Impression smears of the neoplasms prepared at necropsy will provide the opportunity to examine the lymphocytes in more detail. Immunohistochemical techniques have been used to characterize the T- or B-cell origin of spontaneous lymphoid tumors in laboratory mice. *Differential diagnoses* include histiocytic sarcoma and granulocytic (myelogenous) leukemia. In mice with granulocytic leukemia with splenic involvement, the splenic follicles are usually intact, unlike lymphoblastic lymphoma.

HISTIOCYTIC SARCOMA. Neoplasms of primitive mononuclear cell origin are especially common in certain strains of laboratory mice, such as B6 and SJL mice. These tumors were initially classified by Dunn as "type A" tumors and composed primarily of reticulum-type (histiocytic) cells. Neoplasms of this type have been produced experimentally using retroviruses or carcinogens in intact or thymectomized mice. Based on immunohistochemistry, these neoplasms arise from mononuclear phagocytic cells, such as Kupffer cells and tissue macrophages. At necropsy, there may be marked enlargement of the spleen, with nodular involvement of other tissues, such as liver, uterus, vagina, kidney, lung, and ovaries. In some cases, only one organ (e.g., uterine wall) may be involved. On microscopic examination, there are circumscribed nodular to multifocal infiltrates in tissues such as liver, spleen, lymph nodes, intestine, bone marrow, female reproductive tract, and lung. Neoplastic infiltrates consist of large histiocytic cells with irregular basophilic nuclei, fibrillar, eosinophilic cytoplasm, and indistinct cytoplasmic outlines. Neoplasms may vary in composition, from elongated fibrillar cells forming pallisading patterns to rounded cell types. Large nuclei and multinucleated giant cells are a common finding (Fig. 1.85). The neoplastic cells tend to be particularly elongated in those arising in the uterine wall, and they have on occasion been

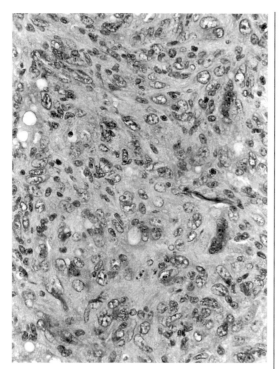

FIG. 1.85—Histiocytic sarcoma (Dunn's type A reticulum cell sarcoma). Cells have large, irregular, indented nuclei, poorly delineated cytoplasmic borders, and scattered multinucleated giant cells.

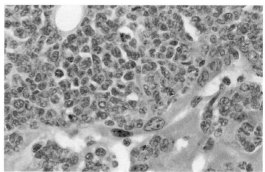

FIG. 1.86—Liver from mouse with myelogenous leukemia. Infiltrating cells have distinct indented to doughnut-shaped nuclei.

diagnosed as malignant shwannomas. Erythrophagocytosis may be associated with the neoplastic infiltrates, particularly in the liver. Occasionally tumors of this type involve a solitary lymph node or multiple ones. They consist of a prominent stromal component interspersed within a dense population of well-differentiated lymphocytes.

DIAGNOSIS. The nodular pattern and the nature of the indented to fusiform cells are useful diagnostic aids. *Differential diagnoses* include lymphoma, so-called shwannomas of the uterine wall, fibrosarcomas, leiomyosarcomas, and granulomatous inflammatory processes.

MYELOGENOUS LEUKEMIA. Spontaneous myelogenous (granulocytic) leukemias are occasionally observed in some strains of older laboratory mice. They have been associated with retroviral infections and may be produced experimentally with chemical carcinogens or irradiation. The neoplastic process appears to originate in the spleen, with subsequent involvement of a variety of tissues, including bone marrow, liver, lung, adrenal, and kidney. Clinically, animals are anemic and depressed, and peripheral leukocyte counts may approach 200,000/mm^3. At necropsy, frequently there is marked splenomegaly, with variable involvement of liver, kidneys, and other organs. On microscopic examination, there is usually massive infiltration of the splenic red pulp with malignant myeloid cells, with sparing of the splenic follicles. Diffuse infiltration of the bone marrow commonly occurs. Focal to diffuse infiltration of lung, liver, kidney, and adrenal may also occur (Fig. 1.86). Myeloid cells have large, vesicular nuclei that vary in shape from round to indented to ring forms.

DIAGNOSIS. The presence of diffuse neoplastic infiltrates, particularly in the bone marrow, with the characteristic nuclear morphology and the presence of splenic infiltrates with the sparing of the splenic follicles are useful diagnostic criteria. *Differential diagnoses* include lymphoid neoplasms and hyperplasia of the cells of the granulocytic series secondary to a suppurative disease process.

Mammary Tumors

EPIZOOTIOLOGY AND CLASSIFICATION. There is a great variation in the incidence of mammary tumors in different strains of mice. For example, while the incidence of mammary tumors in the BALB/c strain is low, up to 100% of C3H females may have mammary tumors by the time they reach 9 mo of age. There is general agreement that endogenous mammary tumor viruses (MMTVs) play an important role in mammary neoplasia in this species. Chemical carcinogens and hormones also influence the incidence of mammary tumors in laboratory mice. Prolactin, progesterone, and estrogens may all play a role in the development of hormone-responsive mammary tumors. Stress due to conditions such as intensive breeding or overcrowding may have a significant influence on the incidence of neoplasia. In one study in C3H/He mice evaluated at 400 d of age, a high percentage of the stressed females had mammary tumors, compared with those housed under optimum conditions.

Mammary neoplasia is an important facet of genetically altered mice as models for human breast cancer. A recent meeting of veterinary and medical pathologists resulted in a consensus recommendation for nomenclature and classification of mouse mammary tumors (Cardiff et al. 2000), which is recommended reading. Spontaneous mouse tumors were originally classified under a scheme developed by Thelma Dunn, using letter designations (A, B, AB, L, P, Y, etc.). Subsequently, a tissue-based system (alveolar, ductal, myoepithelial) was used, but both of these schemes were fraught with anthropomorphism and were not effective at defining the new types of tumors that are arising in genetically altered mice. Since these schemes are now effete, they are not described. The new scheme is based upon descriptors and modifiers, as shown in Tables 1.1 and 1.2.

PATHOLOGY/PATHOGENESIS. The earliest discernable lesions are focal and multifocal hyperplasias within the terminal ductule or alveolar buds. Two types of precancerous lesions arise in MMTV-infected mice. Hyperplastic alveolar nodules resemble prelactating mammary gland but stand out from the background of the nonlactating gland as nodules. Plaques are circumscribed ductal proliferations that appear during pregnancy and regress on parturition. As either of these lesions evolve and become autonomous of hormonal influences, some progress into mammary intraepithelial neoplasias (MINs) (high- or low-grade), adenomas, or carcinomas. Mammary glands of mice with spontaneous (MMTV-

TABLE 1.1—Descriptors of mouse mammary tumors

Glandular	Composed of glands
Acinar	Composed of small glandular clusters with small lumina. This is a subclass of glandular that is typical of MMTV-induced tumors.
Cribriform	Composed of sheets or nests of cells forming lumina with round, punched out spaces
Papillary	Composed of fingerlike projections of epithelium covering a central nonneoplastic fibrovascular stroma
Solid	Composed of solid sheets of epithelial cells with little or no glandular differentiation
Squamous	Composed solely of squamous cells with or without keratinization and without glandular pattern
Fibroadenoma	Composed of both myxoid fibrous stroma and glands
Adenomyoepithelioma	Composed of myoepithelium and lands
Adenosquamous	Composed of both glandular and squamous elements

associated) tumors most frequently have low-grade adenomas of acinar and papillary types. At necropsy, one or more mammary glands can be enlarged, firm, and lobulated. The lobulated pattern is best demonstrated on a cut surface (Fig. 1.87). The neoplasms are usually circumscribed and may occur anywhere along the mammary chain from the axillary to the inguinal region. There are a variety of patterns seen histologically (Figs. 1.88 and 1.89).

Mammary tumors in genetically altered mice follow predictable behaviors. Remarkably, models generated with oncogenes originally identified by MMTV insertional mutagenesis generally develop tumors reminiscent of MMTV-induced natural neoplasia. Other genetically altered mice have tumors of unique phenotype, but they, too, fall within discernable phenotypic (signature) categories, represented by *myc, c-erbB2, ras,* and *ret1* (among others) phenotypes that do not resemble MMTV-induced tumors. The skilled pathologist can accurately predict the causative transgene, based upon tumor morphology.

TABLE 1.2—Modifiers of mouse mammary tumor descriptors

Biological potential

Carcinoma	Neoplasm of epithelium with malignant biological behavior (invasion, metastasis)
Adenocarcinoma	Neoplasm of glandular epithelium with proven malignant biological behavior
Adenoma	Neoplasm of glandular epithelium without proven malignant biological behavior
Mammary intraepithelial neoplasia (MIN)	Intraluminal epithelial proliferations with cytologic atypia, including in situ carcinomas
Hyperplasia	Any increase in cell number without cytologic atypia
Tumor	Any space occupying mass with unknown biological potential

Property

Atypia	Cells with abnormal nuclear morphology
Necrosis	Cell death generally not applied to apoptosis
Fibrosis	Increased or abnormal deposition of connective tissue
Secretory	Tissues or glands producing or exporting lipid or protein
Metaplasia	A change from one adult cell type to another adult cell type

Topography

Diffuse	All of the mammary gland is involved.
Focal	One area of the mammary gland is involved.
Multifocal	Multiple foci of the mammary gland are involved.

Inducer

Gene-induced	Tumors that have morphological or cytological patterns characteristic of specific transgenes or specific mutations
MMTV-induced	Tumors known to be induced by MMTV
Chemically-induced	Tumors known to be induced by a chemical carcinogen
Hormone-induced	Tumors known to be induced by exogenous hormones

Biological/Experimental Context

Biological	Parity, pregnancy, lactation, involution, hormones
Experimental	Promoter, exogenous hormones or chemicals

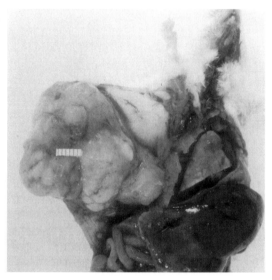

FIG. 1.87—Mammary adenocarcinoma in aged female mouse. Note the lobulated appearance of the mass.

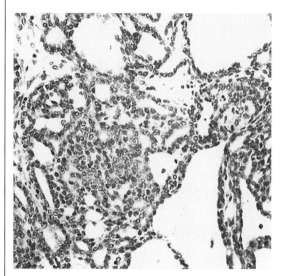

FIG. 1.88—Mammary acinar adenocarcinoma, illustrating variation in the morphology of the acini.

DIAGNOSIS. The location of the neoplasms in female mice and the typical histological pattern are useful diagnostic aids.

SIGNIFICANCE. Mammary tumors can be locally invasive and may metastasize hematogenously to the lung, but most spontaneous tumors are adenomas.

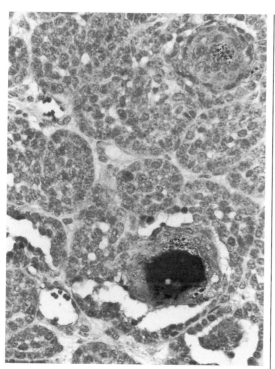

FIG. 1.89—Adenosquamous mammary carcinoma. Note the solid trabecular formation formed by squamous epithelial cells in some regions and the presence of keratinized material.

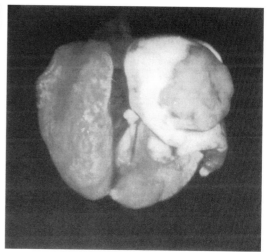

FIG. 1.90—Pulmonary carcinoma in aged laboratory mouse. There is a large, raised, circumscribed mass in the cranial regions of the right lung, with displacement of the normal pulmonary parenchyma.

Pulmonary Tumors

EPIZOOTIOLOGY AND PATHOGENESIS. Primary pulmonary tumors are some of the most common tumors seen in older mice, particularly in strains such as GR, BALB, and A mice. B6 mice are relatively resistant to their spontaneous development. Tumors are not normally virus-induced but can be produced experimentally in mice with certain carcinogens. Depending on the histological pattern, pulmonary tumors have been classified as alveolar cell or bronchiolar tumors. The classification remains controversial, and other terms suggested include alveolar/bronchiolar and alveolar tumors. The use of techniques such as electron microscopy and in situ hybridization have provided additional and sometimes conflicting interpretations on the cell of origin of these tumors. Based on one ultrastructural study, alveolar cell tumors were interpreted to arise from type II pneumocytes, while bronchiolar tumors originated from Clara cells. However, other elec-

tron microscopic studies have suggested that there is not necessarily a good correlation between the cell type of origin and the patterns seen by light microscopy. Based on in situ hybridization studies, surfactant typical of type II pneumocytes was identified in all primary pulmonary neoplasms studied, regardless of whether their histologic patterns were primarily solid or tubulopapillary in type. It was proposed that they all be classified as either alveolar adenomas or alveolar carcinomas. The term "alveolar/bronchiolar tumor" appears to be the most appropriate term, regardless of the nature of the architecture seen microscopically.

PATHOLOGY. At necropsy, the tumors appear as circumscribed, firm to resilient, pearl-gray nodules approximately 0.5–5.0 mm in diameter, located in the subpleural regions or deep within the parenchyma of the lung. Malignant tumors may be large, with bulging contours (Fig. 1.90). There may be evidence of pleural invasion, with seeding of the visceral and parietal pleura. On microscopic examination, typical *alveolar adenomas* consist of a circumscribed mass, with compression of the adjacent structures (Fig. 1.91). They are composed of closely packed cuboidal to columnar cells lining remnants of alveolar septa, with a sparse stroma of collagenous tissue. Tumor

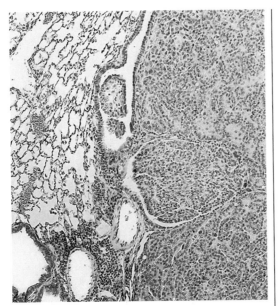

FIG. 1.91—Pulmonary adenoma, bronchioloalveolar cell type. Cuboidal epithelial cells are lining alveolar septa. There is a distinct line of demarcation between the tumor and the adjacent histologically normal lung tissue.

cells are relatively uniform in size, with round, hyperchromatic nuclei and acidophilic cytoplasm. Cells are nonciliated, and mitotic figures are rare. *Pulmonary adenomas of bronchioloalveolar origin* (previously referred to as bronchiolar tumors) are frequently adjacent or protruding into bronchioles. They consist of tubular to papillary patterns composed of columnar epithelial cells with convoluted to folded basal nuclei. There is compression of the adjacent alveolar structures. *Pulmonary carcinomas* tend to invade the adjacent parenchyma, including the pleura; frequently form papillary structures; and consist of large, pleomorphic epithelial cells with irregular, polygonal, hyperchromatic nuclei (Fig. 1.92). There may be extensive invasion of the adjacent pleural surface and occasionally extension into the intercostal muscles.

DIAGNOSIS. The presence of epithelial tumors with the typical histological features in older mice is a useful criterion. *Differential diagnoses* include metastatic tumors from sites such as mammary gland or liver and focal alveolar epithelial cell hyperplasia, as seen occasionally in older mice.

Hepatocellular Tumors. Mice develop a variety of detectable changes in the liver, particularly in older animals. These may be altered foci. *Eosinophilic cell foci* are areas present in the lobules and consist of large eosinophilic hepatocytes with granular cytoplasm. *Basophilic cell foci* are composed of small hepatocytes with distinctly basophilic cytoplasm, and *clear cell foci* are composed of hepatocytes with a central nucleus and clear to lacy cytoplasm. The changes are primarily due to alterations in staining properties, and there are no obvious alterations in liver architecture, nor is there compression of the adjacent parenchyma. Therefore, these are not true tumors; they must be differentiated from proliferative processes, which may vary from foci of hyperplasia to hepatoma to hepatocellular carcinoma. Primary hepatic tumors readily occur in mice treated with a variety of hepatocarcinogens, but spontaneous hepatocellular tumors also occur in untreated animals.

PATHOLOGY. At necropsy, the tumors may vary from circumscribed, raised, moderately firm, gray to tan nodules up to 5 mm or more in diameter to large, poorly delineated, pale to dark red fleshy masses. On microscopic examination, *hepatomas* occur as distinct nodules that compress the adjacent tissue. They are composed of well-differentiated cells and occasionally have prominent, eosinophilic, cytoplasmic globules. *Hepatocellular carcinomas* are usually large and poorly delineated, and they frequently have a characteristic trabecular pattern (Fig. 1.93). Frequently prominent are anisokaryosis, karyomegaly, and cytomegaly. Occasionally, malignancies of the liver consist of small, poorly differentiated hepatocytes, and hepatocellular carcinomas may also form adenoid or glandular patterns. The larger hepatocellular tumors may have areas of necrosis and hemorrhage, and frequently there are large vascular spaces within the mass. Metastases to the lung may occur.

Harderian Gland Tumors. Naturally occurring tumors of the Harderian lacrimal gland normally

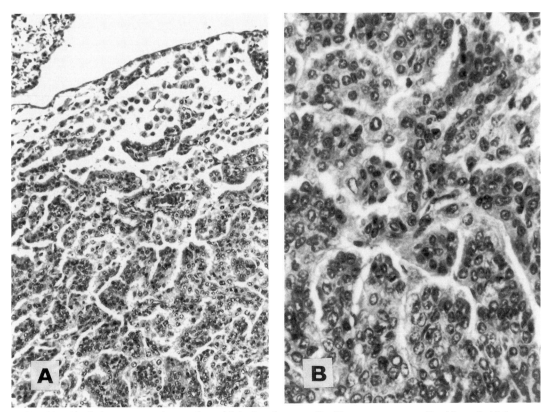

FIG. 1.92—(**A**) Pulmonary carcinoma, bronchioloalveolar type. Papillary structures are lined by cuboidal epithelial cells. (**B**) Higher magnification of **A,** demonstrating the papillary patterns and the prominent cuboidal epithelial cells.

appear late in life and are slowly growing neoplasms. The incidence of Harderian gland tumors can be increased with irradiation or the administration of chemical carcinogens.

PATHOLOGY. At necropsy, there is usually protrusion of the eye on the affected side. The mass typically consists of a lobulated, resilient, light tan to white structure in the orbital space. Microscopically, the tumors are usually papillary cystadenomas and are composed of relatively well-differentiated epithelial cells with vacuolated cytoplasm (Fig. 1.94). Invasive Harderian gland adenocarcinomas also occur (Fig. 1.95). They tend to be less well differentiated and invasive and may metastasize to other sites, such as lung.

Myoepitheliomas. Myoepitheliomas arise infrequently in most strains of mice but are relatively more common in other strains, such as BALB mice, especially females. They most frequently arise from submaxillary and parotid salivary glands but can also be associated with mammary, preputial, and Harderian glands. These tumors can become very large, with cystic chambers containing serous fluid. Microscopically, tumors are composed of large, pleomorphic spindle cells with epithelial and mesenchymal features (Fig. 1.96). Cystic areas form as a result of necrosis. Metastasis to the lung may occur with large tumors. A curious feature is concomitant myeloid hyperplasia of bone marrow and spleen, apparently related to a secretory product of the tumor.

Other Neoplasms in the Laboratory Mouse. It is beyond the scope of this summary to include descriptions of all the spontaneous neoplasms that occur in this species. Included

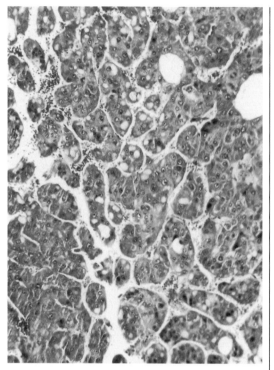

FIG. 1.93—Hepatocellular carcinoma, trabecular type. The neoplasm consists of cords of poorly differentiated hepatocytes in a trabecular pattern.

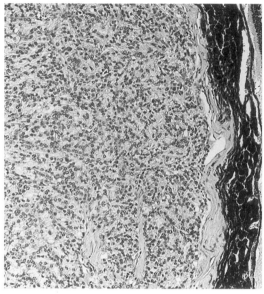

FIG. 1.95—Harderian gland adenocarcinoma. The neoplasm consists of poorly differentiated fusiform to cuboidal epithelial cells, with displacement of the adjacent sclera and retina.

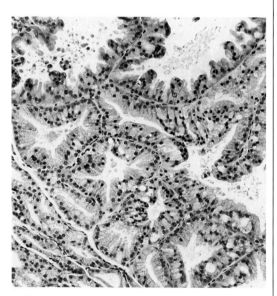

FIG. 1.94—Harderian gland adenoma. The tumor is composed of relatively well-differentiated acinar structures, with compression of the adjacent, histologically normal, Harderian gland tissue.

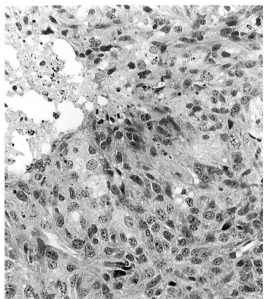

FIG. 1.96—Myoepithelial carcinoma of the parotid salivary gland of laboratory mouse. The mass is composed of densely packed bands of fusiform cells. There are foci of necrosis containing cellular debris within the mass.

in the *neoplasms of the female reproductive tract* are tubular adenomas, granulosa cell–thecal cell tumors, and papillary adenocarcinomas of the ovary; and adenocarcinomas and leiomyosarcomas of the oviduct and uterus. *Neoplasms of the male reproductive tract* are relatively rare. Occasionally adenocarcinomas and carcinomas occur in the preputial or other accessory sex glands. *Neoplasms of the endocrine organs* include pituitary gland adenomas, adrenocortical adenomas, pheochromocytomas, and follicular cell adenomas of the thyroid gland.

BIBLIOGRAPHY FOR NEOPLASMS

Neoplasms of the Hematopoietic/Lymphoreticular System

Dunn, T.B. 1954. Normal and pathologic anatomy of the reticular tissue of laboratory mice, with a classification and discussion of neoplasms. J. Natl. Cancer Inst. 19:1281–1433.

Foster, H.L., et al., eds. 1982. *The Mouse in Biomedical Research. IV. Experimental Biology and Oncology.* New York: Academic.

Fredrickson, T.N., et al. 1995. Classification of mouse lymphomas. Curr. Top. Microbiol. Immunol. 194:109–16.

Frith, C.H. 1990. Histiocytic sarcoma, mouse. In *Monographs on Pathology of Laboratory Animals: Hematopoietic System,* ed. T.C. Jones et al., pp. 58–65. New York: Springer-Verlag.

Frith, C.H., and Ward, J.M. 1988. *Color Atlas of Neoplastic and Non-Neoplastic Lesions in Aging Mice.* New York: Elsevier.

Frith, C.H., et al. 1993. The morphology, immunohistochemistry, and incidence of hematopoietic neoplasms in mice and rats. Toxicol. Pathol. 21:206–18.

———. 1985. *A Color Atlas of Hematopoietic Pathology of Mice.* Little Rock, Ark.: Toxicology Pathology Associates.

Furmanski, P., and Rich, M.A. 1982. Neoplasms of the hematopoietic system. In *The Mouse in Biomedical Research. IV. Experimental Biology and Oncology,* ed. H.L. Foster et al., pp. 352–71. New York: Academic.

Krueger, G.R.F. 1990. Lymphoblastic lymphoma, mouse. In *Monographs on Pathology of Laboratory Animals: Hematopoietic System,* ed. T.C. Jones et al., pp. 264–75. New York: Springer-Verlag.

Pascal, R.R., et al. 1973. Glomerulonephritis associated with immune complex deposits and viral particles in spontaneous murine leukemia: An electron microscopic study with immunofluorescence. Lab. Invest. 29:159–65.

Pattengale, P.K., and Frith, C.H. 1983. Immunomorphologic classification of spontaneous lymphoid cell neoplasms occurring in female BALB/c mice. J. Natl. Cancer Inst. 70:169–79.

Pattengale, P.K., and Taylor, C.R. 1983. Experimental models of lymphoproliferative disease: The mouse as a model for human non-Hodgkin's lymphomas and related leukemias. Am. J. Pathol. 113:237–65.

Ward, J.M., and Sheldon, W. 1993. Expression of mononuclear phagocyte antigens in histiocytic sarcoma of mice. Vet. Pathol. 30:560–65

Ward, J.M., et al. 1999. Thymus, spleen, and lymph nodes. In *Pathology of the Mouse: Reference and Atlas,* ed. R.R. Maranpot et al., pp. 332–60. Vienna, IL: Cache River Press.

Mammary Tumors

Cardiff, R.D., et al. 2000. The mammary pathology of genetically engineered mice: The consensus report and recommendations from the Annapolis meeting. Oncogene 19:968–88.

DeOme, K.B., et al. 1959. Development of mammary tumors from hyperplastic alveolar nodules transplanted into gland-free mammary fat pads of female C3H mice. Cancer Res. 19:515–20.

Dunn, T.B. 1959. Morphology of mammary tumors in mice. In *Pathophysiology of Cancer,* ed. F. Homberger, pp. 38–84. New York: Harper (Hoeber).

Harbell, J.W., et al. 1982. Hormone requirements of the pregnancy-dependent mammary tumor of GR/A mice: An in vitro study. J. Natl. Cancer Inst. 69:1391–1402.

Lee, A.E., et al. 1989. Reinfection of virus free mice with mouse mammary tumor virus. Lab. Anim. 23:133–37.

Medina, D. 1982. Mammary tumors. In *The Mouse in Biomedical Research. IV. Experimental Biology and Oncology,* ed. H.L. Foster et al., pp. 373–96. New York: Academic.

Riley, V. 1975. Mouse mammary tumors: Alteration of incidence as apparent function of stress. Science 189:465–67.

Seely, J.C., and Boorman, G.A. 1999. Mammary gland and specialized sebaceous glands. In *Pathology of the Mouse: Reference and Atlas,* ed. R.R. Maronpot et al. pp. 612–35. Vienna, Ill.: Cache River Press.

Pulmonary Tumors

Dixon, D., et al. 1999. Lungs, pleura, and mediastinum. In *Pathology of the Mouse: Reference and Atlas,* ed. R.R. Maronpot et al. pp. 293–332. Vienna, Ill.: Cache River Press.

Kauffman, S.L., et al. 1979. Histologic and ultrastructural features of the Clara cell adenoma of the mouse lung. Lab. Invest. 40:708–16.

Pilling, A.M., et al. 1999. Expression of surfactant protein mRNA in normal and neoplastic lung of B6C3F$_1$ mice as demonstrated by in situ hybridization. Vet. Pathol. 36:57–63.

Stewart, H.L., et al. 1979. Tumors of the respiratory tract. IARC Sci. Publ. 23:251–61.

Hepatocellular Tumors

Becker, F.F. 1982. Morphological classification of mouse liver tumors based on biological characteristics. Cancer Res. 42:3918–23.

Frith, C.H., and Ward, J.M. 1980. A morphologic classification of proliferative and neoplastic hepatic lesions in mice. J. Environ. Pathol. and Toxicol. 3:329–51.

Harderian Gland Tumors

Holland, J.M., and Fry, R.J.M. 1982. Neoplasms of the integumentary system and Harderian gland. In *The Mouse in Biomedical Research. IV. Experimental Biology and Oncology,* ed. H.L. Foster et al., pp. 513–28. New York: Academic.

Ihara, M., et al. 1994. Morphology of spontaneous Harderian gland tumors in aged B6C3F$_1$ mice. J. Vet. Med. Sci. 56: 775–78.

Myoepitheliomas

Burger, G.T., et al. 1985. Myoepithelioma, salivary glands, mouse. In *Monographs on Pathology of Laboratory Animals: Digestive System,* ed. T.C. Jones et al., pp. 185–89. New York: Springer-Verlag.

Sundberg, J.P., et al. 1991. Myoepitheliomas in inbred laboratory mice. Vet. Pathol. 28:313–23.

General Bibliography and Other Neoplasms

Booth, C.J., and Sundberg, J.P. 1995. Hemangiomas and hemangiosarcomas in inbred laboratory mice. Lab. Anim. Sci. 45:497–502

Goodman, D.G., and Strandberg, J.D. 1982. Neoplasms of the female reproductive tract. In *The Mouse in Biomedical Research. IV. Experimental Biology and Oncology,* ed. H.L. Foster et al., pp. 397–411. New York: Academic.

Holland, J.M., and Fry, R.J.M. 1982. Neoplasms of the integumentary system and Harderian gland. In *The Mouse in Biomedical Research. IV. Experimental Biology and Oncology,* ed. H.L. Foster et al., pp. 513–28. New York: Academic.

Mostofi, F.K., and Sesterhenn, I. 1982. Neoplasms of the male reproductive system. In *The Mouse Biomedical Research. IV. Experimental Biology and Oncology,* ed. H.L. Foster et al., pp. 414–38. New York: Academic.

Percy, D.H., and Jonas, A.M. 1971. Incidence of spontaneous tumors in CD(R)-1 HaM/ICR mice. J. Natl. Cancer Inst. 46:1045–65.

Russfield, A.B. 1982. Neoplasms of the endocrine system. In *The Mouse in Biomedical Research. IV. Experimental Biology and Oncology,* ed. H.L. Foster et al., pp. 465–75. New York: Academic.

Squire, R.A., et al. 1978. Tumors. In *Pathology of Laboratory Animals,* ed. K. Benirschke, et al., pp. 1052–1283. New York: Springer-Verlag.

Laboratory rats are represented by a fewer number of outbred stocks and inbred strains than laboratory mice. Small numbers of transgenic rats now exist, and it is likely that transgenic rats will become more prevalent, but never to the degree of mice. Genetic background of rats is as important a consideration as in mice for expression of disease. Rats are subject to infection with fewer viruses than mice but seem to make up for this with more clinically significant bacterial infections.

ANATOMIC FEATURES

Hematology. The predominant peripheral blood leukocyte in rats is the lymphocyte, which makes up approximately 80% of the cell population. Eosinophils tend to possess annular, ring-shaped nuclei without lobation. Nuclear ring forms are common among granulocytes in tissues, as in the mouse. Basophils are rare. Mature male rats have higher total leukocyte counts than do females, in both lymphocytes and granulocytes.

Gastrointestinal System. The rat is anatomically similar to the mouse. Salivary gland sexual dimorphism also occurs in rats. Intestinal Paneth cells have smaller granules than do mice. Unlike mice, the rat liver is consistently lobated into four major lobes and lacks a gallbladder. Hepatocytes are more uniform in size than in the mouse. However, polyploidy is a common morphological feature in adult animals, and the number of binucleate cells increases with age. Bile is not concentrated. The liver may also reflect general disease states. Marked atrophy of hepatic cords is a common manifestation of reduced (or absence of) food intake (Fig. 2.1). The rat pancreas is diffuse.

Genitourinary System. The male and female rat reproductive organs are basically similar to those

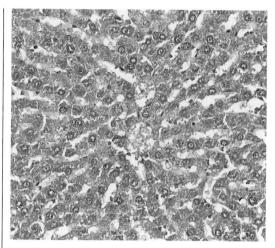

FIG. 2.1—Liver from adult rat with marked atrophy of hepatic cords. Note the reduction in cytoplasmic volume of hepatocytes, indicative of reduced food intake and seen in disease states.

of the mouse. Adult female rats develop cyclic uterine infiltrates of eosinophils, which can be misconstrued as abnormal. Rats have three pairs of pectoral and three pairs of inguinal mammary glands. As in the mouse, mammary tissue extends throughout much of the subcutis of the sides and necks of rats. Proteinuria is normal in rats, due to tubular production of alpha globulins. Proteinuria due to loss of serum proteins is not normal (see Chronic Progressive Glomerulonephropathy).

Skeletal System. As in mice and hamsters, bones lack Haversian systems. Adult rats, particularly males of some strains, continue to grow, and epiphyseal ossification is not complete until after 1 yr of age. Hematopoiesis remains active in long bones throughout life.

Lymphopoietic System. The rat thymus remains prominent into young adulthood and involutes

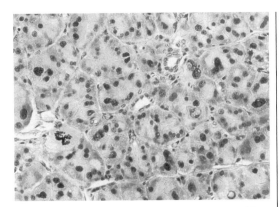

FIG. 2.2—Exorbital gland from mature male rat. Note the marked anisokaryosis of epithelial cells lining acini, a normal finding in males.

thereafter. Occasionally the thymus has involuted to the point where it is no longer identifiable by as early as 1 yr of age, particularly in males. Splenic hematopoiesis occurs in the adult rat, but not to the extent seen in mice. Prominent hematopoietic activity usually denotes an underlying disease state. In pathogen-free rats, splenic hematopoiesis is minimal, with only a few megakaryocytes present. Hemosiderin progressively accumulates in splenic macrophages throughout life, particularly in breeding females.

Respiratory System. The rat is similar anatomically to the mouse (see Chap. 1). Rats possess serous cells in respiratory epithelium, which are unique to this species.

Other Anatomic Features. Adrenals of wild rats are remarkably larger than in their domesticated cousins. Adrenals of females are larger than those of males. Rats are endowed with prominent brown fat, as in mice. The exorbital lacrimal glands of rats display striking epithelial megalokarya, particularly in older males (Fig. 2.2). This increases with age and should not be confused with a disease state. The fur of male albino rats tends to yellow with age.

BIBLIOGRAPHY
FOR ANATOMIC FEATURES

Bailey, Y., and Duprat, P. 1990. Normal blood cell values, rat. In *Monographs on Pathology of Laboratory Animals: Hematopoietic System*, ed. T.C. Jones et al., pp. 27–38. New York: Springer-Verlag.

Bannasch, P. et al. 1997. Foci of altered hepatocytes, rat. In *Monographs on Pathology of Laboratory Animals*, ed. T.C. Jones. New York: Springer-Verlag.

Bivin, W.S., et al. 1979. Morphophysiology. In *The Laboratory Rat. I. Biology and Diseases*, ed. H.J. Baker et al., pp. 74–103. New York: Academic.

Boorman, G.A., et al. 1990. *Pathology of the Fischer Rat: Reference and Atlas.* New York: Academic.

Gaertner, D.J., et al. 1988. Cytomegalic changes and inclusions in lacrimal glands of laboratory rats. Lab. Anim. Sci. 38:79–82

Greene, E.C. 1963. *Anatomy of the Rat.* New York: Hafner.

Jones, T.C., et al., eds. 1997. *Monographs on Pathology of Laboratory Animals: Digestive System.* New York: Springer-Verlag.

Kuper, C.F., et al. 1990. Development and aging, thymus, rat. In *Monographs on Pathology of Laboratory Animals: Hematopoietic System*, ed. T.C. Jones et al., pp. 257–63. New York: Springer-Verlag.

———. 1986. Spontaneous pathology of the thymus in aging Wistar (Cpb:WU) rats. Vet. Pathol. 23:270–77.

Richter, C.P. 1954. The effects of domestication and selection on the behavior of the Norway rat. J. Natl. Cancer Inst. 15:727–28.

Ringler, D.H., and Dabich, L. 1979. Hematology and clinical biochemistry. In *The Laboratory Rat. I. Biology and Diseases*, ed. H.J. Baker et al., pp. 105–21. New York: Academic.

Sanderson, J.H., and Phillips, C.E. 1981. *An Atlas of Laboratory Animal Haematology.* Oxford: Clarendon.

Valli, V.E., et al. 1990. Evaluation of blood and bone marrow, rat. In *Monographs on Pathology of Laboratory Animals: Hematopoietic System*, ed. T.C. Jones et al., pp. 9–26. New York: Springer-Verlag.

VIRAL INFECTIONS

DNA VIRAL INFECTIONS

Adenoviral Infection. Laboratory rats have an uncertain relationship with adenoviruses. Serological surveys indicate that they seroconvert to adenoviruses that are antigenically related to mouse adenovirus K87 (see Chap. 1). Under experimental conditions, rats could not be infected with mouse adenovirus of either type, suggesting that rats are naturally infected with serologically related but rat-specific adenovirus(es). Disease due to adenovirus in rats is absent. Lesions represent incidental findings and resemble those of enterotropic mouse adenovirus K87, with intranuclear inclusions in scattered small intestinal enterocytes (Fig. 2.3). Discernable intranuclear inclusions have been induced by treatment of rats with chemotherapeutic agents,

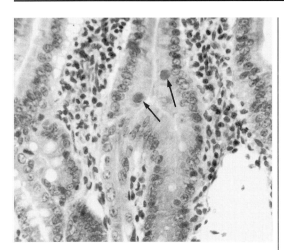

FIG. 2.3—Section from small intestine from rat, illustrating intranuclear inclusion bodies in enterocytes (*arrows*) typical of spontaneous adenovirus infection.

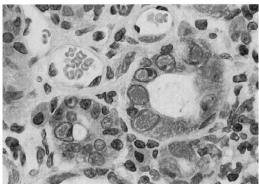

FIG. 2.4—Submandibular salivary gland of rnu nude rat naturally infected with rat papovavirus. Note prominent intranuclear inclusions.

presumably activating subliminal infection. Attempts to isolate the rat adenovirus have failed.

Herpesviral Infection: Rat Cytomegalovirus Infection. Rats are host to their own rat cytomegalovirus (RCMV), which is antigenically distinct from mouse CMV. Based upon presence of lesions in salivary glands, RCMV is common in wild rats but nonexistent in laboratory rats. RCMV infects the salivary and lacrimal glands, causing typical cytomegaly with both intracytoplasmic as well as intranuclear inclusions in ductal epithelium, with nonsuppurative interstitial inflammation. Intracerebral inoculation of suckling rats with RCMV will produce a nonsuppurative encephalitis with karyomegaly, intranuclear and intracytoplasmic inclusion bodies in neural tissue, and polykaryocyte formation. Serological tests are available but not generally applied because of its rarity in laboratory rat populations.

Papovaviral Infection. A polyoma virus, serologically distinct from polyoma and K viruses of mice, can infect rats, but its prevalence is unknown. This agent became apparent in a colony of athymic nude (rnu) rats, in which 10–15% developed a wasting disease with pneumonia and parotid sialoadenitis. Intranuclear inclusions were present in duct epithelium and, to a lesser extent, acini of parotid glands. Euthymic rats did not develop disease. Viral antigen was found in salivary glands, larynx, and, less often, bronchial epithelium and kidney. Since the virus has not been isolated, serological screens of rat populations for this agent are not performed. Recent examination of diagnostic material from rnu rats by the authors has revealed striking intranuclear inclusions in salivary gland epithelium (Fig. 2.4), bronchiolar epithelium, and alveolar lining cells, resulting in interstitial pneumonia and weight loss. Other organs examined were histologically normal.

Parvoviral Infections: Rat Virus, H-1 Virus, Rat Parvovirus. Parvoviruses are small, single-stranded, nonenveloped DNA viruses of the family Parvoviridae, with nuclear replication. They are relatively resistant and remain infectious at room temperature for a considerable period of time. Naturally occurring parvoviruses in the laboratory rat are represented by three major genetic/antigenic groups. Kilham's rat virus (RV), the prototype virus for one group, includes isolates RV, H-3, X-14, RV-Y, and HER virus; Toolan's H-1 is the prototype for the second group, which includes H-1 and HT viruses. RV and H-1 groups are related and share partial antigenic cross-reactivity. A third type, which is distantly related to RV and H-1, has been recently discovered. This agent (or agents) was originally called rat orphan parvovirus (ROPV) but is now referred to as rat parvovirus (RPV). RPV has gone undetected serologically because of the hemagglutination inhibition (HI) method of assay. RPV does not share homologous cross-reacting structural antigens (VP1 and VP2) with RV or H-1 virions but possesses conserved cross-reacting nonstructural antigens (NS1 and NS2) that are expressed in infected cells during virus replication. Thus, serological methods such as HI, which rely on virus, do not detect antibody to RPV, whereas methods like indirect fluorescent antibody (IFA) testing, which use infected cells as a substrate (which contain both virus structural and nonstructural antigens), detect antibody to all rat parvoviruses. RPV seems to be nonpathogenic and is distinct from mouse parvovirus (MPV).

EPIZOOTIOLOGY AND PATHOGENESIS. Serological surveys show infections with members of the RV and H-1 groups to be relatively common in laboratory rats, with a lower incidence of antibodies to the H-1 group. RPV also seems to be common among laboratory rats. Wild rats have been found to be seropositive for RV. Transmission appears to occur primarily by oronasal contact with infected animals, or by contaminated fomites. Virus shedding has been documented in urine, feces, and oropharynx. RV is recognized to be the most pathogenic of these parvoviruses under both field and experimental conditions and may be the only strain that produces clinical disease under natural conditions. Transplacental transmission of RV has been demonstrated in pregnant rats inoculated orally with high doses of RV, resulting in infertility and fetal resorption. RV may persist in colonies for long periods of time. Rats born to seropositive dams receive maternal antibodies during the neonatal period and usually acquire RV at 2–7 mo of age. Virus may also be shed in the milk during lactation and in the feces. In seronegative 2-d-old suckling rats inoculated oronasally with RV, inoculated animals were able to transmit virus for up to 10 wk, and for at least 7 wk after seroconversion had occurred. Rats inoculated as juveniles shed RV for at least 3 wk postinoculation. Virus may be reactivated by immunosuppression, resulting in acute systemic disease. Although persistence can theoretically occur in individual rats, persistence of parvoviral infections in colonies of rats is dependent on the continuous availability of new

susceptible animals to permit propagation of the virus. The widespread distribution of parvoviruses and their requirements for dividing cells for replication results in the frequent contamination of tumor cell lines and tumor virus stocks that have been passaged in laboratory rats.

In the experimentally induced disease in newborn rats, target tissues for RV replication include primordial cells of the cerebellar cortex, periventricular region, hepatocytes, endothelial cells, and bone marrow. Other target organs include kidney, lung, and genital tract. The multiple hemorrhages seen in the experimental and naturally occurring disease are attributed to the endothelial cell and megakaryocyte damage associated with viral replication in these tissues. Intestinal mucosal lesions, which are so prominent in feline and canine parvoviral infections, do not occur in rats and may be due to a lack of receptors in the intestinal tract. Documented descriptions of spontaneous outbreaks of parvoviral infections in rats are rare. In one report, juvenile rats were clinically affected. Clinical signs included dyspnea, ruffled hair coat, muscular weakness, and cyanotic scrotums. In this outbreak, rats seroconverted to RV, and later to H-1, suggesting that H-1 may have potentiated the development of the disease.

Naturally occurring disease has not been attributed to H-1 viruses or RPVs. Experimental studies indicate that both of these types of parvovirus are also prone to persistence, and RPV has a strong tropism for lymphoid tissue.

PATHOLOGY. In the adult form of RV disease, there is congestion of lymph nodes, loss of body fat, scrotal hemorrhage, and peritesticular fibrinous exudation (Fig. 2.5). Splenomegaly, icterus, and ascites are variable findings. Microscopic changes may be present in the brain, liver, and testes. Disseminated foci of hemorrhage occur in the cerebrum and cerebellum in a random distribution involving gray and white matter with malacia and obliteration of the normal architecture (Fig. 2.6). In the testes and epididymis, there may be multifocal coagulation necrosis and hemorrhage consistent with infarction, with thrombosis of regional vessels. Focal hepatocellular necrosis may occur, and amphophilic, intranuclear inclusions may be present in hepatocytes, endothelial cells, and bile duct epithelium

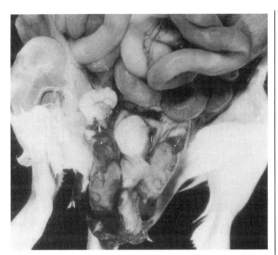

FIG. 2.5—Spontaneous rat virus (RV) infection in young rat. Note the marked hemorrhage and fibrinous exudation in the peritesticular region. (Courtesy Coleman et al. 1983, reprinted from Coleman, G.L., et al. Vet Pathol. 20:49–56, 1983.)

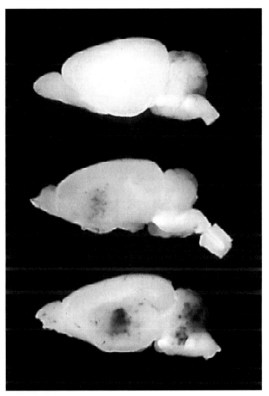

FIG. 2.6—Brains of rats experimentally infected with RV, depicting hemorrhagic encephalopathy. (Courtesy R.O. Jacoby)

(Fig. 2.7). Neonatal or infant rats can develop classic cerebellar hypoplasia, hepatitis, and jaundice. Recovered rats can be found with peliosis hepatis and nodular hyperplasia with portal scarring. Infertility, fetal resorption, and abortion may occur in pregnant females.

DIAGNOSIS. The provisional diagnosis, based on the presence of typical lesions and inclusions, can be confirmed by the demonstration of viral antigen by immunohistochemistry. Seroconversion may be detected by various procedures such as the complement fixation (CF), HI, virus neutralization (NT), or IFA. The CF, HI, and NT tests will permit the differentiation of members of the RV from the H-1 group. RPV antibody has been detected only with IFA. *Differential diagnoses* include bacterial septicemias such as pseudomoniasis, chronic wasting due to agents such as *Mycoplasma pulmonis,* and trauma. Infertility and fetal resorption must be differentiated from conditions such as nutritional disorders and mycoplasmal infections.

SIGNIFICANCE. Enzootic infections with parvoviruses are common in conventional breeding

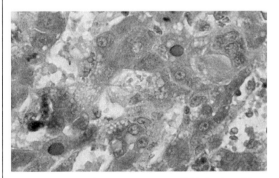

FIG. 2.7—Liver from spontaneous RV infection, illustrating typical intranuclear inclusions in hepatocytes. (Courtesy R.O. Jacoby)

colonies of laboratory rats. They are normally carried as an inapparent infection for long periods of time. Some parvoviruses represent a potential cause of clinical disease, particularly when rats are subjected to procedures that may result in immunosuppression. Subclinically infected laboratory rats also are a potential source of contamination for transplantable tumors, tissue-culture cell lines, and virus stocks.

Poxviral Infection. Poxviral infections have been reported to occur in laboratory rats from Eastern Europe and the former Soviet Union. The agent (or agents) is Turkmenia rodent poxvirus, which is closely related to cowpox virus and distinctly different from ectromelia virus. Clinical signs resembled mousepox in mice, ranging from inapparent infections to dermal pox and tail amputation with high mortality. Both dermal and respiratory tract lesions occur. Microscopically, rats with respiratory signs had severe interstitial pneumonia with edema, hemorrhage, and pleural effusion. Focal inflammatory lesions occur in the upper respiratory tract. Felids and human contacts are susceptible to infection with this poxvirus.

RNA VIRAL INFECTIONS

Coronaviral Infection: Sialodacryoadenitis. Based upon serological surveys, antibodies to coronaviruses are common in both laboratory and wild rats. The two naturally occurring coronaviruses isolated from this species are Parker's rat coronavirus (PRC) and sialodacryoadenitis virus (SDAV). PRC is the name given to a single coronavirus isolate, which was the first coronavirus isolated from rats. SDAV is a morphological designation and represents any and all subsequent coronavirus isolates that produced sialodacryoadenitis. PRC was first isolated from the lungs of rats. Intranasal inoculation of newborn and weanling rats with PRC produced rhinitis, tracheitis, and interstitial pneumonitis, with focal atelectasis and high mortality in infants. PRC also induces salivary and lacrimal gland lesions, but these were overlooked in the original descriptions. SDAV isolates produce lacrimal and salivary gland lesions but also produce pulmonary disease in young rats. Thus, these viruses should be considered part of a single biological grouping (rat

coronaviruses). Nevertheless, this dichotomy and terminology continues because of historical precedent. Like the mouse hepatitis virus (MHV), the rat coronavirus group is likely to contain numerous, constantly changing strains that vary in virulence.

EPIZOOTIOLOGY AND CLINICAL SIGNS. Based on early serological surveys, the percentage of colonies seropositive for rat coronavirus was relatively high. However, rat coronaviruses are now relatively uncommon in well-managed facilities, but these facilities continue to experience periodic outbreaks. Transmission is primarily by infected nasal secretions or saliva, and the virus spreads rapidly following introduction into a susceptible population of rats. In epizootics, there can be subclinical to high morbidity and virtually no mortality, except through anesthetic deaths. Typical clinical signs associated with SDA during the acute stages of the disease include sniffling, blepharospasm, epiphora, and intermandibular swelling. Dark red encrustations may be present around the eyes and external nares. These porphyrin-containing substances are released from damaged Harderian glands and emit a characteristic pink fluorescence under an ultraviolet light source. Other complications sometimes seen during the convalescent period may include unilateral or bilateral glaucoma/megaloglobus, hyphema, and corneal ulceration. Ocular changes that occur are secondary to the destructive lesions and impaired function of the lacrimal glands. This may result in failure to lubricate the cornea properly, corneal drying, impaired intraocular drainage, hemorrhage, and subsequent permanent damage to the eye. Reproductive disorders, including neonatal mortality and aberrations in the estrous cycle, have also been associated with SDA.

PATHOLOGY. Acutely infected rats can display excessive lacrimation or have red encrustations around the external nares and eyelids. Reflection of the skin of the ventral neck can reveal subcutaneous, periglandular, and interlobular edema of the parotid and/or the submandibular (submaxillary) salivary glands. In contrast to normal glands, affected glands are enlarged and blanched (Fig. 2.8). Similar changes are frequently evident in the exorbital lacrimal glands.

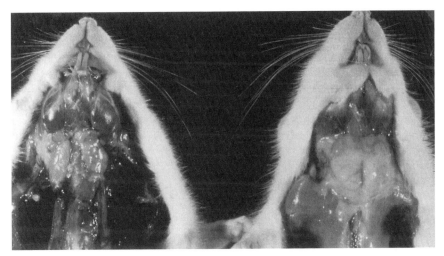

FIG. 2.8—Gross lesions typical of sialodacryoadenitis viral infection when necropsied during the acute stages of the disease (6 d postexposure). There is marked swelling of the submandibular glands, with interlobular and periglandular edema in the animal on the right, compared with the control rat on the left. (Courtesy Percy and Wojcinski 1986, reprinted by permission)

Harderian glands (and other lacrimal glands) can also be enlarged and blanched with periglandular and interstitial edema. Harderian glands often have blotchy brown pigmentation.

MICROSCOPIC CHANGES. During the acute stage of the disease, affected parotid and submandibular salivary glands and lacrimal glands (infraorbital, exorbital, Harderian) have coagulation necrosis of the ductal structures, with variable involvement of adjacent acini and effacement of the normal architecture. Interstitial edema, with mononuclear and polymorphonuclear cell infiltration, frequently occurs (Fig. 2.9). During the reparative stages of the disease, beginning at 7–10 d postexposure, there is nonkeratinizing squamous metaplasia of ductal and acinar structures of salivary and lacrimal glands, with reactive hyperplasia of cervical lymph nodes. Cellular infiltrates in affected glands at this stage are primarily lymphocytes, plasma cells, and macrophages (Fig. 2.10). Squamous metaplasia can be marked in the Harderian glands (Fig. 2.11). In salivary glands, regeneration of acinar and ductal epithelial cells is usually essentially complete by 3–4 wk postexposure. There may be isolated ducts or acini lined by poorly differentiated epithelial cells, with scattered aggregations of mononuclear cells, including mast

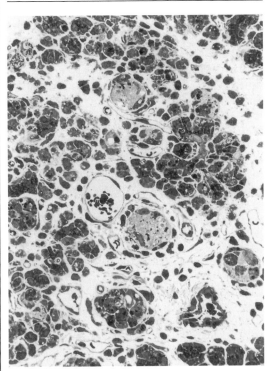

FIG. 2.9—Submandibular salivary gland from Wistar rat collected at 6 d postexposure to SDA virus. Note the marked necrosis of ductal and acinar epithelial cells, with effacement of the normal architecture.

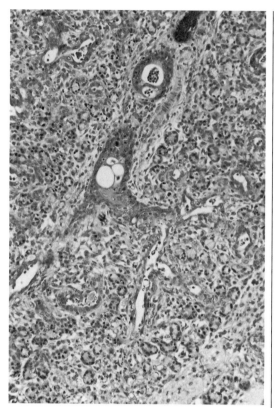

FIG. 2.10—Submandibular salivary gland at 8 d post-exposure to SDA virus. Ducts and acini are lined by poorly differentiated epithelial cells, with marked mononuclear cell infiltration.

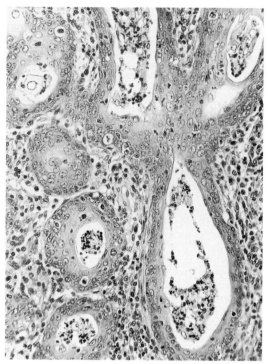

FIG. 2.11—Harderian gland from rat at 3 wk postexposure to SDA virus. There is a persistent dacryoadenitis, with squamous metaplasia and mononuclear cell infiltration. Dilated ducts and acini contain leukocytes and cellular debris.

cells, but usually the salivary glands are essentially normal histologically at this stage postexposure. On the other hand, focal residual inflammatory lesions may persist in the Harderian glands for several weeks. Reactive foci are frequently associated with interstitial deposition of pigmented material.

In the respiratory tract, necrotizing rhinitis, with mononuclear and polymorphonuclear cell infiltration, occurs during the acute stages of the disease. Both respiratory and olfactory epithelium are affected. The majority of the repair is complete by 14 d postexposure, although residual lesions may persist longer in specialized areas such as the vomeronasal organ. In the lower respiratory tract, there is transient tracheitis, and focal bronchitis and bronchiolitis, with leukocytic infiltration, hyperplasia of respiratory epithelial cells, and

flattening and loss of ciliated cells (Fig. 2.12). Focal alveolitis, when present, is characterized by hypercellularity of alveolar walls and mobilization of alveolar macrophages. Lesions in the lower respiratory tract are transient and usually have disappeared by 8–10 d postexposure.

Athymic nude rats are particularly susceptible to coronaviral infection and develop chronic persistent infections and wasting disease. Chronic suppurative rhinitis, bronchopneumonia, and chronic inflammatory lesions in the salivary and lacrimal glands have been described. Viral antigen was evident in affected tissues, including epithelium of the urinary tract.

DIAGNOSIS. The presence of the typical lesions of the salivary and lacrimal glands confirmed on microscopic examination is sufficient to make the diagnosis. Viral antigen may be demonstrated in the respiratory tract and affected salivary and

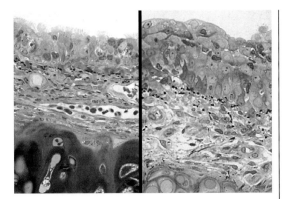

FIG. 2.12—Trachea from rat examined at 4 d postexposure to SDA virus. Note the hyperplasia of respiratory epithelium, loss of ciliated epithelial cells, and submucosal edema in affected animal (*right*) compared with control trachea.

lacrimal glands at 4–6 d postexposure. Initially, strains of rat coronavirus were replicated only on primary rat kidney cells, although isolates have now been adapted to replicate on selected cell lines such as L-2 cells. In general, viral isolation is not a practical procedure in most circumstances. Serological testing is the recommended and practical method to confirm prior exposure to SDA virus. Either the IFA test, using mouse coronavirus-infected cells as a source of antigen, or the enzyme-linked immunosorbent assay (ELISA) method is most frequently used for the serodiagnosis of SDA. *Differential diagnoses* include nasal and ocular discharge associated with mycoplasma, Sendai virus, or pneumonia virus of mice (PVM) infections; subcutaneous edema of the head associated with *Pseudomonas aeruginosa* infections; ocular and nasal irritation associated with high environmental ammonia levels; and stress-associated chromodacryorrhea. The presence of porphyrin-containing red encrustations around the eyes and nose (chromodacryorrhea) is not diagnostic for SDA. Chronic disease states (e.g., chronic respiratory disease) and recent stress-associated events may also result in the release of porphyrins from the Harderian glands.

SIGNIFICANCE. SDA is a disease of high morbidity and negligible mortality that occasionally occurs in conventional colonies of laboratory rats.

Permanent ocular damage may occur in a small percentage of rats as a result of dacryoadenitis and impaired function of Harderian glands. Transient respiratory tract damage and hypersecretion may result in unexpected deaths in rats anesthetized during the acute stages of SDA. In addition, there is evidence that the virus has a significant additive effect in rats previously infected with *Mycoplasma pulmonis,* and possibly the cilia-associated respiratory (CAR) bacillus. There is a significant depletion of epidermal growth factor (EGF) in affected submandibular salivary glands during the convalescent stages of the disease. In view of the demonstrated effects of EGF on functions such as reproduction and carcinogenesis, there may be significant effects on certain types of research. Behavioral changes and reproductive disorders including aberrations of the estrous cycle and neonatal mortality have also been associated with epizootics of the disease. Active infection also precipitated graft-vs.-host disease in the salivary and lacrimal glands of rats with allogenic bone marrow grafts. Prior exposure to the virus appears to provide protection against the development of the typical disease on reinfection for up to 15 mo. In facilities housing infected animals, the use of seropositive noncontagious rats has been one method recommended to establish a coronavirus-free breeding colony. Athymic rats are particularly susceptible to the virus.

Hantaviral Infection. Rats are susceptible to infection with hantaviruses, and thereby pose a zoonotic hazard to human contacts. The genus *Hantavirus* belongs to the family Bunyaviridae and contains at least 14 rodent-borne viruses. Members of this genus are spread by aerosol and contact, in contrast to other bunyaviruses, which are arthropod-borne. Phylogenetic trees comparing nucleotide sequences show two major lineages of hantaviruses. One represents viruses associated with hemorrhagic fever and renal syndrome (HFRS) in humans, and the other represents recently discovered but widespread viruses of the New World that are associated with hantavirus pulmonary syndrome (HPS) in humans. It is now apparent that hantaviruses originally evolved in the Old World, then spread by rodents to the New World across the Bering land bridge. Humans are incidental hosts.

EPIZOOTIOLOGY AND PATHOGENESIS. Rats (*Rattus norvegicus* and *R. rattus*), several species of the genus *Peromyscus,* and other rodents are susceptible to natural infection with hantaviruses. In the rat, Hantaan virus (a member of the HFRS group) produces no clinical evidence of disease. In experimentally inoculated animals, viremia and virus shedding may occur in the saliva, and intracage transmission may occur up to 2 mo postinoculation. There is no evidence of transplacental transmission. Immunohistochemistry, PCR, and histopathology of naturally infected *Peromyscus* mice revealed antigen and viral nucleic acid in lung, liver (portal macrophages and sinusoidal cells), kidney (glomeruli), and spleen (both red and periarteriolar white pulp). With the caveat that these were wild-caught, microbiologically undefined animals, histopathology consisted of pulmonary septal edema and nonsuppurative portal hepatitis. Histopathology of laboratory rats has not been evaluated, but lesions are likely to be present, despite commonly accepted dogma of subliminal infection. Antibodies to the virus have been demonstrated in rats and/or human contacts in Asia, Europe, Africa, and North America. The source of the virus in human infections is considered to be by contact with infected rodents and their urine. In human cases of HFRS, clinical symptoms include fever, thrombocytopenia, and capillary leakage resulting in myalgia, headache, petechiation, with prominent retroperitoneal and renal hemorrhage. Humans infected with HPS develop fever and capillary leakage that is localized to the lungs. Death occurs from shock and cardiac complications.

DIAGNOSIS. Serologic assays are available and should be used as part of routine safety precautions in laboratory animal programs using wild rodents or laboratory rats.

SIGNIFICANCE. Hantaviruses are important zoonotic pathogens of laboratory rodents with potentially serious consequences for humans. Hantaviruses have caused several laboratory-associated outbreaks of HFRS in Asia and Europe, and these have been traced to infected rats from breeders, wild rodents, and experimentally infected rodents. The ubiquity of these viruses in wild rodents of North America, including *R. norvegicus,* dictates constant awareness of the hazard.

Paramyxoviral Infections

PNEUMONIA VIRUS OF MICE (PVM) . PVM is a paramyxovirus in the genus *Pneumovirus* with an affinity for the respiratory tract. It infects mice, rats, hamsters, and possibly guinea pigs and gerbils. In addition to the prevalence of seropositive laboratory mice, antibodies to PVM have also been demonstrated in gerbils and in wild rodents.

EPIZOOTIOLOGY AND PATHOGENESIS. Based on serological surveys, enzootic infections with PVM commonly occur in laboratory rats. The percentage of colonies of rats positive for PVM varies but may be up to 80% or more. Intranasal inoculation of F344 rats with PVM has resulted in the production of gross and microscopic lesions by 6 d postinoculation, although animals showed no clinical evidence of disease. In experimental infections, complement-fixing antibodies to PVM peaked at 14 d postinoculation and dropped sharply by 19 d.

PATHOLOGY. Acute, multifocal, nonsuppurative vasculitis and interstitial pneumonitis with necrosis are typical lesions seen during the acute stages of the disease. There are prominent perivascular infiltrates, with hyperplasia of bronchus-associated lymphoid tissue, perivasculitis, and multifocal interstitial pneumonitis. These lesions tend to persist for several weeks in the rat.

DIAGNOSIS. The presence of interstitial pneumonitis and perivasculitis attributed to PVM will require confirmation by seroconversion, and this is the most practical method used to make the diagnosis. In laboratories with the appropriate facilities and personnel, the recovery of the virus from the respiratory tract during the acute stages of the disease or the demonstration of viral antigen by immunohistochemistry may be attempted. *Differential diagnoses* include pneumonitis due to other viral agents such as Sendai virus or the rat coronaviruses.

SIGNIFICANCE. PVM is now a recognized pathogen of the respiratory tract in the laboratory rat, and represents a potential complication in enzootically infected colonies. Based on serological surveys, the virus exists as an enzootic infection in many colonies of laboratory rats. PVM may also be a copathogen in other respiratory diseases, such as mycoplasmal infections. The possibility of interspecies transmission to other laboratory animals, such as mice, hamsters, and gerbils, is another consideration.

SENDAI VIRUS INFECTION. Sendai virus (parainfluenza 1) is an RNA virus of the family Paramyxoviridae. Indigenous to mice, Sendai virus is recognized to cause respiratory disease in the laboratory rat and hamster, and seroconversion also occurs in guinea pigs.

EPIZOOTIOLOGY AND PATHOGENESIS. Although clinical disease and lesions of the respiratory tract are rarely attributed to Sendai virus infection in the rat, serological surveys indicate that the virus has been relatively widespread in colonies of rats. Transmission may occur by direct contact or by aerosols. Following exposure by inhalation, the virus replicates in the upper respiratory tract, then extends down the trachea and smaller airways in a stepwise manner. Viral antigen is detectable from approximately 1 to 7 d. Virus has been recovered from the lung for up to 7 d postinoculation (pi), and for up to 12 d when inoculated as young rats. Peak interferon levels have been detected in the lung by 6 hr pi. Serum antibody levels may be present for 7 or more mo, dropping to low or nondetectable levels by 9 mo pi. Clinical signs are usually not detected in epizootics of the disease. The pathogenesis of Sendai virus infection in the rat is analogous to Sendai in genetically resistant strains of mice.

HISTOPATHOLOGY. In rats necropsied during the acute stages of the disease, there is rhinitis, with focal to diffuse necrosis of respiratory epithelial cells. Leukocytic infiltrates consist of neutrophils, lymphocytes, and plasma cells. Residual lesions may persist in the nasal mucosa for 3 or more weeks. In the lower respiratory tract, there is a multifocal hyperplastic to suppurative bronchitis and bronchiolitis; in severe cases a necrotizing bronchitis and bronchiolitis, and frequently a focal alveolitis. Alveolar septa are hypercellular,

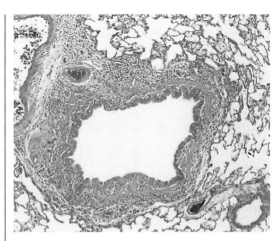

FIG. 2.13—Bronchitis/bronchiolitis associated with recent Sendai virus infection in rat. Note the marked mononuclear cell infiltration around the affected airway.

and infiltrating cells consist of alveolar macrophages, neutrophils, and lymphocytes. At the alveolar level, viral replication occurs in type I and type II pneumocytes and in alveolar macrophages. In the subacute and resolving stages, there is prominent perivascular and peribronchial cuffing with lymphocytes and plasma cells (Fig. 2.13). Mononuclear cell infiltrates may persist for up to several weeks in alveolar septa, and there may be some evidence of residual interstitial fibrosis in alveolar walls.

DIAGNOSIS. Animals are usually asymptomatic; thus the detection of pulmonary lesions on microscopic examination is frequently the first indication of a possible infectious disease. The changes are not specific for Sendai, and confirmation will require demonstration of a rise in antibody. Necrotizing bronchitis and bronchiolitis are features of the disease. In suspected epizootics of Sendai viral infection, *differential diagnoses* must include PVM, rat coronavirus, and *Mycoplasma pulmonis* infections. Therefore serological testing for PVM, rat coronavirus, and *Mycoplasma,* and culture for bacteria and *Mycoplasma,* are required in order to exclude other possible respiratory pathogens.

SIGNIFICANCE. Sendai virus is an important respiratory pathogen in the laboratory rat and is recognized to have an additive effect on respiratory infections with *M. pulmonis*. Sendai virus infection may also impair the normal immune response and has been associated with impaired fetal development and neonatal mortality by indirect means. In enzootically infected colonies, there is a danger of transmission to other susceptible species, including mice, guinea pigs, and hamsters.

Picornaviral Infection: Rat Cardiovirus. Seroconversion of rats to TMEV (a mouse cardiovirus) occurs occasionally in laboratory rats. A single mouse encephalomyelitis virus (MEV) - type agent, MHG virus, which has been isolated from adult laboratory rats, induced neurological disease in experimentally inoculated suckling rats and mice. This agent is closely related to MEV (see Chap. 1) and can be isolated from intestine, lung, and brain of infected rats. No natural disease has been found in rats associated with MEV-like agents. Another isolate from Wistar rats in Japan was characterized by reverse-transcriptase polymerase chain reaction (RT-PCR), and gene sequences were compared with TMEV-GDVII. There were significant differences. The name "rat cardiovirus" (RCaV) was proposed. Rats and mice inoculated intracerebrally with RCaV remained asymptomatic throughout the study.

Rotaviral Infection: Infectious Diarrhea of Infant Rats (IDIR). An epizootic of diarrhea in infant rats has been attributed to a rotaviruslike agent that is morphologically identical but antigenically distinct from most previously characterized rotaviruses. The agent is probably of human origin. Following oral inoculation of suckling rats with the virus, recipients develop diarrhea within 24–36 hr. Transient growth retardation, cracking and bleeding in the perianal region, and drying and flaking of skin are typical clinical signs. Rats are susceptible to experimental infection at all ages and to disease up to 12 d of age. They are resistant to clinical disease after 2 wk.

PATHOLOGY. The stomach usually contains milk curd, with watery contents in the proximal small intestine. The distal small intestine and large intestine contain yellow-brown to green fluid and gas. Microscopic changes include intestinal villous attenuation, necrosis of enterocytes, and

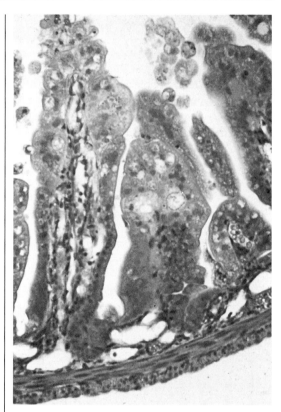

FIG. 2.14—Distal small intestine from suckling rat postinoculation with rotavirus (IDIR). Note pathognomonic syncytia. (Courtesy S.L. Vonderfecht)

pathognomonic epithelial syncytia (Fig. 2.14). Changes are most evident in the ileal region. Eosinophilic intracytoplasmic inclusions may be present in syncytia. Viral antigen can be demonstrated in affected enterocytes. Viral precursor material and rotaviral particles may be visualized in cells by electron microscopy.

DIAGNOSIS. Identification of the characteristic gross and microscopic findings and the demonstration of typical rotaviral particles in tissue sections or intestinal contents are sufficient to confirm the diagnosis. To date, a reliable immunoassay procedure has not been developed for the disease. *Differential diagnoses* include possible bacterial infections of the intestinal tract such as *Escherichia coli* or streptococci.

SIGNIFICANCE. IDIR represents one cause of diarrhea and transient growth retardation in suckling rats. The virus may be antigenically identical to a rotavirus associated with human patients. Suckling rats inoculated with the human isolate developed diarrheal disease identical to IDIR.

Reoviral Infection. Rats frequently seroconvert to reovirus 3, but natural or experimental disease does not occur in this species. Mice are the only laboratory animals that are susceptible to reovirus-induced disease (see Chap. 1).

Retroviral Infection. Rats, like mice, hamsters, guinea pigs, and other species, are infected with endogenous retroviruses, which are transmitted vertically as provirus sequences in the genome. These viruses are of minimal practical significance but have been manipulated experimentally by combining with murine leukemia viruses and other rat leukemia viruses to form defective rat sarcoma viruses. Common laboratory sarcoma viruses of rat origin include the Harvey and Kirsten sarcoma agents.

BIBLIOGRAPHY FOR VIRAL INFECTIONS

DNA Viral Infections

Adenoviral Infection
Smith, A.L., and Barthold, S.W. 1987. Factors influencing susceptibility of laboratory rodents to infection with mouse adenovirus strains K87 and FL. Arch. Virol. 95:143–48.
Smith, A.L., et al. 1986. Comparative biological characterization of mouse adenovirus strains FL and K87 and seroprevalence in laboratory rodents. Arch. Virol. 91:233–46.
Ward, J.M., and Young, D.M. 1976. Latent adenoviral infection of rats: Intranuclear inclusions induced by treatment with a cancer chemotherapeutic agent. J. Am. Vet. Med. Assoc. 169:952–53.

Herpesviral Infection:
Cytomegaloviral Infection
Kilham, L., and Margolis, G. 1975. Encephalitis in suckling rats induced with rat cytomegalovirus. Lab. Invest. 33:200–206.
Lyon, H.W., et al. 1959. Cytomegalic inclusion disease of lacrimal glands in male laboratory rats. Proc. Soc. Exp. Biol. Med. 101:164–66.
Priscott, P.K., and Tyrell, D.A.J. 1982. The isolation and partial characterization of a cytomegalovirus from the brown rat, *Rattus norvegicus*. Arch. Virol. 73:145–60.

Papovaviral Infection
Ward, J.M., et al. 1984. Papovaviral sialoadenitis in athymic nude rats. Lab. Anim. 18:84–89.

Parvoviral Infections
Ball-Goodrich, L.J., et al. 1998. Rat parvovirus type 1: the prototype for a new rodent parvovirus serogroup. J. Virol. 72:3289–99.
Coleman, G.L., et al. 1983. Naturally occurring lethal parvovirus infection of juvenile and young-adult rats. Vet. Pathol. 20:49–56.
Gaertner, D.J., et al. 1995. Persistent rat virus infection in juvenile athymic rats and its modulation by immune serum. Lab. Anim. Sci. 45:249–53.
Jacoby, R.O., et al. 1996. Rodent parvovirus infections. Lab. Anim. Sci. 46:370–80.
———. 1987. The pathogenesis of rat virus infection in infant and juvenile rats after oronasal inoculation. Arch. Virol. 95:251–70.
Kilham, L. 1966. Viruses of laboratory and wild rats. In *Viruses of Laboratory Rodents*, ed. R. Holdenried, pp. 117–46. NCI Monograph 20. Washington, D.C.: U.S. Government Printing Office.
Kilham, L., and Margolis, G. 1969. Transplacental infection of rats and hamsters induced by oral and parenteral inoculations of H-1 and rat viruses (RV). Teratology 2:111–24.
———. 1966. Spontaneous hepatitis and cerebellar "hypoplasia" in suckling rats due to congenital infection with rat virus. Am. J. Pathol. 49:457–75.
Margolis, G., and Kilham, L. 1972. Rat virus infection of megakaryocytes: A factor in hemorrhagic encephalopathy? Exp. Mol. Pathol. 16:326–40.
Robinson, G.W., et al. 1971. Seroepidemiological study of rat virus infection in a closed laboratory colony. Am. J. Epidemiol. 96:443–46.
Tattersall, P., and Cotmore, S.F. 1986. The rodent parvoviruses. In *Viral and Mycoplasmal Infections of Laboratory Rodents: Effects on Biomedical Research,* ed. P. N. Bhatt et al., pp. 305–48. New York: Academic.
Ueno, Y., et al. 1997. Epidemiological characterization of newly recognized rat parvovirus, a rat orphan parvovirus. J. Vet. Med. Sci. 59:265–69.

Poxviral Infections
Iftimovici, R., et al. 1976. Enzootic with ectromelia symptomatology in Sprague-Dawley rats. Rev. Roum. Med. Virol. 27:65–66.
Kraft, L.M., et al. 1982. Morphological evidence for natural poxvirus infection in rats. Lab. Anim. Sci. 32:648–54.
Krikun, V.A. 1977. Pox in rats: Isolation and identification of pox virus. Vopr. Virusol. 22:371–73.
Marennikova, S.S., and Shelukhina, E.M. 1976. White rats as a source of pox infection in carnivora of the family Felidae. Acta Virol. 20:422.
Marennikova, S.S., et al. 1978a. Identification and study of a poxvirus isolated from wild rodents in Turkmenia. Arch. Virol. 56:7–14.
———. 1978b. Pox infection in white rats. Lab. Anim. 12:33-36.

RNA Viral Infections

Coronaviral Infection

Bhatt, P.N., and Jacoby, R.O. 1977. Experimental infection of axenic rats with Parker's rat coronavirus. Arch. Virol. 54:345–52.

Bhatt, P.N., et al. 1972. Characterization of the virus of sialodacryoadenitis of rats: A member of the coronavirus group. J. Infect. Dis. 126:123–30.

Bihun, C.G., and Percy, D.H. 1995. Morphologic changes in the nasal cavity associated with sialodacryoadenitis virus infection in the Wistar rat. Vet. Path. 32:1–10.

Brammer, D.W., et al. 1993. Elimination of sialodacryoadenitis virus from a rat production colony by using seropositive breeding animals. Lab. Anim. Sci. 43:633–34

Caseboldt, D.B., et al. 1988. Prevalence rates of infectious agents among commercial breeding populations of rats and mice. Lab. Anim. Sci. 38:327–29.

Hajjar, A.M., et al. 1991. Chronic sialodacryoadenitis virus (SDAV) infection in athymic rats. Lab. Anim. Sci. 41:22–25.

Harkness, J.E., and Ridgeway, M.D. 1980. Chromodacryorrhea in laboratory rats (*Rattus norvegicus*): Etiologic considerations. Lab. Anim. Sci. 30:841–44.

Jacoby, R.O., et al. 1975. Pathogenesis of sialodacryoadenitis virus in gnotobiotic rats. Vet. Pathol. 12:196–209.

Lussier, G., and Descoteaux, J-P. 1986. Prevalence of natural virus infections in laboratory mice and rats used in Canada. Lab. Anim. Sci. 36:145–48.

Macy, J.D., et al., 1996. Reproductive abnormalities associated with coronavirus infection in rats. Lab. Anim. Sci. 46:129–32.

Maru, M., and Sato, K. 1982. Characterization of a coronavirus isolated from rats with sialoadenitis. Arch. Virol. 73:33–43.

Parker, J.C., et al. 1970. Rat coronavirus (RCV): A prevalent naturally occurring pneumotropic virus of rats. Arch. Gesamte Virusforsch. 31:293–302.

Percy, D.H., and Williams, K.L. 1990. Experimental Parker's rat coronavirus infection in Wistar rats. Lab. Anim. Sci. 40:603–7.

Percy, D.H., et al. 1990. Duration of protection following reinfection with sialodacryoadenitis virus. Lab. Anim. Sci. 40:144–49.

———. 1989a. Sequential changes in the Harderian and exorbital lacrimal glands in Wistar rats infected with sialodacryoadenitis virus. Vet. Pathol. 26:238–45.

———. 1989b. Replication of sialodacryoadenitis virus in mouse L-2 cells. Arch. Virol. 104:323–33.

———. 1988. Depletion of salivary gland epidermal growth factor by sialodacryoadenitis virus infection in the Wistar rat. Vet. Pathol. 25:183–92.

Rossie, K.M., et al. 1988. Graft-versus-host disease and sialodacryoadenitis viral infection in bone marrow transplanted rats. Transplantation 45:1012–16.

Schoeb, T.R., and Lindsey, J.R. 1987. Exacerbation of murine respiratory mycoplasmosis by sialodacryoadenitis virus infection in gnotobiotic F344 rats. Vet. Pathol. 24:392–99.

Schunk, M.K., et al. 1995. Effect of time of exposure to rat coronavirus and *Mycoplasma pulmonis* on respiratory tract lesions in the Wistar rat. Can. J. Vet. Res. 59:60–66.

Utsumi, K., et al. 1980. Infectious sialoadenitis and rat breeding. Lab. Anim. 14:303–7.

Weir, E.C., et al. 1990a. Persistence of sialodacryoadenitis virus in athymic rats. Lab. Anim. Sci. 40:138–43.

———. 1990b. Infection of SDAV-immune rats with SDAV and rat coronavirus. Lab. Anim. Sci. 40:363–66.

Wojcinski, Z.W., and Percy, D.H. 1986. Sialodacryoadenitis virus-associated lesions in the lower respiratory tract of rats. Vet. Pathol. 23:278–86.

Hantavirus Infection

Childs, J.E., et al. 1987. Epizootiology of Hantavirus infections of Baltimore: Isolation of a virus from Norway rats and characteristics of infected rat populations. Am. J. Epidemiol. 126:55–68.

Johnson, K. 1986. Hemorrhagic fever-Hantaan virus. In *Viral and Mycoplasmal Infections of Laboratory Rodents: Effects on Biomedical Research,* ed. P.N. Bhatt et al., pp. 193–215. New York: Academic.

Leduc, J.W., et al. 1984. Hantaan-like viruses from domestic rats captured in the United States. Am. J. Trop. Med. Hyg. 33:992–98.

Lee, P.W., et al. 1986. Pathogenesis of experimental Hantaan-like viruses from domestic rats captured in the United States. Am. J. Trop. Med. Hyg. 33:992–98.

Schmaljohn, C., and Hjelle, B. 1997. Hantaviruses: A global disease problem. Emerging Infect. Dis. 3:95–104.

Pneumonia Virus of Mice (PVM)

Brownstein, D.G. 1985. Pneumonia virus of mice infection, lung, mouse and rat. In *Monographs on Pathology of Laboratory Animals: Respiratory System,* ed. T.C. Jones et al., pp. 206–10. New York: Springer-Verlag.

Vogtsberger, L.M., et al. 1982. Histological and serological response of B6C3F1 mice and F344 rats to experimental pneumonia virus of mice infection. Lab. Anim. Sci. 32:419.

Sendai Virus Infection

Burek, J.D., et al. 1977. A naturally occurring epizootic caused by Sendai virus in breeding and aging rodent colonies. II. Infection in the rat. Lab. Anim. Sci. 27:963–71.

Carthew, P., and Aldred, P. 1988. Embryonic death in pregnant rats owing to intercurrent infection with Sendai virus and *Pasteurella pneumotropica.* Lab. Anim. 22:92–97.

Castleman, W.L. 1983. Respiratory tract lesions in weanling outbred rats infected with Sendai virus. Am. J. Vet. Res. 44:1024–31.

Castleman, W.L., et al. 1987. Pathogenesis of bronchiolitis and pneumonia induced in neonatal and weaning rats by parainfluenza (Sendai) virus. Am. J. Pathol. 129:277–96.

Coid, R., and Wardman, G. 1971. The effect of parainfluenza type 1 (Sendai) virus infection on early pregnancy in the rat. J. Reprod. and Fertil. 24:39–43.

Garlinghouse, L.E., and Van Hoosier, G.L., Jr. 1978. Studies on adjuvant-induced arthritis, tumor transplantability, and serologic response to bovine serum albumin in Sendai virus–infected rats. Am. J. Vet. Res. 39:297–300.

Garlinghouse, L.E., et al. 1987. Experimental Sendai virus infection in laboratory rats I. Virus replication and immune response. Lab. Anim. Sci. 37:437–41.

Giddens, W.E., et al. 1987. Experimental Sendai virus infection in laboratory rats. II. Pathology and histochemistry. Lab. Anim. Sci. 37:442–48.

Jakob, G.J., and Dick, E.C. 1973. Synergistic effect in viral-bacterial infection: Combined infection of the murine respiratory tract with Sendai virus and *Pasteurella pneumotropica.* Infect. Immun. 8:762–68.

Schoeb, T.R., et al. 1985. Exacerbation of murine respiratory mycoplasmosis in gnotobiotic F344/N rats by Sendai virus infection. Vet. Pathol. 22:272–82.

Picornaviral Infection: Rat Cardiovirus

McConnell, S.J., et al. 1964. Isolation and characterization of a neurotropic agent (MHG virus) from adult rats. Proc. Soc. Exp. Biol. Med. 115:362–67.

Ohsawa, K., et al. 1998. Genetic analysis of TMEV-like virus isolated from rats: Nucleic acid characterization of 3-D protein region. Contemp. Top. 37(4):113.

Rotaviral Infection

Vonderfecht, S.L. 1986. Infectious diarrhea of infant rats (IDIR) induced by an antigenically distinct rotavirus. In *Viral and Mycoplasmal Infections of Laboratory Rodents: Effects on Biomedical Research,* ed. P.N. Bhatt et al., pp. 254–52. New York: Academic.

Vonderfecht, S.L., et al. 1984. Infectious diarrhea of infant rats produced by a rotavirus-like agent. J. Virol. 52:94–98.

General Bibliography

Bhatt, P.N., et al., eds. 1986. *Viral and Mycoplasmal Infections of Laboratory Rodents: Effects on Biomedical Research,* ed. P.N. Bhatt et al. New York: Academic.

Caseboldt, D.B., et al. 1988. Prevalence rates of infectious agents among commercial breeding populations of rats and mice. Lab. Anim. Sci. 38:327–29.

Lindsey, J.R. 1986. Prevalence of viral and mycoplasmal infections in laboratory rodents. In *Viral and Mycoplasmal Infections of Laboratory Rodents: Effects on Biomedical Research,* ed. P.N. Bhatt et al., pp. 801–8. New York: Academic.

Lussier, G., and Descoteaux, J-P. 1986. Prevalence of natural virus infections in laboratory mice and rats used in Canada. Lab. Anim. Sci. 36:145–48.

Van Nunen, M.E.J., et al. 1978. Prevalence of viruses in colonies of laboratory rodents. Z. Versuch. 20:201–8.

BACTERIAL INFECTIONS

GRAM-NEGATIVE ENTERIC BACTERIAL INFECTIONS

***Campylobacter/Lawsonia* Infections.** *Campylobacter* infects a wide range of host species and is emerging as an important intestinal pathogen. *Campylobacter* has been isolated from young rats with mild diarrhea or soft feces, and its frequency may be higher than suspected if it is searched for among colonies of laboratory rats. Intracellular *Campylobacter*-like organisms have been associated with the epithelium of intestinal adenocarcinomas in a colony of Wistar rats. Based upon morphology, the agent was interpreted to be *Lawsonia intracellularis.*

***Clostridium piliforme* Infection: Tyzzer's Disease.** The etiologic agent of Tyzzer's disease is a filamentous, weakly gram-negative, spore-forming, obligate intracellular bacterium. For years, it has been named *Bacillus piliformis,* but recent genetic information has required its reclassification as *Clostridium piliforme.*

EPIZOOTIOLOGY AND PATHOGENESIS. The Tyzzer's bacillus has a wide host range and may remain infectious in contaminated bedding for up to 1 yr. Despite the wide host range, *C. piliforme* isolates tend to be host-specific, with minimal antigenic cross-reactivity among isolates (for additional information on epizootiology and pathogenesis, see the section on Tyzzer's disease in Chap. 6). Outbreaks in laboratory rats usually occur in adolescent rats during the postweaning period. Ingestion of spores is the likely source of the infection. Transplacental transmission has been demonstrated in seropositive rats treated with prednisolone during the last week of pregnancy. However, the organism can be eliminated from immunocompetent rats by cesarean section and appropriate disinfection techniques. Subclinically infected rats can transmit the organism to naive rats via contaminated bedding. Tyzzer's disease is typically an enterohepatic disease, with secondary involvement of the heart. In naturally occurring outbreaks of the disease, clinical signs may include depression, ruffled hair coat, abdominal distension, low morbidity, and high mortality in clinically affected animals. Clinical disease with low mortality has also been reported.

PATHOLOGY. Rats with Tyzzer's disease often develop a unique, marked dilation of the terminal small intestine (megaloileitis). The flaccid ileum may be distended up to 3–4 times the normal diameter, with variable involvement of the jejunum and cecum. Megaloileitis does not always occur in rats with Tyzzer's disease. Enteritis may be evident only at the microscopic level. The mesenteric lymph nodes are swollen and edematous. Disseminated pale foci of necrosis up to several millimeters in diameter are scattered throughout the parenchyma of the liver. There may also be circumscribed to linear pale foci present on the heart (Fig. 2.15). Microscopic changes are confined primarily to the ileum, liver, and myocardium. In the intestine, there is frequently a necrotizing transmural ileitis, with segmental involvement of affected areas. There is necrosis and sloughing of enterocytes and edema of the lamina propria and submucosa, frequently with fragmentation and hypercellularity of the muscular layers. Infiltrating inflammatory cells are primarily mononuclear cells, with a sprinkling of neutrophils. In the liver, the histological characteristics vary from foci of acute coagulation necrosis to focal hepatitis, with polymorphonuclear and mononuclear cell infiltration (Fig. 2.16). Hepatic lesions interpreted to be of some duration are characterized by fibrosis, with the presence of multinucleated giant cells and mineralized debris in reparative foci. In the heart, lesions may vary from necrosis of isolated myofibers to destruction of relatively large segments of myocardium. There is vacuolation to fragmentation of the sarcoplasm, with interstitial edema and mononuclear and polymorphonuclear cell infiltration. Giemsa, Warthin-Starry, or PAS stains are used to demonstrate bundles of slender bacilli in the cytoplasm of enterocytes in ileal lesions, in hepatocytes sur-

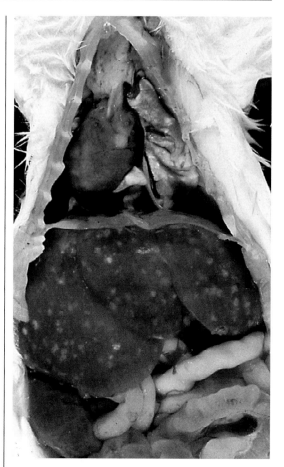

FIG. 2.15—Tyzzer's disease in a young rat. Note the multifocal hepatitis and focal myocarditis.

rounding necrotic foci, and scattered in the sarcoplasm in myocardial lesions. In many cases, finding typical fascicles of intracytoplasmic bacilli, particularly in liver, may require arduous searching.

DIAGNOSIS. Confirmation of the diagnosis requires the demonstration of the typical organisms in tissue sections. The triad of organs usually affected in Tyzzer's disease (intestine, liver, and heart) are also useful diagnostic features. Serologic tests are now widely used, but use of a single isolate as antigen may not detect seroconversion among different host species (including between mice and rats) due to significant antigenic heterogeneity. *Differential diagnoses* include salmonellosis and ileus following the

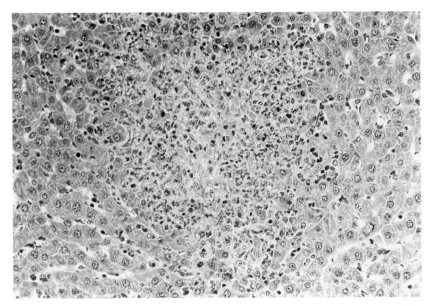

FIG. 2.16—Focal hepatitis in Tyzzer's disease in juvenile rat. There is necrosis of hepatocytes with polymorphonuclear cell infiltration.

intraperitoneal administration of chloral hydrate for general anesthesia.

SIGNIFICANCE. Although now uncommon in laboratory rats, Tyzzer's disease can be a cause of disease and mortality in this species. Following confirmation of the diagnosis, investigations should include husbandry and sanitation, as well as the possibility of interspecies transmission from other rodents or rabbits. Tyzzer's disease occurs in a wide variety of mammals, including a recently documented case in an AIDS patient. Clinically normal seropositive rats have been identified in colonies, indicating that inapparent infections may occur.

***Helicobacter* Infection.** Proliferative and ulcerative typhlitis has been observed in athymic nude rats naturally infected with *Helicobacter colis*. Similar lesions appeared upon experimental inoculation. Another helicobacter, *H. trogontum*, has been isolated from the large intestine of Wistar and Holtzman rats. Experimental inoculation of NIH Swiss germ-free mice with this agent resulted in inflammation of the gastric and intestinal mucosa.

***Salmonella* Infection.** During the early years of this century *Salmonella* infections represented an important infectious disease in laboratory rodents in North America. However, with improved sanitation, health-monitoring methods, and feeding practices, the disease now rarely occurs in laboratory animal facilities.

EPIZOOTIOLOGY AND CLINICAL SIGNS. Of the multitude of serotypes of *Salmonella enteritidis* capable of causing disease in the laboratory rat, serotypes *enteritidis* and *typhimurium* were most frequently implicated. In the period 1895–1910, serotype *enteritidis* was used as a rodenticide to control populations of wild rats in Europe and the United States. Enthusiasm waned when the public health implications became apparent. Clinical signs include depression, ruffled hair coat, hunched posture, weight loss, and variations in the nature of the feces from softer, lighter, formed stool to fluid contents. There may be porphyrin-containing red encrustations around the eyes and nose in clinically affected animals.

PATHOLOGY. Subclinical infections without discernible lesions are frequent. In clinically affected rats, the ileum and cecum are frequently distended with liquid contents and flecks of blood, and there is thickening of the gut wall in affected areas. Focal ulcerations may be present in the mucosa of the cecum and ileum. Splenomegaly frequently occurs. On microscopic examination, lesions in the ileum and cecum are characterized by hyperplasia of crypt epithelial cells, edema of the lamina propria, and leukocytic infiltration with focal ulceration. There is hyperplasia of the mesenteric lymph nodes, spleen, and Peyer's patches, with focal necrosis and leukocytic infiltration. In acute cases, lesions in other viscera are consistent with a gram-negative septicemia. In the spleen, focal necrosis and hemorrhage occur in the red pulp. Sinusoidal congestion and focal coagulation necrosis are frequent findings in the liver. Focal embolization may occur in tissues such as spleen, liver, and lymph nodes. Emboli consist of bacteria, fibrinous exudate, and cellular debris.

DIAGNOSIS. Isolation and identification of the organism from animals with lesions or from inapparent carriers are necessary to confirm the diagnosis of *Salmonella* infection. Salmonellae are intermittently present in the intestine, especially in carrier animals. One recommended procedure is to incubate fecal pellets or macerated tissue in selenite-F plus cystine broth overnight, followed by streaking onto brilliant green to promote the growth of the organism. Mesenteric lymph nodes may yield *Salmonella* in rats with negative fecal culture. *Differential diagnoses* include pseudomoniasis, rotaviral enteritis, cryptosporidiosis, management-related problems due to failure to provide feed or water, and Tyzzer's disease.

SIGNIFICANCE. Following the diagnosis of salmonellosis, the zoonotic potential should be emphasized. Possible sources of the organism include contaminated feed or fomites and transmission from other species, including human carriers, and from wild rodents. Corrective steps should include the identification of the source of the infection, improved sanitation, and if feasible, immediate slaughter. Repeated fecal samplings may be required in order to detect inapparent carrier animals.

GRAM-NEGATIVE RESPIRATORY INFECTIONS

Bordetella bronchiseptica Infection. *B. bronchiseptica* is an uncommon, typically opportunistic pathogen in laboratory rats, but it can cause significant disease.

EPIZOOTIOLOGY AND PATHOGENESIS. The organism is a relatively common inhabitant of the upper respiratory tract of species such as the guinea pig and domestic rabbit. It is recognized to be an important pathogen in the guinea pig and has been associated with respiratory tract infections in the rabbit. The organism tends to colonize on the apices of respiratory epithelial cells, resulting in impaired clearance by ciliated epithelial cells.

PATHOLOGY. Aerosol exposure to *B. bronchiseptica* in laboratory rats has resulted in lesions characterized by supurative rhinitis; multifocal bronchopneumonia, with polymorphonuclear cell and lymphocytic infiltration; and peribronchial lymphoid hyperplasia. In animals examined at 2 or more weeks postinoculation, there were fibroblast proliferation and mononuclear cell infiltration. In spontaneous cases of bronchopneumonia associated with *Bordetella* infection, there has been a suppurative bronchopneumonia with consolidation of affected anteroventral areas of the lung. Frequently there is an identifiable concurrent infection, such as rat coronaviral infection.

DIAGNOSIS. The isolation of the organism in large numbers from affected tissues is required. It is a small, motile, gram-negative bacillus that grows readily on conventional laboratory media, producing small blue-gray colonies.

SIGNIFICANCE. *B. bronchiseptica* is a bona fide opportunistic pathogen in the laboratory rat. When isolated from the respiratory tract in rats with lesions, it is likely that there are concurrent infections with other pathogens, such as mycoplasmal or viral agents.

Cilia-Associated Respiratory (CAR) Bacillus Infection. Naturally occurring respiratory disease has been associated with a filamentous, argyrophilic bacillus with gliding motility that colonizes the ciliated epithelium of airways. The organism stains gram-negative and is difficult to grow on conventional cell-free media. It has also been demonstrated on respiratory epithelium in mice, rabbits, cattle, and pigs. The first reported outbreak in rats was associated with prior exposure to Sendai virus and *Mycoplasma pulmonis* infection in the context of chronic respiratory disease (CRD). However, there have been spontaneous CRD outbreaks in animals apparently free of concurrent mycoplasmal infections, and the lesions were similar to those seen in primary mycoplasmal infection. In addition, lesions similar to those seen in confirmed cases of murine respiratory mycoplasmosis (MRM) have been produced in *Mycoplasma*-free rats inoculated intranasally with the CAR bacillus. Although the organism was first described in 1980, based on retrospective staining of tissue sections, there is evidence that the organism has been associated with some outbreaks of respiratory disease for decades.

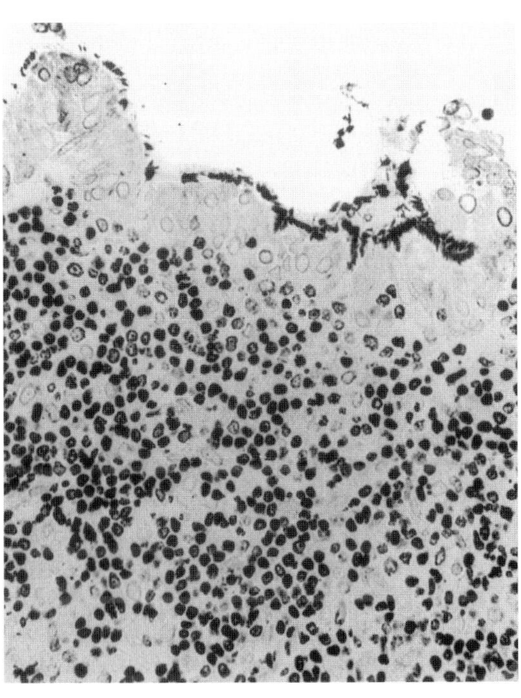

EPIZOOTIOLOGY AND PATHOGENESIS. The organism survives freezing and thawing and remains viable in allantoic fluid at room temperature for at least 1 wk. Infections have been established in rats that were inoculated intranasally with the organism grown in embryonated chick eggs. The CAR bacillus has also been transmitted from infected dams to their pups, and there is evidence that contaminated bedding is another means (albeit inefficient) of spread to other rats. In a sequential study in young Wistar rats inoculated intranasally with the organism, colonization of the upper respiratory tract and airways was evident by 14 d pi. Mucopurulent bronchopneumonia, progressing to bronchiectasis, was observed beginning at 3 wk pi. Lesions were similar to those observed in *Mycoplasma*-associated CRD.

PATHOLOGY. Chronic suppurative bronchitis and bronchiolitis, with peribronchiolar cuffing with lymphocytes and plasma cells, are typical microscopic findings. There is marked leukocytic infiltration in the lamina propria of affected airways. In sections stained with the Warthin-Starry method, slender, argyrophilic bacilli are inserted along the apices of the ciliated respiratory epithelium (Figs. 2.17 and 2.18).

FIG. 2.17—Bronchus from rat infected with the cilia-associated respiratory (CAR) bacillus (Warthin-Starry stain). Note the marked peribronchiolar mononuclear cell infiltration and the presence of organisms on the surface of bronchial epithelium.

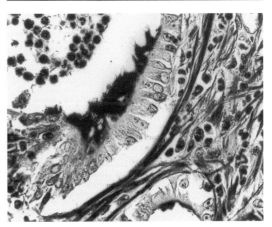

FIG. 2.18—Higher magnification of bronchus from CAR bacillus–infected rat stained by the Warthin-Starry method. Dark-staining bacilli are oriented along the apices of respiratory epithelial cells.

DIAGNOSIS. The typical slender bacteria are best demonstrated by silver stains, such as the Warthin-Starry impregnation technique. The organisms are also readily evident as electron-dense bacilli oriented between the cilia of respiratory epithelial cells by electron microscopy. A quantitative micro-ELISA procedure is available to detect seropositive animals. However, the use of CAR bacillus whole cell lysates as antigen for serology is problematic, in that this bacterium has a number of cross-reacting antigens among other bacteria. Other diagnostic techniques include the demonstration of the CAR bacillus in silver-stained tracheal scrapings using Steiner's silver stain, or in nasal swabs using the polymerase chain reaction (PCR) method. The organism has been grown in embryonated chick eggs, cell culture, and more recently, in cell-free media. *Differential diagnoses* include mycoplasmal infections and pneumonia due to conventional bacteria, with possible complications due to concurrent infections with Sendai or rat coronavirus.

SIGNIFICANCE. The relative importance and prevalence of the CAR bacillus in spontaneous outbreaks of chronic respiratory disease require further study. Although similar morphologically, there appear to be distinct antigenic differences between rodent and rabbit strains studied to date. Based on current information, it is evident that the CAR bacillus can be an important contributing factor in some outbreaks of respiratory disease, either as a primary or secondary pathogen.

Haemophilus **Infection.** A hitherto unknown species of *Haemophilus* has been isolated from the nasal cavity, trachea, lungs, and female genital tract. In rats sampled from one vendor, the organism was recovered from a significant percentage of animals, and antibodies to the *Haemophilus* sp. was detected in close to 50% of animals tested. On microscopic examination, mild inflammatory cell infiltrates were present in the lower respiratory tract. The organism was categorized as a member of the family Pasteurellaceae, *Haemophilus* sp. Co-infection with other respiratory pathogens was not fully investigated.

SIGNIFICANCE. The prevalence of this organism has not been determined. In view of the sites of colonization and the presence of lesions in the respiratory tract, this unclassified *Haemophilus* sp. represents a possible complicating factor in the laboratory rat under experiment.

Mycoplasmal Infection: Murine Respiratory Mycoplasmosis (MRM). Chronic respiratory disease (CRD) in rats has undergone an interesting historical evolution, in which it was initially believed to be multifactorial. As knowledge grew, *Mycoplasma pulmonis* was associated with CRD, and *M. pulmonis* was shown to produce CRD in experimentally infected rats. This gave rise to the term MRM as the preferred terminology over CRD. However, CRD is now known to be multifactorial. It is usually associated with concomitant infection with *M. pulmonis,* CAR bacillus, and respiratory viruses, with environmental effectors, such as ammonia. Nevertheless, *M. pulmonis* is the major component of CRD. *Mycoplasma pulmonis* is a member of the order Mycoplasmatales, small bacteria devoid of cell walls. They are usually fastidious in their growth requirements and require selective media for optimum growth. There are a variety of pleomorphic forms, and specialized tip structures appear to play a key role in the attachment of mycoplasmas to the host cell. Some antigenic heterogeneity occurs among strains of *M. pulmonis*. There are demonstrable common cross-reactive antigens between two other naturally occurring murine mycoplasmas, *M. neurolyticum* (mice) and *M. arthritidis*. As discussed in Chapter 1, *M. pulmonis* is the only clinically significant *Mycoplasma* sp.

EPIZOOTIOLOGY AND PATHOGENESIS. Thanks to responsible quality control and health-monitoring programs, there has been a marked reduction in the incidence of myocoplasmosis (and CRD) in rats. However, based on serological surveys, the incidence of seropositive colonies may be over 50%. Some of the positive animals may be due to cross-reacting antigens due to exposure to *M. arthritidis*. Reports of naturally occurring infections with clinical disease due to *M. arthritidis* are rare. However, the organism has been isolated from sites such as the respiratory tract and middle ear. Arthritis has been produced experimentally in mice and rats inoculated intravenously with *M. arthritidis* (as well as *M. pulmonis*), but there is little evidence that the organism is the cause of clinical disease under natural conditions.

Transmission of *M. pulmonis* among cage mates and to adjacent cages probably occurs primarily by aerosols. It may require up to several months to establish an infection in contact animals, and clinical disease may not occur until up to 6 mo postinfection. Intrauterine transmission may also occur, although newborn pups appear to be frequently infected by exposure to the infected dam during the postnatal period. Placentitis and fetal bronchopneumonia have been produced in pregnant rats inoculated intravaginally with *M. pulmonis* prior to breeding. The incidence and intensity of the disease are influenced by a variety of factors, such as strain of rat, concurrent infections, and environmental conditions. For example, LEW rats develop a more severe disease than do F344 rats postexposure to *M. pulmonis*. Concurrent infections with organisms such as Sendai virus, rat coronavirus, or CAR bacillus have an additive effect on the disease. Similarly, other opportunistic secondary bacterial invaders frequently play a role in the progression of the disease. Regarding environmental conditions, ammonia concentrations at the cage level of greater than 25 ppm may also enhance the progression of the disease.

The organism has an affinity for the epithelial cells of the respiratory tract, middle ear, and endometrium. Invasion of the middle ear probably occurs via the eustachian tube. This usually results in a chronic infection, since the eustachian tube opens into the tympanic bulla on the dorsal aspect, affording poor drainage to the nasopharynx. Rats have cartilaginous rings only around primary bronchi. Thus damage to respiratory epithelium with ciliostasis, and the resulting accumulation of lysozyme-rich inflammatory exudate in airways, frequently results in weakening of bronchiolar walls and subsequent bronchiectasis and bronchiolectasis. *Mycoplasma*-associated host cell damage may occur by a variety of means including uptake of essential cell metabolites and release of cytotoxic substances such as H_2O_2. Damage to ciliated epithelial cells and impairment of cilial activity results in impaired airway clearance and subsequent respiratory disease. Both the intact organisms and the cell membranes are nonspecifically mitogenic for lymphocytes. Thus the marked lymphocytic infiltration seen in response to mycoplasmal infections of the respiratory tract does not appear to be due only to a response to an antigenic stimulus. The extensive lesions seen in some strains postexposure to *M. pulmonis* may be due to an exaggerated and misdirected cellular immune response. The organism usually persists in infected rats, even in the presence of relatively high antibody titers.

PATHOLOGY. Clinical signs can include minimal to florid respiratory distress, sniffling, torticollis, and infertility. In severely affected animals, dyspnea, ruffled hair coat, and weight loss may occur. Porphyrin-containing dark red encrustations may be present around the eyes and external nares. At necropsy, serous to catarrhal exudate may be present in the nasal passages, trachea, and major airways. In animals with profuse viscid exudate in the airways, there may be patchy vesicular to bullous emphysema in the lungs. Early pulmonary lesions are usually manifested as pinpoint gray lesions. As peripheral bronchiectasis and bronchioectasis become apparent, varying sized foci are present with clear mucous- or pus-filled lumina. Affected lobes and areas are usually anteroventral in distribution, unilateral or bilateral, often asymmetric in severity, and dark plum-colored to light tan (Fig. 2.19). In advanced cases, there are scattered areas of abscessation involving

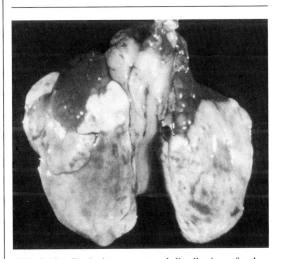

FIG. 2.19—Typical anteroventral distribution of pulmonary lesions in chronic respiratory disease in laboratory rat that was associated with *Mycoplasma pulmonis* infection.

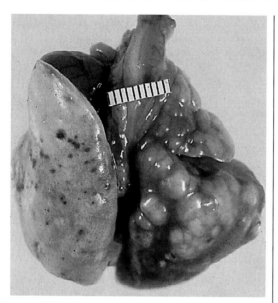

FIG. 2.20—Advanced case of chronic respiratory disease due to *Mycoplasma pulmonis* (MRM). There are multiple abscesses associated with bronchiectatic airways in the right lung.

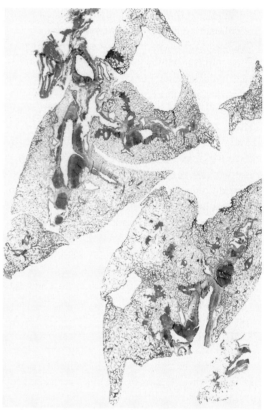

FIG. 2.21—Peribronchial cuffing with lymphocytes and plasma cells, a characteristic histological finding associated with *Mycoplasma pulmonis* infection in laboratory rats.

one or both lungs (Fig. 2.20). One or both tympanic bullae may contain serous to inspissated purulent material, with thickening of the tympanic membrane. The uterine horns, ovarian bursae, and oviducts may contain purulent exudate. However, frequently there is no macroscopic evidence of abnormalities in mycoplasmal perioophoritis or endometritis.

Microscopic changes in the affected tympanic bullae, turbinates, and major airways are characterized by a leukocytic infiltrate in the submucosa consisting of neutrophils, lymphocytes, and plasma cells. Epithelial cells in affected areas are often cuboidal to squamous, and hyperplasia of goblet cells frequently occurs. Leukocytes, mucus, and cell debris are frequently present on the surface in affected areas. Peribronchial and perivascular infiltration with lymphocytes and plasma cells is a prominent feature at all stages of the disease, including the early stages (Fig. 2.21). Chronic bronchitis and bronchiolitis frequently progress to bronchiectasis and bronchiolectasis, which is characterized by dilation of airways and peribronchiolar cuffing with lymphocytes, with variable degrees of hyperplasia and metaplasia of respiratory epithelium (Fig. 2.22). Collections of

mucus, leukocytes, and cellular debris are present in the lumen (Fig. 2.23). There may be rupture of the bronchiolar walls, with release of inflammatory cells, mucus, and debris into the adjacent parenchyma. Frequently the alveolar changes are focal to segmental in distribution. Macrophages, neutrophils, and mucus may be present in alveolar spaces, with lymphocytic infiltration in the alveolar septa. There may be variable degrees of alveolar emphysema, with focal to patchy rupture of alveolar septa. In advanced cases of MRM, the architecture may be completely obliterated by the chronic suppurative process.

Genital tract lesions, when present, consist of perioophoritis and endometritis, with mononuclear and polymorphonuclear cell infiltration in the stratum compactum and endometrium. In some cases, the lumen may be packed with leukocytes (Fig. 2.24).

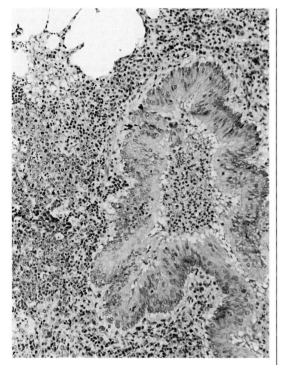

FIG. 2.22—Pulmonary lesions associated with a more advanced case of mycoplasmosis. There is an area of consolidation with hyperplasia of bronchial epithelial cells and leukocytic infiltration into the airway and adjacent parenchyma.

DIAGNOSIS. The typical lesions demonstrated grossly and histologically are sufficient to establish a provisional diagnosis. Using media appropriate for the cultivation of *Mycoplasma* such as the SP-4 formula, the organism can usually be recovered from affected sites such as the upper and lower respiratory tract and uterus. Nasopharyngeal washes, using *Mycoplasma* broth, are frequently used to collect viable organisms. However, cultures may fail to detect the organism in 25–30% of infected animals. The ELISA is the serological test of choice. However, animals may be falsely seropositive due to exposure to *M. arthritidis*. In addition, rats naturally exposed to *M. pulmonis* may be seronegative for up to 4 mo postexposure. Thus there are limitations to relying solely on serology to confirm the diagnosis. The collection of tissues and sera from retired breeders is recommended as a useful means of screening for mycoplasmal infections. Serological testing for antibodies against respiratory viruses such as Sendai and rat coronavirus are recommended, particularly when lower respiratory disease is severe. Both of these agents have been shown to have an additive effect on the progression of respiratory disease associated with

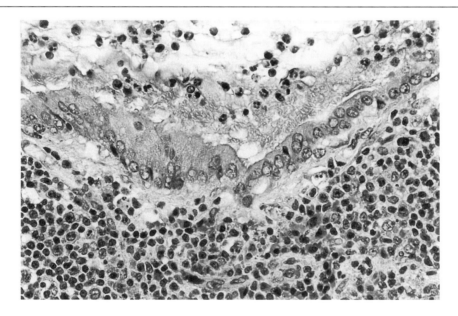

FIG. 2.23—Chronic bronchitis associated with MRM. Note the flattening of respiratory epithelium and loss of cilia in one region, the inflammatory cells on the surface, and the peribronchiolar cuffing with lymphocytes and plasma cells.

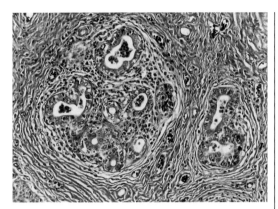

FIG. 2.24—Chronic endometritis associated with *Mycoplasma pulmonis* infection. Leukocytes and cellular debris are present within endometrial glands.

M. pulmonis infection in laboratory rats. Cultures for conventional bacteria are critical, since there are frequently concurrent infections with opportunistic bacteria, such as *Pasteurella,* diplococci, or *Bordetella bronchiseptica.* Co-infection with CAR bacillus can be detected with silver stains of respiratory mucosa or serologically. Infection should be considered chronic, with no merit in antibiotic treatment other than palliating clinical signs. *Differential diagnoses* include pulmonary abscessation due to *Corynebacterium kutscheri* infection, chronic respiratory infections due to the CAR bacillus, otitis media due to conventional bacteria, and suppurative metritis due to *Pasteurella pneumotropica* infection.

SIGNIFICANCE. MRM represents a disease of major importance in the rat, whether kept as pet or in the research laboratory. The disease may seriously compromise the usefulness of affected animals in research, particularly animals used in chronic studies. *M. pulmonis* infections may reduce the normal life span and impair normal respiratory tract function. They are an important cause of infertility in the laboratory rat. Subclinical infections with *M. pulmonis* have been shown to impair other functions, including the humoral immune response. MRM may affect other parameters, including pulmonary carcinogenesis studies. The organism is an important potential contaminant in cell culture and a potential complication for in vitro immunological assays.

***Pasteurella pneumotropica* Infection.** *P. pneumotropica* is a very common, commensal gram-negative coccobacillus that can be an opportunistic pathogen.

EPIZOOTIOLOGY AND PATHOGENESIS. *P. pneumotropica* readily colonizes the intestine, where it may be carried for long periods of time. The organism may be carried in the nasopharynx, conjunctiva, lower respiratory tract, and uterus as an inapparent infection. Transmission probably occurs primarily by direct contact or fecal contamination, rather than by aerosols. The organism is frequently isolated in the absence of disease, and intranasal inoculation has failed to produce lesions in the upper or lower respiratory tract. On the other hand, it may represent an important secondary bacterial invader and opportunistic infection in primary *Mycoplasma pulmonis* or Sendai virus infections. Interstitial pneumonitis and polymorphonuclear cell infiltration has been observed in pregnant rats with primary Sendai virus and secondary *P. pneumotropica* infection. Fetal death and resorption occurred in approximately 30% of fetuses in infected animals. Abundant growth of *P. pneumotropica* was recovered from the lungs of affected dams. An outbreak of chronic necrotizing mastitis in Fischer 344 rats was attributed to the organism.

PATHOLOGY. Lesions associated with pasteurellosis include rhinitis, sinusitis, conjunctivitis, otitis media, suppurative bronchopneumonia, subcutaneous abscessation, suppurative or chronic necrotizing mastitis, and pyometra. On the other hand, the organism may be recovered from various tissues in the absence of lesions.

DIAGNOSIS. Recovery of the organism from lesions in pure culture is an important step in confirming the diagnosis. It has bipolar staining properties and grows on conventional media under aerobic conditions. *Differential diagnosis* includes abscessation due to other pyogenic organisms such as staphylococci, *Corynebacterium,* or *Pseudomonas.*

SIGNIFICANCE. *P. pneumotropica* represents a potential opportunistic infection in the laboratory rat, frequently in association with a recognized primary pathogen such as *M. pulmonis.*

GRAM-POSITIVE BACTERIAL INFECTIONS

Corynebacterium kutscheri **Infection: Pseudotuberculosis; Corynebacteriosis.** *C. kutscheri* is a gram-positive bacillus that can infect mice, rats, and guinea pigs.

EPIZOOTIOLOGY AND PATHOGENESIS. The organism is frequently harbored as an inapparent infection in the absence of concurrent disease, usually in the oropharyngeal, cervical, and submaxillary lymph nodes. Disease and mortality are usually associated with concomitant disease states, such as immunosuppression or nutritional deficiencies. Infections with viral pathogens such as rat coronavirus, Sendai, or rat virus have been shown not to alter the course of the disease experimentally. The organism may be carried for several weeks in the oral cavity and adjacent lymph nodes in the absence of inflammatory lesions. In clinical cases, hematogenous spread probably occurs from these sites, with resultant dissemination to the thoracic and abdominal viscera. Visceral abscesses will eventually heal by scarring and become culture-negative. Clinically, all age groups may be infected.

PATHOLOGY. Weight loss, respiratory distress, and ruffled hair coat are typical clinical signs. At necropsy, dark red encrustations may be present around the eyes and external nares, or there may be a mucopurulent exudate around the nose. In the lung, there frequently are raised pale foci of suppuration of variable size (10 mm to up to 2 cm) with a characteristic hyperemic peripheral zone (Fig. 2.25). Affected areas frequently coalesce with adjacent lesions. Raised foci may be present in other organs, particularly the kidney and liver in the rat (Fig. 2.26). Fibrinous exudate may be present on the pleura and/or pericardial sac.

HISTOPATHOLOGY. Lesions most frequently occur in the lung. There are foci of coagulation to caseation necrosis, with leukocytic infiltration. Neutrophils are the predominant cellular infiltrates in the early stages. Subsequently, there are mononuclear cells composed of macrophages, lymphocytes, and plasma cells (Fig. 2.27).

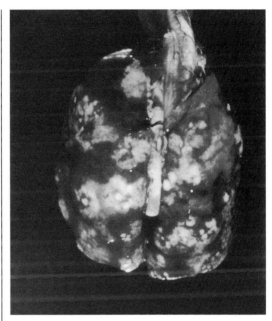

FIG. 2.25—Spontaneous case of *Corynebacterium kutscheri* infection in adult rat. Note the multiple foci of abscessation with peripheral hemorrhage and consolidation in the lung.

Lesions are usually not associated with airways and are interpreted to be hematogenous in origin. There is a concomitant interstitial pneumonitis, with hypercellularity of alveolar septa, perivascular cuffing, and pulmonary edema. Some airways adjacent to affected areas may contain purulent exudate. Focal lesions, when present in parenchymatous organs, are suppurative in nature, with peripheral mononuclear cell infiltration and fibrosis in lesions interpreted to be of several days duration. Bacterial colonies are pathognomonic and appear as amorphous basophilic material in H & E–stained tissue sections and are best demonstrated by tissue Gram stains, or Warthin-Starry or Giemsa stains. The diphtheroid appearance of the bacilli is readily apparent with these stains, with "Chinese letter" configurations (Fig. 2.28). Lymphoid hyperplasia is a frequent finding in chronic cases of corynebacteriosis, and residual scars may be present in target tissues in recovered animals.

DIAGNOSIS. The distribution and nature of the lesions require confirmation by bacterial culture of affected organs or oropharyngeal washings. At

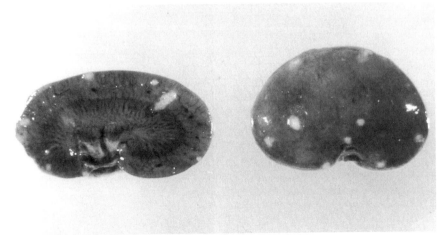

FIG. 2.26—Multifocal suppurative renal lesions due to *Corynebacterium kutscheri* infection. (From McEwen and Percy 1985)

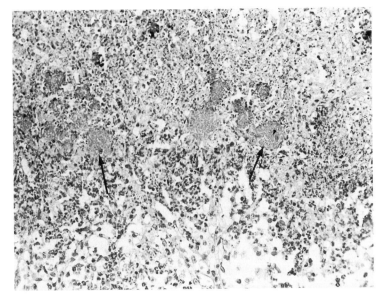

FIG. 2.27—Histological section of lung in case of pseudotuberculosis due to *Corynebacterium kutscheri*. Focal caseating lesion (*arrows*), with infiltrating macrophages, neutrophils, and lymphoid cells.

necropsy, Gram-stained impression smears of abscesses are the best means of demonstrating the typical bacilli and making a provisional diagnosis of corynebacteriosis. Detection of carrier animals is best accomplished by culture of oropharyngeal washes or cervical lymph nodes. An ELISA test is available for detecting seropositive rats. *Differen-tial diagnoses* include pulmonary abscessation associated with advanced cases of chronic respiratory disease, acute to chronic pseudomoniasis, and diplococcal infections.

SIGNIFICANCE. *C. kutscheri* infections represent a potential complicating factor in research. Inap-

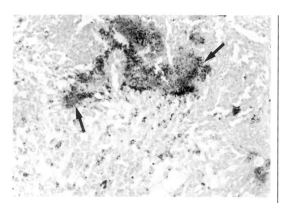

FIG. 2.28—Lung from animal in FIGure 2.27 (Brown and Brenn stain), illustrating the "Chinese letter" arrangement of gram-positive bacilli (*arrows*).

parent carriers may be difficult to detect, although the ELISA test is a useful noninvasive procedure used to identify seropositive carrier animals.

Staphylococcal Infection: Ulcerative Dermatitis. Ulcerative skin lesions have been observed in Sprague-Dawley and other strains of rats ranging in age from 5 wk to 2 yr old. A relatively small percentage of animals are usually affected.

EPIZOOTIOLOGY AND PATHOGENESIS. The incidence of ulcerative dermatitis may vary from 1–2% to over 20% in certain populations of rats. Lesions are most common in males. Coagulase-positive *Staphylococcus aureus* has been isolated both from lesions and the skin of clinically normal animals. *S. aureus* has also been isolated from the feces and oropharynx of some affected animals. Toenail clipping or amputation of the toes of the hind feet has resulted in remission of skin lesions, emphasizing the role of self-trauma in the development of the disease. Subcutaneous inoculation of *S. aureus* resulted in lesions in 25–40% of inoculated rats, usually at a site other than the inoculation site. Trauma with persistent irritation appears to be an important contributing factor. The possibility of the introduction of staphylococci by human carriers has been proposed.

PATHOLOGY. Irregular, circumscribed red ulcerative skin lesions occur over the shoulder and rib cage, submandibular regions, neck, ears, and head, with hair loss in the area (Fig. 2.29). In acute cases, microscopic examination of lesions

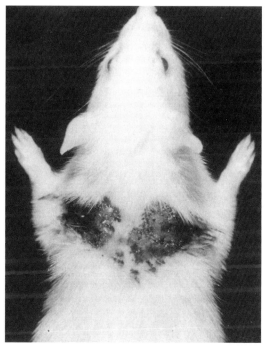

FIG. 2.29—Ulcerative dermatitis in Sprague-Dawley rat, with localization to the dorsal neck and interscapular regions.

reveals an ulcerative dermatitis, with extension into the underlying dermis. In adjacent areas, there is hyperplasia of the epidermis, with leukocytic infiltration into the underlying dermis, neutrophils predominating (Fig. 2.30). Large colonies of gram-positive coccoid bacteria may be present within the proteinaceous material on

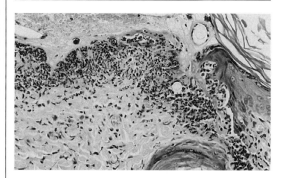

FIG. 2.30—Histological section from rat with ulcerative dermatitis. There is a sharply demarcated area of epidermal coagulation necrosis with underlying leukocytic infiltration. Discrete colonies of darkly staining coccoid bacteria are present on the necrotic epidermis. (Courtesy Tom Forest)

the surface of lesions. There may be variable degeneration and leukocytic infiltration of the adnexae in affected areas. In lesions of some duration, dermal sclerosis and mononuclear cell infiltration are prominent features. Healed lesions frequently have dense collagenous tissue in the dermis, with loss of hair follicles and other adnexae. The lesions are similar to those found in mice associated with this agent. Histopathology suggests a role of epidermolytic toxin, as early stages are reminiscent of burn lesions.

DIAGNOSIS. The presence of the typical ulcerative lesion is a useful diagnostic criterion. Bacterial cultures frequently are positive for coagulase-positive *S. aureus*. *Differential diagnoses* include mycotic infections, fighting injuries, and rarely skin lesions associated with epitheliotropic lymphoid tumors (mycosis fungoides).

Streptococcal Infection: Pneumococcal Infection; Diplococcal Infection. *Streptococcus pneumoniae* has been referred to by a variety of names, including "diplococcus" and "pneumococcus."

EPIZOOTIOLOGY AND PATHOGENESIS. In the past, diplococcal infections were recognized to be a common problem in laboratory rats. In 1969, most conventional commercial sources surveyed had carrier animals, particularly in adolescent rats. Today, outbreaks of clinical disease are rarely recognized in well-managed, barrier-maintained facilities. The organism is carried primarily in the nasoturbinates and tympanic bullae in clinically normal rats. Some of the serotypes isolated from rats are identical to those isolated from human cases, and human carriers have been implicated as a possible source of the organism. *S. pneumoniae* may cause acute primary disease with mortality, but frequently it represents an important secondary invader, particularly in respiratory infections. The abundant polysaccharide capsule is an essential component for bacterial serotyping and also enables the organism to resist phagocytosis by the host cells. Pneumococci are not known to produce soluble toxins. However, several of the recognized serotypes produce tissue damage by activation of the alternate comple-

ment pathway. Clinical signs can include serosanguinous nasal discharge, rhinitis, sinusitis, conjunctivitis, and vestibular signs consistent with middle ear infection. In asymptomatic animals infected with the organism, predisposing factors such as concurrent infections or environmental changes may precipitate an outbreak of the disease.

PATHOLOGY. At necropsy, there may be serous to mucopurulent exudate present in the nasal passages, with variable involvement of the tympanic bullae. In the acute systemic form of the disease, there are variable patterns of characteristic fibrinopurulent polyserositis, including pleuritis, peritonitis, pericarditis, periorchitis, and meningitis (Fig. 2.31). Fibrinopurulent lesions may be confined to the leptomeninges in some fatal cases of streptococcosis. There may be consolidation of one or more lobes of the

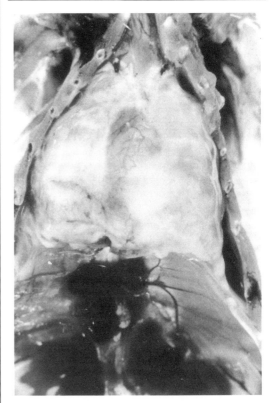

FIG. 2.31—Young rat that succumbed to spontaneous diplococcal (*Streptococcus pneumoniae*) infection. There is an extensive fibrinous pericarditis and pleuritis.

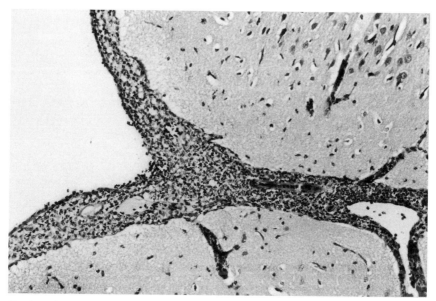

FIG. 2.32—Section of cerebrum of spontaneous diplococcal meningitis. Note the marked polymorphonuclear leukocytic infiltration in the leptomeninges.

lung. Affected areas are dark red to dull tan and relatively firm and nonresilient.

On microscopic examination, in the acute form of the disease fibrinopurulent pleuritis and pericarditis are typical findings. Pulmonary changes vary from localized suppurative bronchopneumonia to acute fibrinopurulent bronchopneumonia, with obliteration of the normal architecture in affected lobes. Fibrinopurulent peritonitis, perihepatitis, and/or leptomeningitis (Fig. 2.32) are frequent findings. Suppurative rhinitis and otitis media may also occur. Embolic suppurative lesions have been observed in organs such as liver, spleen, and kidney. In more chronic, localized disease states, pneumococcal infections have been associated with conditions such as suppurative bronchopneumonia in chronic respiratory disease, as well as otitis media.

DIAGNOSIS. The demonstration of the typical encapsulated diplococci in Gram-stained smears from typical lesions will provide a provisional diagnosis (Fig. 2.33). Confirmation of streptococcosis requires the collection and culture of material from lesions and identification of the organism. The organism grows best aerobically on 5% blood agar in the presence of 10% CO_2 and produces alpha hemolysis. Nasal lavage at necropsy is another recommended procedure to recover the

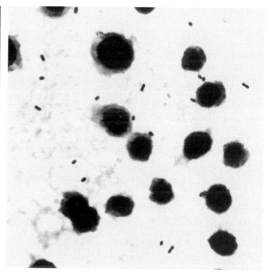

FIG. 2.33—Impression smear from pleura of rat with diplococcal pleuritis (Gram stain). Numerous encapsulated diplococci and mesothelial cells are evident.

organism for bacterial culture. *Differential diagnoses* include corynebacteriosis, salmonellosis, pseudomoniasis, and pasteurellosis.

SIGNIFICANCE. *S. pneumoniae* can be an important cause of disease and mortality, particularly in young rats. Infected animals may harbor the organism in the upper respiratory tract as an inapparent infection. Under the appropriate circumstances, these diplococci may become activated to produce a localized infection or an acute systemic disease, sometimes with significant mortality. *S. pneumoniae* should be considered a potential zoonotic hazard.

Streptococcal (Enterococcal) Infection: Enteropathy in Infant Rats. Epizootics of enteric disease due to enterococcal infections, with high morbidity and mortality, have been observed in suckling rats. The causative agent, which had been identified as a streptococcus, has now been identified as *Enterococcus faecium-durans-2*. The disease was reproduced in suckling rats inoculated with pure cultures of the streptococcus. A similar disease and agent have been seen in other outbreaks in outbred albino rats. Other strains, including *Enterococcus hirae*, have been associated with diarrhea with low mortality in neonatal rats.

PATHOLOGY. Animals are stunted, with distended abdomens and fecal soiling in the perineal region. The stomachs are usually distended with milk, and there is dilation of the small intestine. On microscopic examination, large numbers of gram-positive cocci may be present on the surfaces of histologically normal villi of the small intestine, with minimal or no inflammatory response (Figs. 2.34 and 2.35).

OTHER BACTERIAL INFECTIONS

***Erysipelas* Infection.** Spontaneous *Erysipelas* infections were observed in one outbreak that occurred in laboratory rats in Scandinavia. Lesions included chronic fibrinopurulent polyarthritis, myocarditis, and endocarditis. *Erysipelas rhusiopathiae* was isolated from affected joints.

***Hemobartonella* Infection.** *Hemobartonella muris* infects wild rats and at one time was common in laboratory rats. The organism, an extracellular parasite of erythrocytes, cannot be cultured in vitro. It is transmitted primarily by *Polyplax spinulosa*, which is no longer found in laboratory rats. It can also be transmitted in utero,

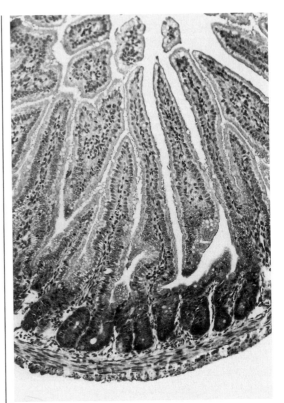

FIG. 2.34—Section of small intestine from case of spontaneous streptococcal enteropathy in suckling rat. The morphology of the villi and enterocytes are essentially normal. Coccoid organisms are adherent to the mucosa. (Courtesy D.M. Hoover)

but apparently inefficiently, since cesarean section is usually successful at eliminating the organism. It can also contaminate biological products derived from infected rodents and is infectious in both rats and mice. Natural infections are invariably inapparent, with mild transient parasitemia, splenomegaly, and reticulosis of erythrocytes. The reticuloendothelial system, especially the spleen, is critical for clearing the parasitemia. Splenectomy of carrier rats may result in hemolytic anemia with hemoglobinuria and death. Splenectomy has been used as a means of diagnosis in suspect populations of rats. Immunosuppression with corticosteroids is ineffective in activating a subclinical infection.

***Klebsiella pneumonia* Infection.** *K. pneumonia* is probably an opportunistic pathogen in the rat, since it can be isolated from feces of normal ani-

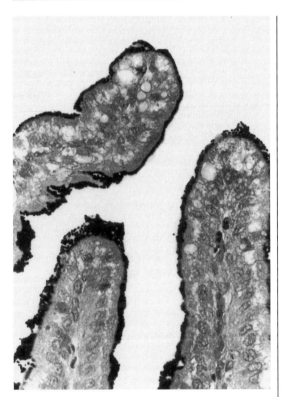

FIG. 2.35—Area in Figure 2.34 (Brown and Brenn stain). Note the aggregations of cocci on the surface of the villi. (Courtesy D. M. Hoover)

mals. However, this organism has been associated with abscesses of cervical, inguinal, and mesenteric lymph nodes and of kidney. This organism has also been associated with mild suppurative rhinitis in otherwise pathogen-free rats.

Leptospira **Infection.** (See the discussion of leptospirosis in Chap. 1.). As in the mouse, leptospirae cause subclinical infection with minimal or no lesions. The most common leptospira in rats is *L. icterohemorrhagiae,* but other species can also infect rats. Human infection is often associated with exposure to infected rats.

Pseudomonas aeruginosa **Infection: Pseudomoniasis.** *P. aeruginosa* is a gram-negative bacillus that is common in the environment, particularly water conduits.

EPIZOOTIOLOGY AND PATHOGENESIS. The organism grows well at room temperature and may be present on a variety of nonsterile fomites, includ-

ing food, bedding, water bottles, bottle stoppers, and sipper tubes. *Pseudomonas* has also been recovered from human carriers, including feces. Ungloved hands are considered to be one source of the organism in animal facilities. The organism transiently localizes in the oropharynx, upper respiratory tract, and large intestine, but maintenance of infection requires continuous exposure, and that exposure is most expeditiously maintained through sipper tubes. Following exposure to *P. aeruginosa,* the incidence of inapparent healthy carriers is usually around 5–20%. However, the incidence of infected animals may approach 100% in lethally irradiated mice and rats. Antibiotic treatment frequently facilitates the colonization of *Pseudomonas,* presumably by reducing the inhibitory effect of normal microflora. Important predisposing factors include any procedure that will result in neutropenia, including irradiation and treatment with steroids or other immunosuppressants. In addition, surgical procedures such as the implantation of indwelling jugular catheters may result in acute to chronic pseudomoniasis. Clinical signs include dyspnea, depression, facial edema, weight loss in animals surviving for more than 24 hr, and high mortality.

PATHOLOGY. In acute cases there may be pulmonary edema, splenomegaly, and visceral ecchymoses consistent with a gram-negative bacterial septicemia. In rats that succumb during the subacute to chronic stages of the disease, multifocal necrosis with abscessation may be present in organs such as lung, spleen, and kidney. In animals with indwelling jugular catheters, vegetative lesions may be present on the tricuspid valves. On microscopic examination, lesions in acute cases are those of an acute bacterial septicemia, with vasculitis, thrombosis, hemorrhage, and polymorphonuclear cell infiltration. In affected foci, changes vary from acute coagulation necrosis to suppuration, with obliteration of the normal architecture. Lesions are usually most extensive in the lung. In addition to thromboembolic changes with hemorrhage, bacterial colonies and proteinaceous fluid are frequently present in alveoli (Fig. 2.36). Necrotizing lesions may also be present in viscera such as spleen and kidney. In subacute to chronic cases of pseudomoniasis,

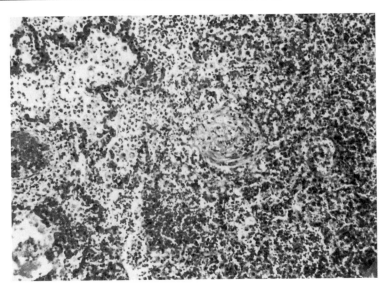

FIG. 2.36—Section of lung from a case of pseudomoniasis. There is a necrotizing pneumonia, with hemorrhage, edema, and leukocytic infiltration.

multiple suppurative lesions with abscessation may be present in tissues, such as lung, kidney, spleen, and lymph nodes. Vegetative endocarditis with septic embolization may be present, particularly in animals with indwelling venous catheters.

DIAGNOSIS. The history of procedures such as those that induce neutropenia or certain surgical manipulations, coupled with typical gross and microscopic changes, should be sufficient to provide a provisional diagnosis. Gram-negative bacilli are usually identifiable in sections stained with tissue Gram stains such as Brown and Brenn. The organism can usually be recovered from heart blood or spleen in septicemic animals. In subacute to chronic cases, *P. aeruginosa* may be isolated from visceral lesions. Blood agar plates and selective media such as Koser's citrate medium are recommended. *Differential diagnoses* include visceral abscessation due to *Corynebacterium kutscheri* or *Pasteurella pneumotropica* infections, salmonellosis, and pulmonary abscessation due to murine respiratory mycoplasmosis.

SIGNIFICANCE. Pseudomoniasis is an important cause of disease and mortality in rats and mice subjected to procedures resulting in leukopenia. Detection of carriers by culturing sipper tubes, improved sanitation, and chlorination or acidification of the drinking water are recommended procedures.

Streptobacillus moniliformis **Infection: Rat Bite Fever.** This bacterium is a commensal organism that inhabits the nasopharynx of rats. Contemporary colonies are usually devoid of this organism, but it is common in wild rats and in some populations of laboratory rats. It can be associated with opportunistic respiratory infections and can cause wound infections and abscesses. It has been found in bronchiolectatic abscesses of rats with chronic respiratory disease, in concert with mycoplasma and CAR bacillus. Of particular concern is its pathogenicity in humans and mice. In humans, it is the cause of rat bite fever. A similar syndrome, called Haverill fever, has been associated with ingestion of rat-contaminated foodstuffs, particularly milk. The bacterium is a gram-negative, pleomorphic rod or filamentous organism that requires blood, serum, or ascites fluid for culture in agar or broth. Another commensal bacterium, *Spirillum muris*, has also been associated with rat bite fever.

Suppurative Pyelonephritis/Nephritis. Suppurative renal lesions are more commonly encountered in male rats and may be associated with a concurrent disease process, such as cystitis or prostatitis. A variety of bacteria have been recovered from affected kidneys, including *Escherichia coli, Klebsiella, Pseudomonas,* and *Proteus* spp. The lower urinary tract is considered to be the most likely portal of entry, particularly in pyelonephritis. However, descending infections may also occur. Lesions are similar to those seen in other species with suppurative disease processes of this system.

BIBLIOGRAPHY
FOR BACTERIAL INFECTIONS

Gram-Negative Enteric Bacterial Infections

Campylobacter/Lawsonia Infections
Vanenberghe, J., et al. 1985. Spontaneous adenocarcinoma of the ascending colon in Wistar rats: The intracytoplasmic presence of a *Campylobacter*-like bacterium. J. Comp. Pathol. 95:45–55.

Clostridium piliforme Infection
Fleischman, R.W., et al. 1977. Adynamic ileus in the rat induced by chloral hydrate. Lab. Anim. Sci. 27:238–43.

Fries, A.S. 1979. Studies on Tyzzer's disease: Transplacental transmission of *Bacillus piliformis* in rats. Lab. Anim. 13:43–46.

Fries, A.S., and Svendsen, O. 1978. Studies on Tyzzer's disease in rats. Lab. Anim. 12:1–4.

Fujiwara, K., et al. 1981. Serologic detection of inapparent Tyzzer's disease in rats. Jap. J. Exp. Med. 51:197–200.

Hansen, A.K., et al. 1992. Rederivation of rat colonies seropositive for *Bacillus piliformis* and subsequent screening for antibodies. Lab. Anim. Sci. 42:444–48.

Jonas, A.M., et al. 1970. Tyzzer's disease in the rat: Its possible relationship with megaloileitis. Arch. Pathol. 90:516–28.

Motzel, S.L., and Riley, L.K. 1992. Subclinical infection and transmission of Tyzzer's disease in rats. Lab. Anim. Sci. 42:439–43.

Riley, L.K., et al. 1990. Protein and antigenic heterogeneity among isolates of *Bacillus piliformis.* Infect. Immun. 58:1010–16.

Smith, K.J., et al. 1996. *Bacillus piliformis* infection (Tyzzer's disease) in a patient infected with HIV-1: Confirmation with 16S ribosomal RNA sequence analysis. J. Am. Acad. Dermatol. 34:342–48.

Tyzzer, E.E. 1917. A fatal disease of the Japanese waltzing mouse caused by a spore-bearing bacillus (*Bacillus piliformis* n.sp.). J. Med. Res. 37:307–8.

Helicobacter Infection
Haines, D.C., et al. 1998. Inflammatory large bowel disease in immunodeficient rats naturally and experimentally infected with *Helicobacter bilis.* Vet. Pathol. 35:202–8.

Mendes, E.N., et al. *Helicobacter trogontum* sp. nov. isolated from the rat intestine. Int. J. Syst. Bact. 46: 916–21.

Moura, S.B., et al. 1999. Microbiological and histological study of gastrointestinal tract of germ-free mice infected with *Helicobacter trogontum.* Res. Microbiol. 150:205–12.

Salmonella Infection
Pappenheimer, A.M., and Von Wedel, H. 1914. Observations on a spontaneous typhoid-like epidemic of white rats. J. Infect. Dis. 14:180–15.

Weisbroth, S.H. 1979. Bacterial and mycotic diseases. In *The Laboratory Rat. I. Biology and Diseases,* ed. H.J. Baker et al., pp. 193–241. New York: Academic.

Gram-Negative Bacterial Infections of the Respiratory Tract

Bordetella bronchiseptica Infection
Bemis, D.A., and Wilson, S.A. 1985. Influence of potential virulence determinants on *Bordetella bronchiseptica*–induced ciliostasis. Infect. Immunol. 50:35–42.

Burek, J.D., et al. 1972. The pathology and pathogenesis of *Bordetella bronchiseptica* and *Pasteurella pneumotropica* infection in conventional and germ-free rats. Lab. Anim. Sci. 22:844–49.

Cilia-associated Respiratory (CAR) Bacillus Infection
Ganaway, J.R., et al. 1985. Isolation, propagation, and characterization of a newly recognized pathogen, cilia-associated respiratory bacillus of rats, an etiological agent of chronic respiratory disease. Infect. Immun. 47:472–79.

Hastie, A.T. et al. 1993. Two types of bacteria adherent to bovine respiratory epithelium. Vet. Pathol. 30:12–19.

Hook, R.R., et al. 1998. Antigenic analyses of cilia-associated respiratory (CAR) bacillus isolates by use of monoclonal antibodies. Lab. Anim. Sci. 48:234–239.

MacKenzie, W.F., et al. 1981. A filamentous bacterium associated with respiratory disease in wild rats. Vet. Pathol. 18:836–39.

Matsushita, S. 1986. Spontaneous respiratory disease associated with cilia-associated respiratory (CAR) bacillus in a rat. Jap. J. Vet. Sci. 48:437–40.

Matsushita, S., and Joshima, H. 1989. Pathology of rats intranasally inoculated with cilia-associated respiratory bacillus. Lab. Anim. 23:89–95.

Medina, L.V., et al. 1996. Rapid way to identify the cilia-associated respiratory bacillus: Tracheal mucosal scraping with a modified microwave Steiner silver impregnation. Lab. Anim. Sci. 46:113–15.

Medina, L.V., et al. 1994. Respiratory disease in a rat colony: Identification of CAR bacillus without other respiratory pathogens by standard diagnostic screening methods. Lab. Anim. Sci. 44:521–25.

Nietfeld, J.C., et al. 1999. Isolation of cilia-associated respiratory (CAR) bacillus from pigs and calves and experimental infection of gnotobiotic pigs and rodents. J. Vet. Diagn. Invest. 11:252–58.

Schoeb, T.R., et al. 1993. Cultivation of cilia-associated respiratory bacillus in artificial medium and determination of the 16S rRNA gene sequence. J. Clin. Microbiol. 31:2751–57.

Van Zwieten, M.J., et al. 1980. Respiratory disease in rats associated with a filamentous bacterium: A preliminary report. Lab. Anim. Sci. 30:215–21.

Haemophilus Infection

Nicklas, W. 1989. Haemophilus infection in a colony of laboratory rats. J. Clin. Microbiol. 27:1636–39.

Mycoplasmal Infection

Aguila, H.N., et al. 1988. Experimental *Mycoplasma pulmonis* infection of rats suppresses humoral but not cellular immune response. Lab. Anim. Sci. 38:138–42.

Brennan, P.C., et al. 1969. The role of *Pasteurella pneumotropica* and *Mycoplasma pulmonis* in murine pneumonia. J. Bacteriol. 97:337–49.

Brunnert, S.R., et al. 1993. Detection of *Mycoplasma pulmonis* in paraffin-embedded tissue by PCR. Lab. Anim. Sci. 43:388.

Broderson, J.R., et al. 1976. Role of environmental ammonia in respiratory mycoplasmosis of the rat. Am. J. Pathol. 85:115–30.

Cassell, G.H. 1982. The pathogenic potential of mycoplasmas: *Mycoplasma pulmonis* as a model. Rev. Infect. Dis. 4:S18–S34.

Cassell, G.H., et al. 1986. Mycoplasmal infections: Disease pathogenesis, implications for biomedical research, and control. In *Viral and Mycoplasmal Infections of Laboratory Rodents: Effects on Biomedical Research,* ed. P.N. Bhatt et al., pp. 87–130. New York: Academic.

Davidson, M.K., et al. 1981. Comparison for methods of detection of *Mycoplasma pulmonis* in experimentally and naturally infected rats. J. Clin. Microbiol. 14:646–55.

Davis, J.K., and Cassell, G.H. 1982. Murine respiratory mycoplasmosis in LEW and F344 rats: Strain differences in lesion severity. Vet. Pathol. 19:280–93.

Lindsey, J.R. 1986. Prevalence of viral and mycoplasmal infections in laboratory rodents. In *Viral and Mycoplasmal Infections of Laboratory Rodents: Effects on Biomedical Research,* ed. P.N. Bhatt et al., pp. 801–8. New York: Academic.

Schoeb, T.R., and Lindsey, J.R. 1987. Exacerbation of murine respiratory mycoplasmosis by sialodacryoadenitis virus infection in gnotobiotic F344 rats. Vet. Pathol. 24:392–99.

Schoeb, T.R., et al. 1985. Exacerbation of murine respiratory mycoplasmosis in gnotobiotic F344/N rats by Sendai virus infection. Vet. Pathol. 22:272–82.

Schreiber, H., et al. 1972. Induction of lung cancer in germ-free, specific-pathogen-free, and infected

rats by ᴺ-nitrosoheptamethyleneimine: Enhancement by respiratory infection. J. Natl. Cancer Inst. 49:1107–14.

Steiner, D.A. et al. 1993. In utero transmission of *Mycoplasma pulmonis* in experimentally infected Sprague-Dawley rats. Infect. Immun. 61: 2985–90.

Tully, J.G. 1986. Biology of rodent mycoplasmas. In *Viral and Mycoplasmal Infections of Laboratory Rodents: Effects on Biomedical Research,* ed. P.N. Bhatt et al., pp. 64–85. New York: Academic.

Pasteurella pneumotropica Infection

Brennan, P.C., et al. 1969. The role of *Pasteurella pneumotropica* and *Mycoplasma pulmonis* in murine pneumonia. J. Bacteriol. 97:337–49.

Burek, J.D., et al. 1972. The pathology and pathogenesis of *Bordetella bronchiseptica* and *Pasteurella pneumotropica* infection in conventional and germ-free rats. Lab. Anim. Sci. 22:844–49.

Carthew, P., and Aldred, P. 1988. Embryonic death in pregnant rats owing to intercurrent infection with Sendai virus and *Pasteurella pneumotropica.* Lab. Anim. 22:92–97.

Hong, C.C., and Ediger, R.D. 1978. Chronic necrotizing mastitis in rats caused by *Pasteurella pneumotropica.* Lab. Anim. Sci. 28:317–20.

Moore, T.D., et al. 1973. Latent *Pasteurella pneumotropica* infection in the intestine of gnotobiotic and barrier-held rats. Lab. Anim. Sci. 23:657–61.

Weisbroth, S.H. 1979. Bacterial and mycotic diseases. In *The Laboratory Rat. I. Biology and Diseases,* ed. H.J. Baker et al., pp. 193–241. New York: Academic.

Gram-Positive Bacterial Infections

Corynebacterium kutscheri Infection

Ackerman, J.I., et al. 1984. An enzyme linked immunoabsorbent assay for detection of antibodies to *Corynebacterium kutscheri* in experimentally infected rats. Lab. Anim. Sci. 34:38–43.

Amao, H., et al. 1995. Natural and subclinical *Corynebacterium kutscheri* infection in rats. Lab. Anim. Sci. 45:11–14.

Barthold, S.W., and Brownstein, D.G. 1988. The effect of selected viruses on *Corynebacterium kutscheri* infection in rats. Lab. Anim. Sci. 38:580–83.

Brownstein, D.G., et al. 1985. Experimental *Corynebacterium kutscheri* infection in rats: Bacteriology and serology. Lab. Anim. Sci. 35:135–38.

Fox, J.G., et al. 1987. Comparison of methods to diagnose an epizootic of *Corynebacterium kutscheri* pneumonia in rats. Lab. Anim. Sci. 37:72–75.

Giddens, W.E., et al. 1969. Pneumonia in rats due to infection with *Corynebacterium kutscheri.* Pathol. Vet. 5:227–37.

McEwen, S.A., and Percy, D.H. 1985. Diagnostic exercise: Pneumonia in a rat. Lab. Anim. Sci. 35:485–87.

Weisbroth, S.H. 1979. Bacterial and mycotic diseases. In *The Laboratory Rat. I. Biology and Diseases,* ed. H.J. Baker et al., pp. 193–241. New York: Academic.

Staphylococcal Infection

Ash, G.W. 1971. An epidemic of chronic skin ulceration in rats. Lab. Anim. 5:115–22.

Fox, J.G., et al. 1977. Ulcerative dermatitis in the rat. Lab. Anim. Sci. 27:671–78.

Kunstyr, I., et al. 1995. Granulomatous dermatitis and mastitis in two SPF rats associated with a slowly growing *Staphylococcus aureus*—a case report. Lab. Anim. 29:177–79.

Wagner, J.E., et al. 1977. Self trauma and *Staphylococcus aureus* in ulcerative dermatitis of rats. J. Am. Vet. Med. Assoc. 171:839–41.

Streptococcal Infection

Borkowski, G.L., and Griffith, J.W. 1990. Diagnostic exercise: Pneumonia and pleuritis in a rat. Lab. Anim. Sci. 40:323–25.

Fallon, M.T., et al. 1988. Inapparent *Streptococcus pneumoniae* type 35 infections in commercial rats and mice. Lab. Anim. Sci. 38:129–32.

Kohn, D.F., and Barthold, S.W. 1984. *Laboratory Animal Medicine.* New York: Academic.

Weisbroth, S.H., and Freimer, E.H. 1969. Laboratory rats from commercial breeders as carriers of pathogenic pneumococci. Lab. Anim. Care 19:473–78.

Yoneda, K., and Coonrod, J.D. 1980. Experimental type 25 pneumococcal pneumonia in rats. Am. J. Pathol. 99:231–42.

Streptococcal (*Enterococcus*) Infection

Etheridge, M.E., and Vonderfecht, S.L. 1992. Diarrhea caused by a slow-growing enterococcus-like agent in neonatal rats. Lab. Anim. Sci. 42:548–50.

Etheridge, M.E., et al. 1988. *Enterococcus hirae* implicated as a cause of diarrhea in suckling rats. J. Clin. Microbiol. 26:1741–44.

Hoover, D., et al. 1985. Streptococcal enteropathy in infant rats. Lab. Anim. Sci. 35:653–41.

Other Bacterial Infections

Erysipelas Infection

Feinstein, R.E., and Eld, K. 1989. Naturally occurring erysipelas in rats. Lab. Anim. 23:256–60.

Klebsiella pneumonia Infection

Harwich, J., and Shouman, M.T. 1965. Untersuchen uber gehauft auftretende *Klebsiella*-infectionen bei versuchsratten. Z. Versuch. 6:141–46.

Jackson, N.N., et al. 1980. Naturally acquired infections of *Klebsiella pneumonia* in Wistar rats. Lab. Anim. 14:357–61.

Pseudomonas aeruginosa Infection

Flynn, R.J. 1963. Introduction: *Pseudomonas aeruginosa* infection and its effects on biological and medical research. Lab. Anim. Sci. 13:1–6.

Johansen, H.K., et al. 1993. Chronic *Pseudomonas aeruginosa* infection in normal and athymic rats. APMIS 101:207–25.

Weisbroth, S.H. 1979. Bacterial and mycotic diseases. In *The Laboratory Rat. I. Biology and Diseases,* ed. H.J. Baker et al., pp. 193–241. New York: Academic.

Wyand, D.S., and Jonas, A.M. 1967. *Pseudomonas aeruginosa* infection in rats following implantation of an indwelling jugular catheter. Lab. Anim. Care 17:261–66.

Streptobacillus moniliformis Infection

Anderson, L.C., et al. 1983. Rat-bite fever in animal research laboratory personnel. Lab. Anim. Sci. 33:292–94.

Wullenweber, M. 1994. *Streptobacillus moniliformis*—a zoonotic pathogen. Taxonomic considerations, host species, diagnosis, therapy, geographical distribution. Lab. Anim. 29:1–15

Suppurative Pyelonephritis/Nephritis

Duprat, P., and Burek, J.D. 1986. Suppurative nephritis, pyelonephritis, rat. In *Monographs on Pathology of Laboratory Animals: Urinary System,* ed. T.C. Jones et al., pp. 219–24. New York: Springer-Verlag.

General Bibliography

Boot, R., et al. 1995. Mutual viral and bacterial infections after housing rats of various breeders within an experimental unit. Lab. Anim. 30: 42–45.

Burek, J.D., et al. 1972. The pathology and pathogenesis of *Bordetella bronchiseptica* and *Pasteurella pneumotropica* infection in conventional and germ-free rats. Lab. Anim. Sci. 22:844–49.

Kohn, D.F., and Barthold, S.W. 1984. Biology and diseases of rats. In *Laboratory Animal Medicine,* ed. J.G. Fox et al., pp. 91–122. New York: Academic.

Lindsey, J.R. 1986. Prevalence of viral and mycoplasmal infections in laboratory rodents. In *Viral and Mycoplasmal Infections of Laboratory Rodents: Effects on Biomedical Research,* ed. P.N. Bhatt et al., pp. 801–8. New York: Academic.

Shultz, L.D., and Sidman, C.L. 1987. Genetically determined murine models of immunodeficiency. Ann. Rev. Immunol. 5:367–403.

Weisbroth, S.H. 1979. Bacterial and mycotic diseases. In *The Laboratory Rat. I. Biology and Diseases,* ed. H.J. Baker et al., pp. 193–241. New York: Academic.

PULMONARY LESIONS OF UNKNOWN ETIOLOGY

Eosinophilic Granulomatous Pneumonia in Brown Norway Rats. The Brown Norway rat has been one animal model used to study the pathogenesis of asthma, since they readily

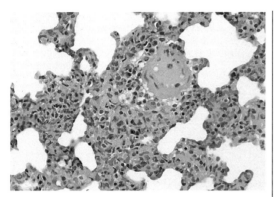

FIG. 2.37—Section of lung from BN rat with spontaneous eosinophilic pneumonitis. Note the marked leukocytic infiltration in interstitium, eosinophils predominating. (Courtesy J. Kwiecien)

develop increased bronchiolar responsiveness and elevated IgE postexposure to allergens. However, animals may develop a spontaneous eosinophil-rich granulomatous pneumonitis in the absence of any experimental procedure. The changes have been attributed to inadvertent exposure to an allergen, but because of the inflammatory nature of the lesions, they could be due to exposure to an unidentified infectious agent (or agents).

The pulmonary lesions are most frequently observed in young female Brown Norway rats under 3 mo of age, although both sexes are susceptible. In affected animals, there is a multifocal to diffuse granulomatous pneumonitis with a cellular infiltrate consisting of epithelioid cells and, in some cases, a prominent multinucleated giant cell component. Frequently there is marked perivascular and peribronchiolar edema with an inflammatory cell infiltrate consisting primarily of eosinophils (Fig. 2.37). The pulmonary perivascular and peribronchiolar edema with infiltrating eosinophils has also been observed on occasion in newly arrived young adult Sprague-Dawley rats. Attempts to demonstrate a parasitic or bacterial agent have been unsuccessful to date. Thus the etiopathogenesis of these changes is yet to be determined.

Other Inflammatory Pulmonary Lesions of Unknown Etiology. Interstitial pneumonitis in the absence of an identifiable infectious agent has been observed in young adult F344 rats involved in toxicity studies. Changes include perivascular lymphocytic infiltration, and alveolitis with infiltration by alveolar macrophages, neutrophils, and lymphocytes, and focal hyperplasia of Type II pneumocytes (Fig. 2.38). Ultrastructural studies revealed sparse numbers of bacilli within alveolar spaces. Mice housed in the same area did not develop these changes. In another report, multifocal granulomatous alveolitis and perivascular lymphocytic infiltration were observed in young Sprague-Dawley rats. An etiologic agent was not identified, although inoculation of cell culture with tissue homogenates produced cytopathic effects. Pathologists in Europe have reported similar findings in young Wistar rats, with no infectious agent identified. Lesions tend to be transient. Microscopically, there are perivascular cellular infiltrates with some involvement of the peribronchiolar regions. The infiltrates consist of mononuclear cells, lymphocytes, and occasionally polymorphonuclear cells. In some cases, similar pulmonary changes have been observed in other rats housed in the same facility, providing evidence that it is a transmissible disease. The search for the causative agent(s) continues.

BIBLIOGRAPHY FOR PULMONARY LESIONS OF UNKNOWN ETIOLOGY

Ellwell, M.R., et al. 1997. Have you seen this? Inflammatory lesions in the lungs of rats. Tox. Pathol. 25:529–31.
Riley, L., et al. 1997. Idiopathic lung lesions in rats: Search for an etiologic agent. Contemp. Top. 36(4):46–47.
Slaoui, M., et al. 1998. Inflammatory lesions in the lungs of Wistar rats. Tox. Pathol. 26:712–13.

MYCOTIC INFECTIONS

***Aspergillus* Infection.** There have been isolated reports of outbreaks of upper respiratory tract infections in laboratory rats due to primary infections with *Aspergillus fumigatus* or *Aspergillus niger.* On microscopic examination, the changes are consistent with a chronic rhinitis with epithelial changes varying from hyperplasia to squamous metaplasia. Fungal hyphae are readily demonstrated on epithelial surfaces of affected nasal passages with PAS or silver stains. Possible predisposing factors include contaminated bed-

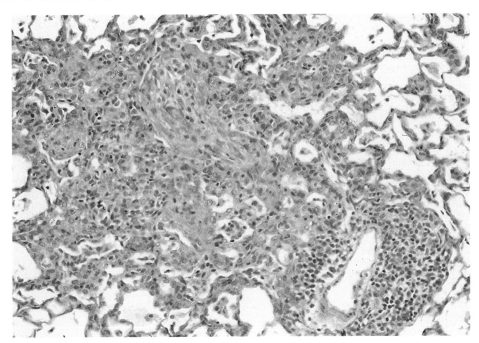

FIG. 2.38—Section of lung from rat with idiopathic pneumonitis. Note the perivascular lymphocytic infiltrates, interstitial pneumonia, and alveolar histiocytosis.

ding, air quality, the presence of concurrent infections, and immune status of the host.

Dermatophyte Infection: Dermatophytosis. Recognized infections with dermatophytes are now relatively rare in laboratory rats, although it appears to occur more frequently in wild rats. The disease is usually caused by *Trichophyton mentagrophytes* in this species. In confirmed outbreaks of the disease, patterns vary from asymptomatic carriers to rats with florid lesions on the skin.

PATHOLOGY. Lesions, when present, are most frequently observed on the neck, back, and at the base of the tail. There is patchy hair loss, and affected areas of skin are usually raised, erythematous, and dry to moist and pustular in appearance. On microscopic examination, hyperkeratosis, epidermal hyperplasia, and leukocytic infiltration in the underlying dermis with folliculitis are typical findings. Arthrospores investing hair shafts may be seen on H & E–stained tissue sections, but the fungi are better demonstrated with PAS or methenamine silver stains (Fig. 2.39).

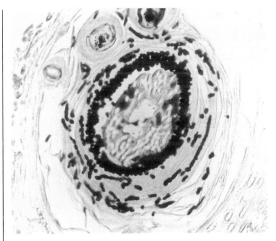

FIG. 2.39—Section of skin from spontaneous case of dermatophytosis (*Trichophyton mentagrophytes*) in laboratory rat (methenamine silver stain). Numerous arthrospores are investing the hair follicle.

DIAGNOSIS. The skin scrapings with wet mount preparations in 10% KOH under a vaseline-ringed coverslip and fungal culture are recommended procedures. Skin biopsies or histological sections collected at necropsy should enable the pathologist to demonstrate the typical arthrospores microscopically.

SIGNIFICANCE. In view of the possibility of interspecies spread, a slaughter policy and thorough disinfection of premises and fomites are recommended. The source of the infection should be investigated, including the possibility that the organism could have been introduced by wild rodents or human contacts.

***Pneumocystis carinii* Infection.** *P. carinii,* an atypical fungus of worldwide distribution, is recognized to be an important cause of disease and mortality in immunocompromised human cases, particularly AIDS patients. Many colonies of conventional rats appear to be naturally infected with *P. carinii,* and there is evidence that laboratory mice and occasionally rabbits may also harbor the fungus. Pneumocystosis has been recognized in other animals, including cats, horses, dogs, and monkeys. Pulmonary lesions associated with pneumocystis infection have been produced in young laboratory rats from infected colonies that are treated for several weeks with immunosuppressants such as cortisone and fed a protein-deficient diet. Steroid-treated female rats may

develop the disease at a faster rate than male rats. Spontaneous pneumocystosis has been recognized in athymic rats. In severely affected animals, clinical signs include weight loss, cyanosis, and dyspnea.

PATHOLOGY. There is diffuse to focal consolidation, and lungs collapse poorly, and frequently, there is an opaque pale pink color. On microscopic examination, there is alveolar flooding with foamy, eosinophilic material, presenting a honeycomb appearance (Fig. 2.40). In athymic rats, pulmonary lesions vary from mild interstitial pneumonitis with scattered alveolar macrophages to severe interstitial pneumonitis with alveoli distended with typical foamy material. In more advanced cases, in addition to the infiltrating inflammatory cells and the foamy alveolar exudate, there is marked proliferation of type II pneumocytes and interstitial fibrosis. In sections stained using procedures such as the Grocott modification of Gomori's methenamine silver technique, numerous black trophozoites and yeastlike cysts 3–5 μm in diameter are present singly or in groups within alveoli. Ultrastructural examination reveals trophozoites with filapodia in close association with type I pneumocytes.

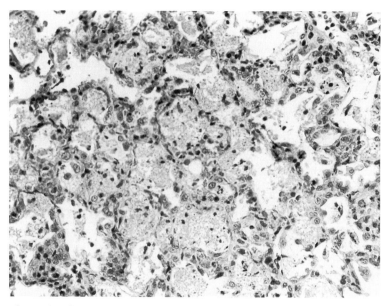

FIG. 2.40—Lung from athymic rat with spontaneous *Pneumocystis carinii* infection. Coccoid organisms are present in the foamy exudate present in alveoli.

Intracystic bodies (nuclei) can be demonstrated within cysts by using impression smears of lung stained with the Giemsa method.

DIAGNOSIS. The demonstration of the typical organisms in pulmonary lesions, using silver-staining procedures on impression smears of lung or in paraffin-embedded specimens, is the recommended method to confirm the diagnosis. A polymerase chain reaction (PCR) has also been used to detect the organism in specimens collected from lung tissue or by bronchioalveolar lavage.

SIGNIFICANCE. Pneumocystosis normally occurs only in rats subjected to significant predisposing factors, such as immunosuppression or dietary deficiency. Some other species are susceptible under similar circumstances. Spontaneous cases of pneumocystosis may occur in athymic nude rats. The strains studied to date appear to be species-specific. Therefore there appears to be little or no danger of interspecies transmission, including transmission of infections between rodents and humans.

BIBLIOGRAPHY
FOR MYCOTIC INFECTIONS

Aspergillus and Dermatophyte Infections
Balsardi, A., et al. 1981. Dermatophytes in clinically healthy laboratory animals. Lab. Anim. 15:75–77.
Rozengurt, N., and Sanchez, S. 1993. *Aspergillus niger* isolated from an outbreak of rhinitis in rats. Vet. Rec. 132:656–57.

Pneumocystis Infections
Armstrong, M.Y., et al. 1991. *Pneumocystis carinii* pneumonia in the rat model. J. Protozool. 38:136S–38S.
Barton, E.G., and Campbell, W.G. 1969. *Pneumocystis carinii* in lungs of rats treated with cortisone acetate: Ultrastructural observations relating to the life cycle. Am. J. Pathol. 54:209–36.
Bauer, N.L., et al. 1993. *Pneumocystis carinii* organisms isolated from rats, ferrets, and mice are antigenically different. Infect. Immun. 61:1315–19.
Cailliez, J.C., et al. 1996. *Pneumocystis carinii:* An atypical fungal micro-organism. J. Med. and Vet. Mycol. 34:227–39.
Cushion, M.T., et al. 1993. Genetic stability and diversity of *Pneumocystis carinii* infecting rat colonies. Infect. Immun. 61: 4801–13.
Feldman, S.H., et al. 1996. Detection of *Pneumocystis carinii* in rats by polymerase chain reaction: Comparison of lung tissue and bronchioalveolar lavage specimens. Lab. Anim. Sci. 46:628–34.
Furuta, T., et al. 1993. Fatal spontaneous pneumocystosis in nude rats. Lab. Anim. Sci 43:551–56.
Oz, H.S., and Hughes, W.T. 1996. Effect of sex and dexamethazone dose on the experimental host for *Pneumocystis carinii.* Lab. Anim. Sci. 46: 109–10.
Pohlmeyer, G., and Deerberg, F. 1993. Nude rats as a model of *Pneumocystis carinii* pneumonia: Sequential morphologic study of lung lesions. J. Comp. Path. 109:217–30.

PARASITIC DISEASES

In addition to the parasitic infestations outlined in this section, there are other parasites that are rarely seen in well-managed facilities. For additional information on the biology and identification of parasites in this species, consult Harkness and Wagner (1995), Hsu (1979), and Flynn (1973).

ECTOPARASITIC INFESTATIONS. Ectoparasites are not an important consideration in laboratory rats, although they are relatively common in the wild rat. They are host to two species of lice, *Polyplax spinulosa* (spined rat louse) and *Hoplopleura pacifica* (tropical rat louse), of which only the former has been described in laboratory rats. *Polyplax* was once an important vector for *Hemobartonella muris* among rats. It can be associated with pruritis, irritability, and anemia, caused directly by feeding and indirectly by *Hemobartonella.* Fleas of several genera, including *Xenopsylla, Leptopsylla,* and *Nosopsyllus,* infest wild rats and, rarely, laboratory rats. Several different types of mites can infest rats, but all are rare in laboratory rats, except *Radfordia ensifera* (*Myobia ratti*), the fur mite, which can be common in some populations. Pruritis, hair loss, and loss of condition are associated with heavy infestations. The mite may be demonstrated in the pellage and may also be evident in tissue sections of affected skin (Fig. 2.41). *Ornithonyssus bacoti* (tropical rat mite) is nonselective in its host range and infests rats on occasion. These mites are associated with rats only while feeding; then they seek refuge in the surrounding environment. Their bites are pruritic, as animal handlers can attest, and they can cause anemia, debility, and infertility. Other mites that reside permanently on the skin or fur of rats include *Demodex* spp., which have been found in follicles as an incidental

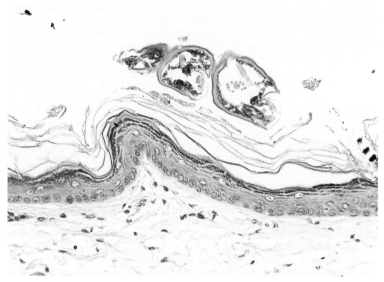

FIG. 2.41—Section of skin from rat with *Radfordia affinis* infestation. Mites are present on the stratum corneum, with minimal reaction in the underlying skin.

finding, and *Notoedres muris*, which burrows in the cornified epithelium of the ear and other hairless skin sites. It is frequently referred to as the ear mange mite. *Notoedres muris* is becoming common among European pet rats and may result in extensive lesions involving the ears and ear canal (Fig. 2.42).

ENDOPARASITIC INFECTIONS

Cryptosporidial Infection: Cryptosporidiosis. An outbreak of diarrhea and high mortality among infant rats of the Rapp hypertensive strain has been described. Surviving pups were runted and their fur was stained with feces. Lesions in

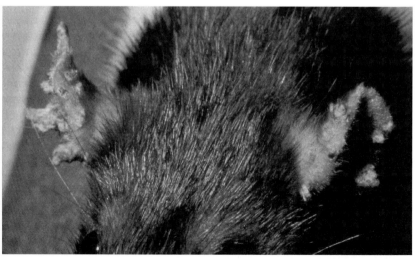

FIG. 2.42—Ear mange in a rat due to infestation with *Notoedres muris*. Note the disfigurement of the ears associated with the proliferative dermatitis. (Courtesy N.J. Schoemaker)

convalescing 21-d-old rats were restricted to the mucosa of the small intestine, primarily jejunum. The mucosa was hyperplastic and villi were shortened and fused, with cryptosporidia attached to the brush borders of enterocytes toward the villus tips. Cryptosporidiosis can be induced experimentally in rats but is transient and mild unless rats are immunosuppressed or athymic.

Other Protozoal Infections. *Giardia muris* and *Spironucleus muris* are flagellates that reside in the small intestine of rats and other rodents. Giardia organisms occur as rounded to crescent-shaped structures situated along the surface of the gut mucosa. *Spironucleus* spp. are visible as pear-shaped organisms in the intestinal crypts approximately $8 \times 2.5 \times 2.5$ μm. These organisms are not considered to be pathogenic in rats under normal conditions, unless there are important predisposing factors such as procedures resulting in immunosuppression. Catarrhal enteritis and weight loss are typical signs, particularly with spironucleosis. Although there have been reports of aberrations in the immune response in mice with spironucleosis, there is no evidence of a similar effect in the rat. Intestinal coccidiosis is found in wild rats but is not seen in laboratory rats.

Helminth Infections: Pinworms (Oxyuriasis). *Syphacia obvelata, S. muris,* and *Aspicularis tetraptera* are all recognized to be infectious for the rat. They are normally found in the cecum and colon in affected animals. *S. muris* commonly occurs in laboratory and wild rats and is transmissible to the laboratory mouse. These parasites have a direct life cycle. Adults have the characteristic morphologic features of oxyurid worms. Eggs are deposited in the colon or on the perianal area. The eggs embryonate and become infectious within a few hours. Rats may become infected by direct ingestion of embryonated eggs from the perianal region; ingestion of eggs in contaminated food and water or from fomites; or direct migration of larvae via the anus to the large intestine. Infected animals are frequently asymptomatic, but younger animals with heavy infections may exhibit various signs, including diarrhea, poor weight gains, impactions, rectal prolapse, and intussusceptions. *Aspicularis tetraptera* frequently occurs in conventional rats and mice. The

life cycle is direct. Eggs are passed in the feces and therefore are not found in the perianal region.

DIAGNOSIS. The microscopic demonstration of the characteristic eggs on touch preparations of the anal region (using transparent adhesive tape) is a useful method for *Syphacia.* The perianal adhesive tape method is of little value in making the diagnosis in *Aspicularis* infections. Eggs can also be demonstrated in stool samples, and adults are visible as small, threadlike worms in the cecum and colon. Adults are also readily visualized in tissue sections of large intestine. Occasionally focal submucosal granulomas may be evident in sections of the large intestine on microscopic examination (Fig. 2.43). *S. obvelata* is primarily a pinworm of mice, but rats are also susceptible to infection by this species. The two species can be differentiated by identifying the characteristic morphologic features of the adults and eggs. Macroscopic identification of the adults in the large intestine and the identification of the

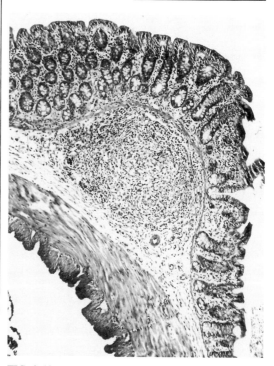

FIG. 2.43—Descending colon from rat with *Syphacia muris* infestation. Note the granuloma in the submucosal region.

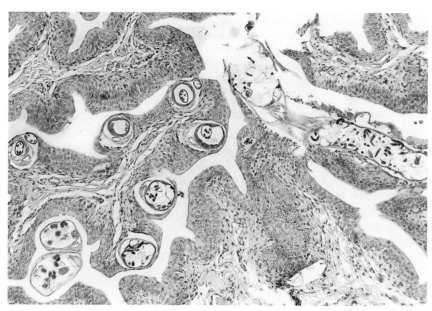

FIG. 2.44—Urinary bladder from rat with *Trichosomoides crassicauda* infestation. Portions of the nematodes are evident in the lumen of the bladder, and anterior portions are embedded in the epithelium, with negligible inflammatory cell response.

eggs on microscopic examination are the recommended methods to make a positive diagnosis.

SIGNIFICANCE OF OXYURIASIS. Except in heavy infections in young rats, clinical signs are usually minimal or absent in affected animals. However, there are concerns regarding possible effects on physiologic processes, such as the immune response. For example, rats infected with *S. obvelata* developed less severe lesions of adjuvant-induced arthritis than did noninfected animals. Transmission to other rodents, particularly mice, may also occur.

Other Helminth Infections

TRICHOSOMOIDES CRASSICAUDA INFECTION. *T. crassicauda* infections occur in the urinary tract of wild rats and, rarely, in laboratory rats. Infected animals are usually asymptomatic, and the thread-like adult worms are found in the lumen and mucosa of the urinary bladder and renal pelvis at necropsy. In tissue sections examined microscopically, migratory-stage larvae and immature worms may be present in multiple tissues, particularly lungs. Adult females reside in the epithelium of the renal pelvis and the urinary bladder, with chronic inflammatory response (Figs. 2.44 and 2.45).

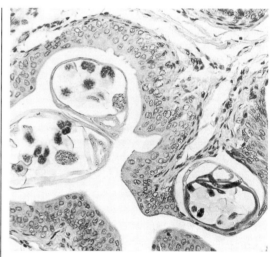

FIG. 2.45—Higher magnification of Figure 2.44, illustrating the uterine contents of the embedded female worms.

Males are much smaller than females and live within the urinary tract lumen or within the uterus of the larger females. Typical double-operculate eggs are passed in the urine, and intracage transmission readily occurs. Urinary calculi and bladder tumors have been associated with this parasitic infection, but to date, an unequivocal causal relationship has not been confirmed.

TAPEWORMS: *HYMENOLEPIS* INFECTIONS. *H. nana* and *H. diminuta* may be present in the small intestine of several species, including rats, mice, hamsters, humans, and nonhuman primates. With *H. nana,* the life cycle may be either direct or indirect. In the indirect life cycle, embryonated eggs are ingested by an arthropod host, such as grain beetles or fleas. Ingestion of these arthropods by a susceptible host will then serve as the source of the parasite eggs. In *H. diminuta* infections, an intermediate host, such as beetles or fleas, is essential for the completion of the life cycle.

DIAGNOSIS. Small, flattened white worms in the small intestine at necropsy may be identified as dwarf tapeworms by microscopic examination. Scoleces or cysticercoids may be identified in smears or in tissue sections of small intestine. Eggs can be demonstrated in the feces in order to confirm the diagnosis.

SIGNIFICANCE. Frequently, affected animals are asymptomatic. In a heavy infection, there may be poor weight gain and sometimes catarrhal enteritis. There is a danger of interspecies transmission, including infection in human contacts.

TAENIA TAENIAFORMIS INFECTION. *Cysticercus fasciolaris* is the larval stage of *T. taeniaformis,* the cat tapeworm. When eggs of this tapeworm are ingested, they migrate through the bowel and often encyst in the liver of rats, mice, and other rodents. Laboratory rats and mice become infected by contamination of food with cat feces. Usually, only one or two cysts will be found in an infected animal. Parasitism in rats can be associated with the development of sarcomas in the reactive tissue around the cyst.

BIBLIOGRAPHY FOR PARASITIC DISEASES

Ectoparasitic Infestations
Flynn, R.J. 1973. *Parasites of Laboratory Animals.* Ames: Iowa State University Press.
Peper, R.L. 1994. Diagnostic exercise: Mite infestation in a laboratory rat colony. Lab. Anim. Sci. 44:172–74

Walberg, J.A., et al. 1981. Demodicidosis in laboratory rats (*Rattus norvegicus*). Lab. Anim. Sci. 31:60–62.

Endoparasitic Infections
Altman, N.H., and Goodman, D.G. 1979. Neoplastic diseases. In *The Laboratory Rat. I. Biology and Diseases,* ed. H.J. Baker et al., p. 346. New York: Academic.
Barthold, S.W. 1997a. *Spironucleus muris* infection, intestine, mouse, rat, hamster. In *Monographs on Pathology of Laboratory Animals: Digestive System,* ed. T.C. Jones et al., pp. 419–21. New York: Springer-Verlag.
————. 1997b. *Giardia muris* infection, intestine, mouse, rat, hamster. In *Monographs on Pathology of Laboratory Animals: Digestive System,* ed. T.C. Jones et al., pp. 422–26. New York: Springer-Verlag.
Hsu, C-K. 1979. Parasitic diseases. In *The Laboratory Rat. I. Biology and Diseases,* ed. H.J. Baker et al., pp. 307–531. New York: Academic.
Moody, K.D., et al. 1991. Cryptosporidiosis in suckling laboratory rats. Lab. Anim. Sci. 41:625–27.
Mullink, J.W.M.A., et al. 1980. Lack of effects of *Spironucleus* (*Hexamita*) *muris* on the immune response to tetanus toxoid in the rat. Lab. Anim. 14:127–28.
Pearson, D.J., and Taylor, G. 1975. The Influence of the nematode *Syphacia obvelata* on adjuvant arthritis in rats. Immunology 29:391–96.
Schwabe, C.W. 1955. Helminth parasites and neoplasia. Am. J. Vet. Res. 16:485.
Zubaidy, A.J., and Majeed, S.K. 1981. Pathology of the nematode *Trichosomoides crassicauda* in the urinary bladder of laboratory rats. Lab. Anim. 15:381–84.

General Bibliography
Flynn, R.J. 1973. *Parasites of Laboratory Animals.* Ames: Iowa State University Press.
Harkness, J.E., and Wagner, J.E. 1995. *The Biology and Medicine of Rabbits and Rodents.* Philadelphia: Lea and Febiger.
Hsu, C-K. 1979. Parasitic diseases. In *The Laboratory Rat. I. Biology and Diseases,* ed. H.J. Baker et al., pp. 307–531. New York: Academic.
Owen, D.G. 1992. Parasites of Laboratory Animals. London: Royal Society of Medicine Services Ltd.

AGING AND DEGENERATIVE DISORDERS

Chronic Progressive Glomerulonephropathy/ Chronic Progressive Nephrosis. The disease has been referred to by a variety of other terms, including glomerulosclerosis, progressive glomerulonephrosis, and "old rat nephropathy."

EPIZOOTIOLOGY AND PATHOGENESIS. The incidence of the disease in older rats varies but may be up to 75% or more in susceptible strains. A variety of predisposing factors may play a role in the development of chronic progressive glomerulonephropathy (PGN). (1) Age: Lesions are usually most extensive in animals at least 12 mo of age. (2) Sex: The disease is considerably more common and more severe in males. (3) Strain: The incidence is usually significantly higher in Sprague-Dawley rats than with most other breeds. (4) Diet: High-protein diets have been considered to be an important contributing factor, although total dietary restriction, rather than protein content, may be more important in reducing the progression of the disease. PGN has been referred to as a "protein leakage disease," due to increased loss of protein in the glomerular filtrate. The eosinophilic droplets present in epithelial cells lining tubules have been associated with increased lysosomal activity and may be a reflection of functional overload of nephrons. (5) Immunological factors: Mesangial deposition of IgM has been observed in affected glomeruli consistent with non–complement-fixing immune complexes, but it does not appear to be primarily an immunologically mediated disease. (6) Endocrine: Prolactin levels have also been implicated as a contributing factor in the development of the disease. Clinical signs associated with the disease include proteinuria, weight loss, and in advanced cases elevated plasma creatinine levels consistent with renal insufficiency.

PATHOLOGY. The renal cortices are usually pitted and sometimes irregular, with variable degrees of enlargement and pallor in some affected animals. On cut surface, there may be irregularities and linear streaks in the cortex and medulla, with varying degrees of brown pigmentation (Fig. 2.46). Microscopic changes are consistent with a chronic glomerulopathy. Glomerular changes vary from minimal thickening of the basement membranes to marked thickening of glomerular tufts, with segmental sclerosis and adhesions to Bowman's capsule (Fig. 2.47). Proteinaceous casts may be present in tubules in the cortex and medulla. Eosinophilic, PAS-positive resorption droplets are frequently present in epithelial cells lining affected nephrons. The droplets may be iron-positive. Tubules are frequently dilated and lined by flattened epithelial cells; contracted and lined by poorly differenti-

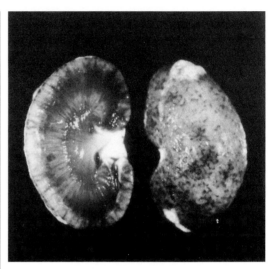

FIG. 2.46—Spontaneous progressive glomerulonephropathy in aged rat. Note the granular appearance to cortical surface and the linear streaks on cut surface.

ated, cuboidal, basophilic epithelial cells; or sclerotic. There may be varying degrees of thickening of proximal tubular basement membranes, interstitial fibrosis, and mononuclear cell infiltration (Fig. 2.48). Macrophages and myofibroblasts appear to play an important role in the development of the interstitial fibrosis associated with PGN. In advanced cases, there may be renal secondary hyperparathyroidism, with mineralized deposits in tissues such as kidney, gastric mucosa, lungs, and the media of larger arteries. Hypercholesterolemia, hypoproteinemia, and elevated blood urea nitrogen consistent with renal insufficiency/failure may be evident in advanced cases, although variations occur. Elevated serum cholesterol and marked proteinuria (>300 mg/dl of urine) are useful diagnostic parameters. *Differential diagnoses:* PGN must be differentiated from other degenerative nephropathies, such as chronic bacterial pyelonephritis, congenital hydronephrosis, and ischemic injury. Nephrosis associated with toxic insults such as overdosing with aminoglycoside antibiotics is another possible cause of renal injury.

SIGNIFICANCE. Chronic progressive glomerulonephropathy or PGN is a common disease associated with the aging process in strains such

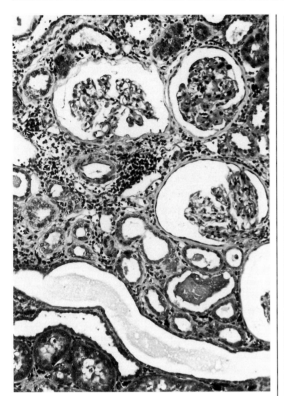

FIG. 2.47—Glomerular changes associated with PGN in aged rat. Note the thickening of glomerular basement membranes and Bowman's capsule. Proteinaceous casts are present in many tubules.

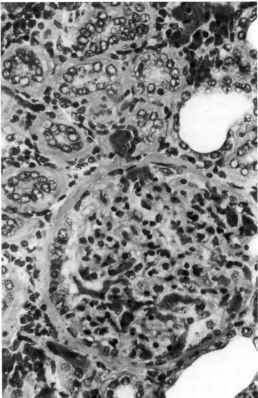

FIG. 2.48—Degenerative changes in tubules in typical case of PGN. There is thickening of basement membranes with flattening of the epithelial cells lining affected tubules.

as the Sprague-Dawley rat. Aside from the proteinuria associated with the disease, there may be weight loss, and severely affected rats may die due to renal failure. It is a major life-limiting disease in the aged rat. Animals with severe disease appear to cope well but may rapidly decompensate and die. Late-stage disease has been associated with hypertension and polyarteritis nodosa.

Nephrocalcinosis. Renal calcification has been observed on occasion in laboratory rats, including animals on regular commercial diets. The disease has been produced by a variety of dietary manipulations, including those with a low-magnesium content, a high-calcium content, high concentrations of phosphorus, and preparations with a low-calcium-phosphorus ratio. Lesions are characterized by the deposition of calcium phos-

phates in the interstitium of the corticomedullary junction, with intratubular aggregations in the same region. In advanced cases, there may be detectable manifestations of renal dysfunction, including albuminuria.

Hydronephrosis. Hydronephrosis is a relatively common incidental finding at necropsy and occurs in a variety of strains and stocks of rats. In some strains, there is a hereditary basis for the disorder. For example, in the brown Norway rat, hydronephrosis appears to be an autosomal polygenetic disorder, with incomplete penetrance. In the Gunn rat, it is apparently inherited as a dominant gene and may be lethal when present in the homozygous state. In studies of hydronephrosis in outbred Sprague-Dawley rats, it was concluded that the condition is a highly heritable trait, probably involving more than one gene. Spontaneous hydronephrosis, particularly of the right kidney, is a well-recognized abnormality, especially in male rats. It has been proposed that the lesion in males may be due to the passage of the internal spermatic vessels across the ureter, resulting in mechanical obstruction to outflow and subsequent hydronephrosis of the affected kidney. However, in one study, sectioning of the right spermatic vessels in young male Wistar-derived rats failed to reduce the incidence of hydronephrosis, compared with control animals.

At necropsy, there may be varying degrees of involvement. In severely affected animals, the kidney consists of a fluid-filled sac containing clear serous fluid. On microscopic examination, there is marked dilation of the renal pelvis, with excavation of the renal medulla, reduction in the length of the collecting tubules, and absence of an inflammatory response. *Differential diagnoses* include pyelonephritis, polycystic kidneys, and renal papillary necrosis. In most strains, unilateral or bilateral hydronephrosis is often an incidental finding at necropsy. There is a hereditary basis in some strains. The defect may be fatal when bilateral. There may be an increased susceptibility to superimposed renal infections due to urine stasis. Functional abnormalities in renal physiology may occur.

Urinary Calculi. The incidence of spontaneous urolithiasis in nonmanipulated laboratory rats is normally low. Calculi when present in the urinary bladder may be associated with hemorrhagic cystitis, hematuria, and sometimes urinary obstruction. Calculi may also be located at other sites (e.g., renal pelvis, ureter, and urethra). The composition of calculi is variable. Analyses have revealed combinations such as ammonium magnesium phosphate, mixed carbonate and oxalate, and mixed carbonate and phosphate with magnesium and calcium. In male rats there are also erroneous reports of a high incidence of mucoid calculi, which are agonally excreted copulatory plugs into the urethra and bladder.

SIGNIFICANCE. Urinary calculi are frequently sporadic in occurrence. A search for specific contributing factors (e.g., estrogen therapy and water restriction) may be unrewarding. They must not be confused with copulatory plugs.

Hematuria/Renal Papillary Hyperplasia. Intermittent hematuria has been reported in hybrid Lewis × Brown Norway rats. The syndrome occurred predominantly in males, but also females. Some, but not all, of the rats had concomitant unilateral or bilateral hydronephrosis. Lesions were confined to the renal papilli and consisted of focal urothelial proliferative change, with hemorrhage and necrosis of the stroma.

Myocardial Degeneration/Fibrosis. Focal to diffuse areas of myocardial degeneration are frequently seen microscopically in conventional and specific-pathogen-free Sprague-Dawley rats, particularly after 1 yr of age. Lesions are more common in male rats. The incidence may be 25% or more in some strains. Endocardial proliferative lesions have also been described.

At necropsy, there may be moderate to marked ventricular hypertrophy, and occasionally pale streaks are evident, but there is usually little evidence of cardiac insufficiency. On microscopic examination, degenerative changes are usually most evident in the papillary muscles of the left ventricle, although the interventricular septum may also be involved. Lesions are characterized by atrophy of myofibers, vacuolation to fragmentation of the sarcoplasm, loss of cross-striations, and mononuclear cell infiltration (Fig. 2.49). Large reactive nuclei are occasionally observed. Interstitial fibrosis, with proliferation of fibrous tissue, is an important microscopic feature of the disease. Although this condition is a frequent microscopic finding in older rats, there may be little or no evidence

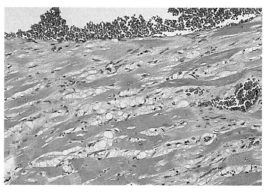

FIG. 2.49—Segmental myocardial degeneration and interstitial fibrosis in aged rat with cardiomyopathy.

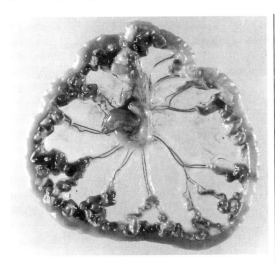

FIG. 2.50—Small intestine and mesenteric attachments in aged Sprague-Dawley rat with polyarteritis nodosa. Note the tortuosity and dilation of mesenteric arterioles, especially along the mesenteric attachments. (Courtesy B.S. Jortner)

of cardiac insufficiency. Degenerative myocardial lesions may be secondary to ischemic change.

Polyarteritis Nodosa. This chronic progressive degenerative disease most frequently occurs in aging rats. The incidence is higher in males. Arterial lesions most frequently occur in medium-size arteries of the mesentery, pancreas, pancreaticoduodenal artery, and testis. The pathogenesis has not been resolved, but an immunologically mediated process is one possible explanation. The spontaneous disease most frequently occurs in the Sprague-Dawley and spontaneous hypertensive rat (SHR) strains and in rats with late-stage chronic nephropathy.

At necropsy, affected vessels are enlarged and thickened in a segmental pattern, with marked tortuosity, particularly in the mesenteric vessels (Fig. 2.50). On microscopic examination, vascular lesions may be present in various tissues, such as mesentery, pancreas, testis, kidney, and most other organs except the lung. There is fibrinoid degeneration and thickening of the media of affected arteries, with smudging of the normal architecture. Infiltrating leukocytes consist of mononuclear cells, with a few neutrophils. There are marked variations in the size and contours in the lumen of affected vessels, and thromboses, occasionally with recanalization, occur (Fig. 2.51).

The presence of the characteristic lesions, particularly in the Sprague-Dawley and SHR strains, is diagnostic for the disease. Drug-induced vascular lesions may resemble the spontaneous disease.

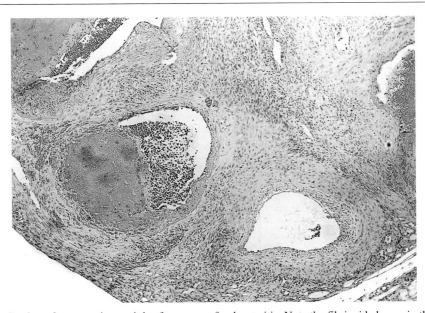

FIG. 2.51—Section of mesenteric arterioles from case of polyarteritis. Note the fibrinoid change in the media of the vessels, with leukocytic infiltration.

Degenerative Changes in the Nervous System. Age-related abnormalities seen in aged rats include Wallerian degeneration in focal areas of the spinal cord and segmental demyelination of the peripheral nervous system, particularly in the sciatic nerves. Wallerian degeneration in the cord is characterized by the presence of enlarged axons containing eosinophilic material. In the brain and spinal cord, there may be degeneration of scattered neurons, with astrogliosis. Lipochrome pigment may be present in some neurons in the brain and spinal cord.

Spontaneous radiculoneuropathy is a degenerative disease of the spinal roots, with concurrent atrophy of skeletal muscle in the lumbar region and hind limbs. Vacuolation and demyelination occur primarily in the lumbosacral roots, particularly the ventral spinal regions. This syndrome is manifest clinically as posterior weakness or paresis in the aged rat.

Aging Lesions of the Liver. Rats develop polyploidy, megalokarya, binuclear hepatocytes, intranuclear cytoplasmic invagination, and intracytoplasmic inclusions of hepatocytes that are similar to but not as striking as in the aging mouse. Although not remarkable in younger animals, the shift to increased ploidy occurs relatively early in life. There is strain-related variation in the incidence of polyploidy in rats. Foci of sinusoidal dilatation and peliosis, either spontaneous or drug-induced, do occur, especially in older animals. Foci of cytoplasmic alteration vary phenotypically from areas of clearing to acidophilic to basophilic staining. These changes are of particular interest to the toxicologic pathologist. A striking lesion that is frequently observed in aging rats is bile ductular proliferation. Initially there are increased numbers of bile ductules in portal tracts, which become dilated, lined by atrophic epithelium, and surrounded by collagenous connective tissue, resulting in a cirrhotic appearance (Fig. 2.52). Extramedullary hematopoiesis may be seen in older rats with conditions such as severe chronic renal disease.

Degenerative Osteoarthritis. Erosion of the articular cartilage occurs in sites such as the sternum and femur in aged rats, with degeneration of cartilaginous matrix, clefting, and cyst formation.

Other Age-related Lesions. For additional information on age-related changes seen in the laboratory rat, consult Burek (1978) and Coleman et al. (1977).

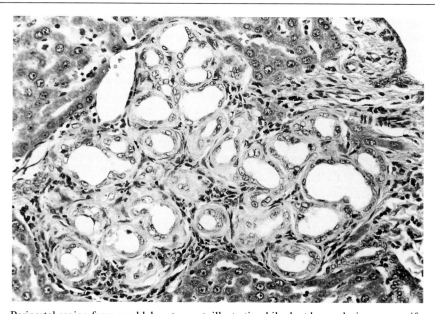

FIG. 2.52—Periportal region from aged laboratory rat, illustrating bile duct hyperplasia, one manifestation of the aging process seen in some strains.

MISCELLANEOUS
AND ENVIRONMENTAL DISORDERS

Malocclusion. Overgrowth of the incisor teeth occurs sporadically in this species. The condition occurs secondary to poor alignment of the upper and lower incisor teeth, with resultant failure to wear in the normal manner. The condition may be secondary to a broken upper or lower incisor tooth but is more often a spontaneous event and in many cases is considered to be due to genetic factors. Depending on the duration and severity of the problem, affected animals are frequently thin due to their inability to prehend and masticate food normally, and in advanced cases, severely affected lower or upper incisors may penetrate into the soft tissues of the palate or jaw (Fig. 2.53). Cellulitis and increased salivation are frequent sequelae in advanced cases.

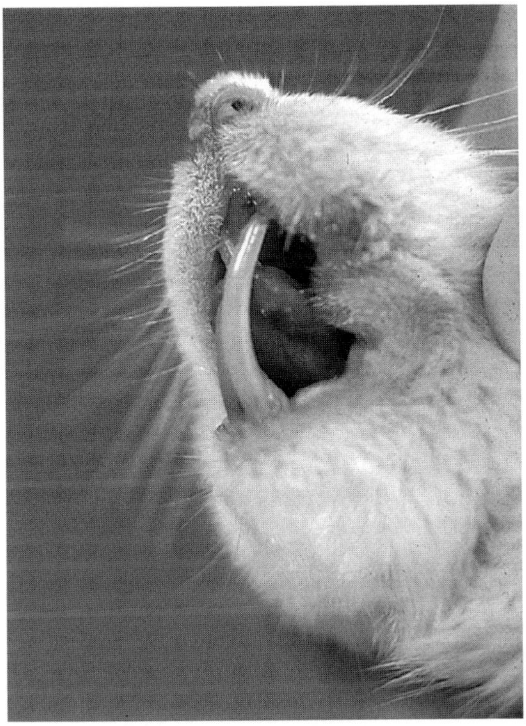

Environmental Disorders

"RINGTAIL." Rats adapt to cold but do not tolerate heat well. Low humidity may predispose young rats to "ringtail," with annular constrictions of the skin of the tail, leading to dry gangrene of the distal tail (Fig. 2.54). This syndrome is most apt to occur in preweaning rats. Traditionally ringtail has been attributed to low environmental humidity (e.g., less than 25%). However, other factors, such as genetic susceptibility, low environmental temperatures, degree of hydration, and nutrition may be involved. A detailed histological study may serve to shed light on the etiopathogenesis of this disease.

Other Environmental Disorders

DEHYDRATION. Rats become dehydrated easily, usually from malfunction of water bottle sipper tubes. Dehydration is often accompanied by por-

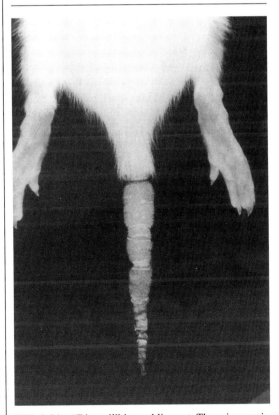

FIG. 2.53—Advanced case of malocclusion in laboratory rat. Note overgrowth of lower incisor into anterior palate.

FIG. 2.54—"Ringtail" in suckling rat. There is prominent annular ridging and contraction, a characteristic feature of the disease.

phyrin staining around the eyes, a sign of general stress.

HIGH ENVIRONMENTAL TEMPERATURE. High environmental temperature can easily cause infertility, particularly in male rats.

LIGHT CYCLES. The female estrous cycle is sensitive to light cycles. For example, exposure to constant light for as little as 3 d may induce persistent estrus, hyperestrogenism, polycystic ovaries, and endometrial hypertrophy.

INTENSITY OF LIGHT. Marked retinal degeneration can occur in albino rats subjected to light intensities that would be relatively harmless to animals with pigmented uveal tracts. Retinal changes can occur in rats exposed to cyclic light with an intensity of 130 lux or higher at the cage level. Typically, the changes are most severe in rats housed on the top shelves of racks nearest the ceiling light fixtures. There is a progressive reduction of the photoreceptor cell nuclei in the outer nuclear layer of the central retina. Advanced disease has marked depletion and alteration of the retinal layers, with concomitant cataract formation. This must be differentiated from peripheral retinal degeneration, which occurs in some strains of rats as a genetically inherited disorder. Degenerative changes may also occur in the Harderian glands of rats exposed to high-intensity light.

QUALITY OF BEDDING. Dusty bedding material can result in inhalation of foreign material into the lungs, with focal aspiration pneumonia (Fig. 2.55). High mortality has been observed in Sprague-Dawley rats housed on aromatic cedar wood shavings. Reduced weight gains were also observed. The mechanism(s) of the disease was not determined.

Chloral Hydrate Ileus. Intraperitoneal injection of chloral hydrate or related compounds causes peritonitis and ileus. The ileus may not be apparent until up to 5 wk after administration of the drug. Rats develop distended abdomens due to segmental atony and distension of the jejunum, ileum, and cecum (Fig. 2.56). Focal serosal

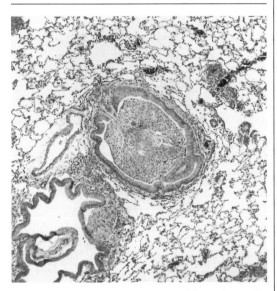

FIG. 2.55—Lung from laboratory rat illustrating aspiration of plant fiber. Note the presence of the aspirated material in the lumen of one airway, the chronic inflammatory response, and the subsequent airway obstruction.

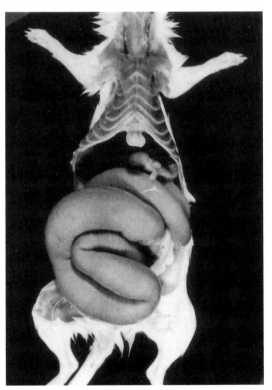

FIG. 2.56—Paralytic ileus in juvenile rat typical of the change associated with the intraperitoneal administration of chloral hydrate as an anesthetic agent. There is marked dilation and ileus of the intestinal tract.

hyperemia can also occur. This must be differentiated from ileus/ileitis due to Tyzzer's disease.

Auricular Chondritis. The disease has been observed in several strains, including Sprague-Dawley and Wistar rats. Nodular lesions are present in the pinnae of the ears. Microscopic lesions are characterized by multinodular, granulomatous inflammatory foci with chondrolysis and invasion by mesenchymal cells. Trauma and infectious agents have been considered as possible underlying causes, but it may be an immunologically mediated disease.

BIBLIOGRAPHY FOR AGING AND DEGENERATIVE DISORDERS

Renal Disorders
Anver, M.R., and Cohen, B.J. 1979. Lesions associated with aging. In *The Laboratory Rat. I. Biology and Diseases,* ed. H.J. Baker et al., pp. 377–99. New York: Academic.

Cohen, B.J., et al. 1970. Veritable hydronephrosis in a mutant strain of brown Norway rats. Lab. Anim. Care 20:489–93.

Couser, W.G., and Stilmant, M.M. 1975. Mesangial lesions and focal glomerular sclerosis in the aging rat. Lab. Invest. 33:491–501.

Gray, J.E. 1986. Chronic progressive nephrosis, rat. In *Monographs on Pathology of Laboratory Animals: Urinary System,* ed. T.C. Jones et al., pp. 174–79. New York: Springer-Verlag.

Gray, J.E., et al. 1982. Early light microscopic changes in chronic progressive nephrosis in several strains of aging laboratory rats. J. Gerontol. 37:142–50.

Lalich, J.J., and Allen, J.R. 1971. Protein overload nephropathy in rats with unilateral nephrectomy. Arch. Pathol. 91:372–82.

Lozzio, B.B., et al. 1967. Hereditary renal disease in a mutant strain of rats. Science 156: 1742–44.

Magnusson, G., and Ramsay, C.H. 1971. Urolithiasis in the rat. Lab. Anim. 5:153–62.

Maronpot, R.R. 1986. Spontaneous hydronephrosis, rat. In *Monographs on Pathology of Laboratory Animals: Urinary System,* ed. T.C. Jones et al., pp. 268–71. New York: Springer-Verlag.

Natatsuji, S., et al. 1998. Macrophages, fibroblasts, and extracellular matrix accumulation in interstitial fibrosis of chronic progressive nephropathy in aged rats. Vet. Pathol. 35:352–60.

O'Donaghue, P.N., and Wilson, M.S. 1977. Hydronephrosis in male rats. Lab. Anim. 11:193–94.

Owen, R.A., and Heywood, R. 1986. Age-related variations in renal structure and function in Sprague-Dawley rats. Toxicol. Pathol. 14:158–67.

Paterson, M. 1979. Urolithiasis in the Sprague-Dawley rat. Lab. Anim. 13:17–20.

Richardson, B., and Luginbuhl, H. 1976. The role of prolactin in the development of chronic progressive nephropathy in the rat. Virchows Arch. Pathol. Anat. 370:13–19.

Ristskes-Hoitinga, J., et al. 1989. Nutrition and kidney calcification in rats. Lab. Anim. 23:313–18.

Tapp, D.C., et al. 1989. Food restriction retards body growth and prevents end-stage renal pathology in remnant kidneys regardless of protein intake. Lab. Invest. 60:184–95.

Treloar, A.F., and Armstrong, A. 1993. Intermittent hematuria in a colony of Lewis × Brown Norway hybrid rats. Lab. Anim. Sci. 43:640–41.

Van Winkle, T.J., et al. 1988. Incidence of hydronephrosis among several production colonies of outbred Sprague-Dawley rats. Lab. Anim. Sci. 38:402–6.

Weaver, R.N., et al. 1975. Urinary proteins in Sprague-Dawley rats with chronic progressive nephrosis. Lab. Anim. Sci. 25:705–10.

Liver
Bannasch, P., et al. 1997. Foci of altered hepatocytes, rat. In *Monographs on Pathology of Laboratory Animals: Digestive System.* ed. T.C. Jones et al. pp. 3–37. New York: Springer-Verlag.

Van Zweiten, M.J., and Hollander, C.F. 1997. Polyploidy, liver, rat. In *Monographs on Pathology of Laboratory Animals: Digestive System.* ed. T.C. Jones et al., pp. 130–33. New York: Springer-Verlag.

———. 1997. Intranuclear and intracytoplasmic inclusions, liver, rat. In *Monographs on Pathology of Laboratory Animals: Digestive System.* ed. T.C. Jones et al., pp. 133–39. New York: Springer-Verlag.

Myocardial Degeneration/Fibrosis
Anver, M.R., and Cohen, B.J. 1979. Lesions associated with aging. In *The Laboratory Rat. I. Biology and Diseases,* ed. H.J. Baker et al., pp. 377–99. New York: Academic.

Burek, J.D. 1978. *Pathology of Aging Rats.* Boca Raton, Fla.: CRC.

Novilla, M.N., et al. 1991. A retrospective study of endocardial proliferative lesions in rats. Vet. Pathol. 28:156–65.

Polyarteritis Nodosa
Bishop, S.P. 1989. Animal models of vasculitis. Toxicol. Pathol. 17:109–17.

Yang, Y.H. 1965. Polyarteritis nodosa in laboratory rats. Lab. Invest. 14:81–88.

Degenerative Changes in the Nervous System
Berg, B.N., et al. 1962. Degenerative lesions of spinal roots and peripheral nerves of aging rats. Gerontology 6:72–80.

Krinke, G.J. 1988. Spontaneous radioneuropathology, aged rats. In *Monographs on Pathology of Laboratory Animals: Nervous System,* ed. T.C. Jones et al., pp. 203–8. New York: Springer -Verlag.

Van Steenis, G., and Kroes, R. 1971. Changes in the nervous system and musculature of old rats. Vet. Pathol. 8:320–32.

Witt, C.J., and Johnson, L.K. 1990. Diagnostic exercise: Rear limb ataxia in a rat. Lab. Anim. Sci. 40:528–29.

Degenerative Osteoarthritis

Burek, J.D. 1978. *Pathology of Aging Rats.* Boca Raton, Fla.: CRC.

Coleman, G.L., et al. 1977. Pathological changes during aging in barrier-reared Fischer F344 male rats. J. Gerontol. 32:258–78.

Yamasaki, K., and Inui, S. 1985. Lesions of articular, sternal and growth plate cartilage in rats. Vet. Pathol. 22:46–50.

Miscellaneous and Environmental Disorders

Burkhart, C.A., and Robinson, J.L. 1978. High rat pup mortality attributed to the use of cedar-wood shavings as bedding. Lab. Anim. 12:221–22.

Kurisu, K. et al. 1996. Sequential changes in the Harderian gland of rats exposed to high intensity light. Lab. Anim. Sci. 46:71–76.

Lawson, P.T., and Churchman, P.R. 1993. Ringtail in a breeding colony of rats due to malfunction of the heating, ventilating, and air conditioning system. Contemp. Top. 32:22.

Noell, W.K., et al. 1966. Retinal damage by light in rats. Invest. Ophthalmol. 5:450–73.

Rao, G.N. 1991. Light intensity–associated eye lesions of Fischer 344 rats in long term studies. Toxicol. Pathol. 19:148–55.

Semple-Rowland, S.L., and Dawson, W.W. 1987. Retinal cyclic light damage threshold for albino rats. Lab. Anim. Sci. 37:389–98.

Chloral Hydrate Ileus

Fleischman, R.W., et al. 1977. Adynamic ileus in the rat induced by chloral hydrate. Lab. Anim. Sci. 27:238–43.

Kohn, D.F., and Barthold, S.W. 1984. Biology and diseases of rats. In *Laboratory Animal Medicine,* ed. J.G. Fox et al., pp. 91–122. New York: Academic.

Auricular Chondritis

McEwen, B.J., and Barsoum, N.J. 1990. Auricular chondritis in Wistar rats. Lab. Anim. 24:280–83.

General Bibliography

Anver, M.R., and Cohen, B.J. 1979. Lesions associated with aging. In *The Laboratory Rat. I. Biology and Diseases,* ed. H.J. Baker et al., pp. 377–99. New York: Academic.

Burek, J.D. 1978. *Pathology of Aging Rats.* Boca Raton, Fla.: CRC.

Coleman, G.L., et al. 1977. Pathological changes during aging in barrier-reared Fischer F344 male rats. J. Gerontol. 32:258–78.

Goodman, D.G., et al. 1980. Neoplastic and non-neoplastic lesions in aging Osborne-Mendel rats. Toxicol. Appl. Pharmacol. 55:433–47.

Hackbarth, H. 1983. Strain differences in inbred rats: Influence of strain and diet on haematological traits. Lab. Anim. 17:7–12.

Harkness, J.E., and Wagner, J.E. 1995. *The Biology and Medicine of Rabbits and Rodents.* Philadelphia: Lea and Febiger.

Jones, T.C., et al. 1997. *Monographs on Pathology of Laboratory Animals: Digestive System,* ed. T.C. Jones et al. New York: Springer-Verlag.

Lamb, D. 1975. Rat lung pathology and quality of laboratory animals: The user's view. Lab. Anim. 9:1–8.

Losco, P.E., and Troup, C.M. 1988. Corneal dystrophy in Fischer 344 rats. Lab. Anim. Sci. 38:702–10.

Turton, J.A., et al. 1989. Age-related changes in the haematology of female F344 rats. Lab. Anim. 23:295–301.

Van Steenis, G., and Kroes, R. 1971. Changes in the nervous system and musculature of old rats. Vet. Pathol. 8:320–32.

NEOPLASMS

It is beyond the scope of this chapter to give a detailed description of the neoplasms of this species. For additional information, consult Burek (1978), Squire et al. (1978), Turusov et al. (1976), and MacKenzie and Garner (1973).

Lymphoreticular Tumors

LARGE GRANULAR LYMPHOCYTIC (LGL) LEUKEMIA IN FISCHER 344, WISTAR, AND WISTAR-FURTH RATS. LGL leukemias are a major cause of death in aging F344 rats and occasionally occur in other strains. The neoplastic cells are readily transplantable to rats of the same strain. The malignancy appears to arise in the spleen and then spreads to other organs. Unlike lymphoreticular tumors of mice, retroviruses are not associated with the development of the disease. Although initially considered to be of natural killer (NK) cell origin, studies of cytotoxic activity and surface antigens suggest that these leukemias are of more heterogeneous lymphocytic cell origin. LGL leukemia is characterized by elevated blood leukocyte counts of up to 400,000/ml^3. Morphologically, leukemic cells resemble large granular leukocytes. Clinical signs are characterized by weight loss, anemia, jaundice, and depression. There is usually a concur-

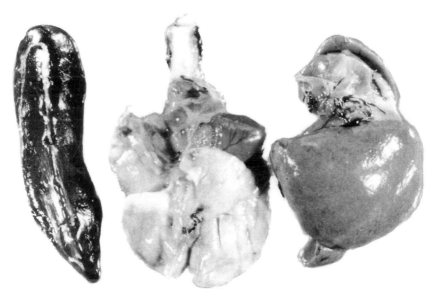

FIG. 2.57—Viscera from a spontaneous case of LGL in Fischer 344 rat. There is marked splenomegaly and hepatomegaly. The carcass was pale and icteric. (Courtesy M.A. Hayes)

rent, immune-mediated hemolytic anemia, with thrombocytopenia and clotting abnormalities suggestive of disseminated intravascular coagulation.

PATHOLOGY. At necropsy, the carcass is usually pale and icteric. The spleen is markedly enlarged, and there may be moderate to marked enlargement of the liver and lymphadenopathy (Fig. 2.57). Petechial hemorrhages are frequently present on the lung and lymph nodes. Stained impression smears of tissues such as spleen reveal lymphocytes 10–15 μm in diameter, with irregular-shaped, frequently indented nuclei; pale cytoplasm; and prominent, azurophilic cytoplasmic granules (Fig. 2.58). On histological examination of tissue sections, there is diffuse infiltration with malignant lymphocytes in organs such as spleen, lymph nodes, liver, and lung. There is frequently marked depletion of lymphoid follicles in the spleen and diffuse infiltration of leukemic cells in the sinusoids. Hepatocellular degeneration commonly occurs, probably a result of the concurrent anemia and neoplastic infiltrates. Erythrophagocytosis may be evident in the liver and spleen.

DIAGNOSIS. The presence of the typical clinical and histological pattern, including anemia, splenomegaly, and icterus, and the characteristic

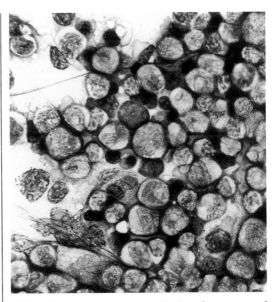

FIG. 2.58—Impression smear of spleen from a case of LGL. There are large numbers of malignant lymphocytes with cytoplasmic granules present in the smear. (Courtesy M.A. Hayes)

lymphocytes in F344 rats are sufficient to confirm the diagnosis. *Differential diagnoses* include lymphosarcoma and histiocytic sarcoma.

SIGNIFICANCE. LGL leukemia is a major cause of disease and mortality in aging F344 rats.

LYMPHOMA/LEUKEMIA. Spontaneous lymphomas and/or lymphocytic leukemias are relatively uncommon in most strains of rats. They are not associated with retroviral infections. At necropsy, splenomegaly, enlarged lymph nodes, and hepatomegaly are characteristic findings. On microscopic examination, there is frequently diffuse infiltration of neoplastic lymphocytes into organs such as spleen and liver, with obliteration of the normal architecture (Fig. 2.59).

CUTANEOUS LYMPHOMA (MYCOSIS FUNGOIDES) . Epidermotropic lymphomas are relatively rare in this species. Clinically, the disease is characterized by the presence of circumscribed erythematous plaques on the skin that may progress to ulceration. Microscopically, in affected areas, there is epidermal hyperplasia with variable ulceration and marked infiltration with neoplastic lymphocytes in the dermis and epidermis. In the epidermis, the infiltrating cells occur singly or in clusters surrounded by a clear halo (Fig. 2.60). Similar changes are present in hair follicles in the region. The infiltrating lymphocytes are medium- to large-size and react with anti-CD3 antibody, providing confirmation that they are of T-cell origin. In cases documented to date, the neoplastic infiltrates have been confined to the skin.

HISTIOCYTIC SARCOMA. Neoplasms of this nature occur most often in Sprague-Dawley rats, but they also have been observed in other strains, including Osborne-Mendel and Wistar rats. The tumors are present primarily in animals over 12 mo of age, and there is no obvious sex predisposition.

PATHOLOGY. At necropsy, sarcomas of this type may be present in the liver, lymph nodes, lung, spleen, mediastinum, retroperitoneum, and subcutaneous tissue. Neoplasms are pale and moderately firm, and they tend to infiltrate and displace normal tissue. Necrotic areas may be scattered in the mass. On microscopic examination, tumors consist of diffuse sheets of neoplas-

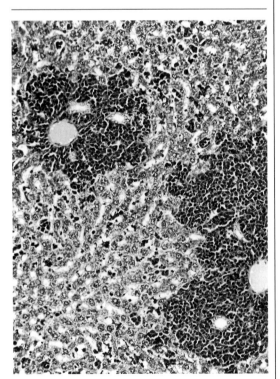

FIG. 2.59—Lymphocytic infiltrate in the liver in a spontaneous lymphosarcoma in mature Wistar rat. Note the marked lymphocytic infiltration in the periportal regions.

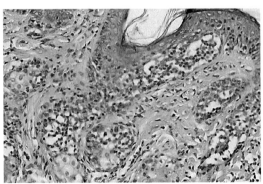

FIG. 2.60—Biopsy of skin from mature pet rat of unknown ancestry, illustrating an example of an epitheliotropic lymphosarcoma. Note the infiltrate of relatively well-differentiated lymphocytes at the dermo-epidermal junction and the dissociation of the adjacent epidermal cells.

tic cells, varying from elongated, pallisading forms to plump, pleomorphic histiocytic cells. The histiocytic cells have vesicular nuclei, prominent nucleoli, and abundant cytoplasm. Multinucleated giant cells are usually present in tumors with a prominent histiocytic component (Figs. 2.61 and 2.62). Based on electron microscopic and immunohistochemical studies, the histiocytic forms are derived from monocytes or histiocytes, while the origin of the fibrous types remains uncertain.

DIAGNOSIS. The presence of diffuse to circumscribed sarcomatous tumors with multinucleated giant cells and a spectrum of cell forms varying from histiocytic to pallisading fusiform cells are typical microscopic findings. *Differential diagnoses* include fibrosarcoma, lymphosarcoma, osteosarcoma, and granulomatous inflammatory tissue.

Mammary Tumors. Mammary tumors are a relatively common occurrence in older female rats, particularly the Sprague-Dawley (S-D) strain.

EPIZOOTIOLOGY AND PATHOGENESIS. The majority of mammary tumors (approximately 80–90%) are the relatively benign fibroadenoma, and most of the remainder are categorized as carcinomas. The benign tumors are particularly common in older S-D females. There are significant variations in the incidence, depending on the source of rats of this strain. Ranges of 7–40% have been recorded in S-D rats studied from different sources. This indicates that there is likely to be significant genetic variations over time, although dietary and environmental factors may have also played a role. In one study, restricting the food intake by 20% reduced the incidence of mammary tumors in female S-D rats by 5-fold, compared with controls. Prolactin levels have also been identified as a key factor. In another study, the serum prolactin values in females with mammary tumors were over 25 times higher than in 6-mo-old virgin females. There have been attempts to equate mammary tumors with the incidence of pituitary adenomas, but unequivocal correlations have not been made. Unlike mammary tumors in mice, retroviruses do not appear to be involved. Based on current knowledge, it appears that sex, age, genetic, dietary, and endocrine factors may all play a role in the incidence of spontaneous mammary tumors. Mammary fibroadenomas also occur occasionally in male rats. The incidence of spontaneous mammary fibroadenomas is markedly reduced in ovarectomized rats.

Regarding their biological behavior, mammary fibroadenomas may become very large and infil-

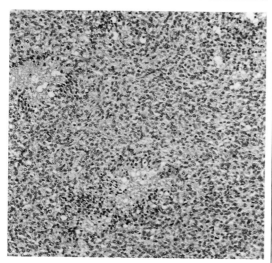

FIG. 2.61—Histiocytic sarcoma in Wistar rat. Note the indistinct cytoplasmic outlines, anisokaryosis, and pleomorphic appearance of the histiocytic cells. (Courtesy Z.W. Wojcinski)

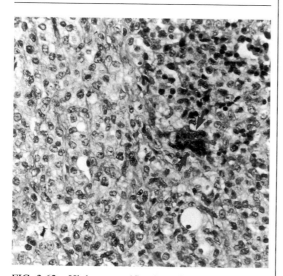

FIG. 2.62—Higher magnification of Figure 2.61, illustrating anisokaryosis and multinucleated giant cells (*arrows*). (Courtesy Z.W. Wojcinski)

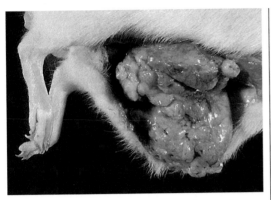

FIG. 2.63—Spontaneous case of fibroadenoma in adult female Sprague-Dawley rat. The prominent lobulations and interlobular fibrous tissue are characteristic gross findings seen with this neoplasm.

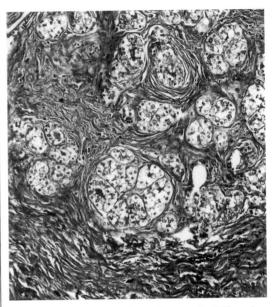

FIG. 2.64—Low-power photomicrograph of fibroadenoma, illustrating the acinar structures and connective tissue components.

trate locally, but they rarely metastasize. They are transplantable by subcutaneous implantation to recipients of the same strain.

PATHOLOGY. At necropsy, a circumscribed, movable, firm, lobulated mass may be located within any of the 12 mammary glands along the mammary chain. They occur occasionally at other sites on the body. In larger tumors, there may be fixation and ulceration of the overlying skin. The lobulated appearance is readily evident on cut surface (Fig. 2.63).

On microscopic examination, there is distinct interlobular and intralobular connective tissue surrounding relatively well-differentiated acinar structures. There are variable proportions of acinar and collagenous tissue. In some cases, the mass may consist primarily of connective tissue, with scattered acinar structures. In other fibroadenomas, epithelial components predominate (Figs. 2.64 and 2.65). Acini are lined by cuboidal epithelial cells, frequently with prominent vacuoles in the cytoplasm.

DIAGNOSIS. The histological pattern and the nature of the tumor, particularly in older female S-D rats, are sufficient to confirm the diagnosis.

SIGNIFICANCE. Mammary fibroadenomas are the most common tumor in female S-D rats. In pet animals, surgical removal is feasible, provided that the mass is not too large for complete excision. However, in both females and males, tumors are likely to recur in another mammary gland.

In the past, **malignant mammary tumors** have represented a relatively small percentage of mammary tumors in the laboratory rat. However, diagnostic pathologists in some laboratories have reported an increase in malignant mammary tumors in this species. Mammary adenocarcinomas have also been produced experimentally by estrogen administration. A variety of patterns may be evident histologically. They have been classified by various terms, including "anaplastic adenocarcinoma" (Fig. 2.66), "cribriform," "tubular," "papillary," and "comedocarcinoma."

Pituitary Gland Tumors. Pituitary adenoma is one of the more common tumors that occur in older animals, particularly in strains such as the Sprague-Dawley and Wistar rat. In addition to age, genetic factors, diet, and breeding history may also play a role. Reduction in food intake reduces the incidence of spontaneous pituitary tumors, and in another study, mated females had a lower incidence of pituitary tumors than did virgin females. In some studies, there is a slightly higher incidence in females, but this is not a consistent finding. Clinical signs vary, from animals

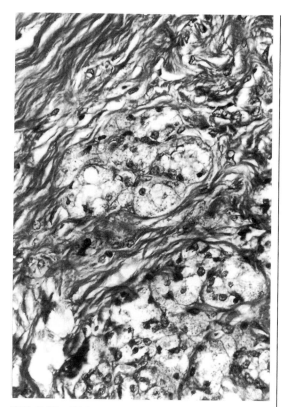

FIG. 2.65—Higher magnification of Figure 2.64, demonstrating the relatively well-differentiated vacuolated epithelial cells lining acini and the prominent intralobular collagenous tissue.

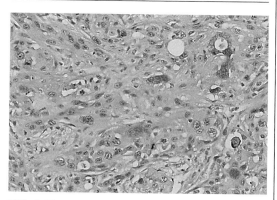

FIG. 2.66—Anaplastic mammary adenocarcinoma in adult female rat. Note the sheets of infiltrating poorly differentiated epithelial cells.

that are asymptomatic to animals with severe depression, frequently with incoordination. The majority of pituitary tumors are interpreted to be chromophobe adenomas. Acidophil and basophil tumors have also been described. However, immunohistochemical techniques are required for positive identification. In pituitary tumors studied by immunocytochemistry, prolactin-producing tumors are the most common type. Most tumors are interpreted to arise from the pars distalis, although tumors of the pars intermedia have also been described. Pituitary carcinomas are relatively uncommon.

PATHOLOGY. At necropsy, the pituitary is enlarged, frequently with prominent lobulations. The tumor is often dark red to brown and hemorrhagic in appearance (Fig. 2.67). In larger tumors, there may be minimal to marked compression of the overlying mesencephalon. On microscopic examination, the anterior pituitary consists of

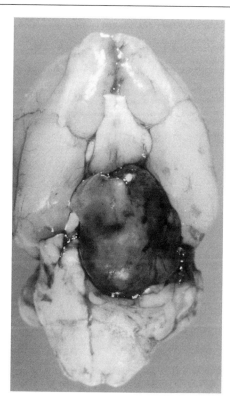

FIG. 2.67—Pituitary gland adenoma in aged female Wistar rat. Note the variable color of the large fleshy mass.

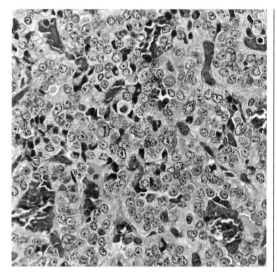

FIG. 2.68—Histological section of spontaneous pituitary adenoma, with prominent cords of epithelial cells interspersed within a vascular stroma.

cords or nests of glandular cells bound by strands of connective tissue, with an abundant cavernous vascular capillary network. The cells typically have large nuclei and prominent nucleoli, with abundant, lightly basophilic to amphophilic cytoplasm consistent with a chromophobe adenoma (Fig. 2.68). Giant nuclei may be present in the mass. Mitotic figures are occasionally observed. A pseudocapsule composed of a fine band of connective tissue separates the tumor from the adjacent, nontransformed pituitary tissue. More than one adenoma may be present in an affected gland. Frequently there is evidence of hemorrhage within the mass, and hemosiderin pigment may be present in some tumors.

DIAGNOSIS. The presence of an enlarged pituitary gland composed of nests and cords of large, relatively uniform glandular cells, with an abundant capillary network and occasionally hemorrhage, is a typical finding, and consistent with a diagnosis of pituitary adenoma. *Differential diagnoses:* It is necessary to distinguish pituitary adenomas from hyperplastic and hypertrophic lesions. Hyperplastic changes are characterized by the proliferation of cells of normal size, with no evidence of pseudo capsule formation or marked compression of adjacent pituitary tissue. Nodules of hypertrophic cells may be present in glands and must be differentiated from adenomas. They occur as islands of large cells, sometimes with mitoses, but there is no evidence of encapsulation.

SIGNIFICANCE. Pituitary adenomas are relatively common in aged female and male rats. Attempts

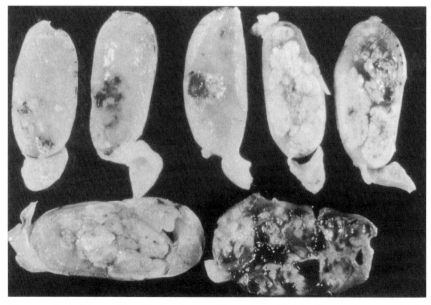

FIG. 2.69—Testes collected from older F344 male rats, illustrating a high incidence of interstitial (Leydig) cell tumors. There are multiple circumscribed masses, with accompanying hemorrhage. (Courtesy M.A. Hayes)

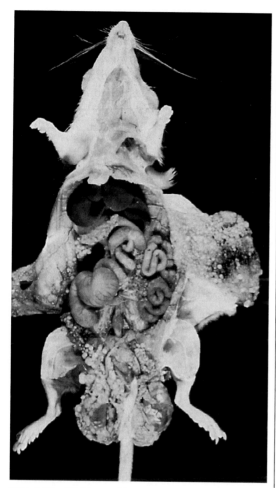

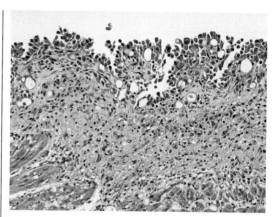

FIG. 2.71—Heart from mesothelioma depicted in Figure 2.70. On the pericardium, note the papillary structures lined by exfoliating mesothelial cells, with fibrous tissue proliferation in the underlying epicardium.

FIG. 2.70—F344 rat with diffuse mesothelioma involving both the abdominal and thoracic cavities. Note the multiple raised circumscribed polypoid lesions on the serosal surfaces.

have been made to correlate prolactin-producing pituitary tumors with an increased incidence of mammary fibroadenomas, but to date this has not been resolved.

Testicular Tumors

INTERSTITIAL CELL TUMORS. These tumors most frequently occur in F344 rats, and they are present in most older males of this strain. On gross examination, they appear as circumscribed, lobulated, light yellow to hemorrhagic single or multiple masses involving one or both testes (Fig. 2.69). Microscopic changes are consistent with tumors of Leydig cell origin.

Masses normally consist of sheets of cells of two types: polyhedral to elongated cells with granular to vacuolated cytoplasm and smaller cells with hyperchromatic nuclei and scanty cytoplasm.

SIGNIFICANCE. In addition to their frequent occurrence in aged male rats, particularly the F344 strain, interstitial cell tumors have been associated with concurrent hypercalcemia.

Mesothelioma. These neoplasms are occasionally encountered in laboratory rats, particularly the F344 strain. Affected rats frequently present with ascites, and at necropsy, usually there are multiple raised circumscribed yellow to brown nodules present in both the peritoneal and pleural cavities (Figs. 2.70 and 2.71). In most cases the primary site is interpreted to be the tunica vaginalis of the testes, with subsequent implantation on the serosal surfaces of the peritoneal and pleural cavities. Microscopically, there are diffuse to nodular aggregations of cuboidal to polyhedral cells on serosal surfaces. *Differential diagnoses* include chronic peritonitis associated with intraperitoneal experimental procedures or chronic bacterial infections, as well as polyarteritis.

Zymbal's Gland Tumors. These tumors occur in the holocrine gland located at the base of the

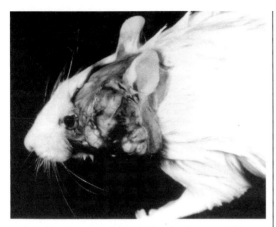

FIG. 2.72—Lobulated Zymbal's gland tumor arising from glands at the external ear canal in adult rat.

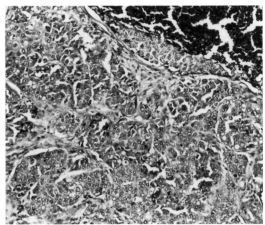

FIG. 2.74—Higher magnification than Figure 2.73 of another Zymbal's gland carcinoma, illustrating the trabecular and acinar patterns formed by the malignant epithelial cells.

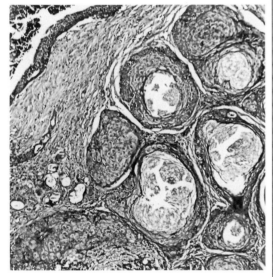

FIG. 2.73—Zymbal's gland adenocarcinoma. Note the polyhedral cells and the formation of acinarlike structures containing keratinized material and debris.

Other Neoplasms. Other neoplasms that occur in the laboratory rat include thyroid tumors, particularly parafollicular cell types, tumors of the skin and adnexae, and neoplastic liver nodules.

BIBLIOGRAPHY FOR NEOPLASMS

Lymphoreticular Tumors

Abbott, D.P., et al. 1983. Mononuclear cell leukemia in aged Sprague-Dawley rats. Vet. Pathol. 20:434–39.

Barsoum, N.J., et al. 1984. Histiocytic sarcoma in Wistar rats. Arch. Pathol. Lab. Med. 108:802–7.

Goodman, D.G., et al. 1980. Neoplastic and non-neoplastic lesions in aging Osborne-Mendel rats. Toxicol. Appl. Pharmacol. 55:433–47.

Graves, P., et al. 1982. Spontaneous rat malignant tumors of fibrohistocytic origin: An ultrastructural study. Vet. Pathol. 19:497–505.

Jones, T.C., et al., eds. 1990. *Monographs on Pathology of Laboratory Animals: Hematopoietic System.* New York: Springer-Verlag.

Prats, M., et al. 1994. Epidermotropic cutaneous lymphoma (Mycosis fungoides) in an SD rat. Vet. Pathol. 31:396–98.

Rosol, T.J., and Stromberg, P.C. 1990. Effects of large granular lymphocytic leukemia on bone in F344 rats. Vet. Pathol. 27:391–96.

Squire, R.A., et al. 1981. Histiocytic sarcoma with a granuloma-like component occurring in a large colony of Sprague-Dawley rats. Am. J. Pathol. 106:21–30.

Stromberg, P.C., et al. 1990. Spleen cell population changes and hemolytic anemia in F344 rats with large granular lymphocytic leukemia. Vet. Pathol. 27:397–403.

external ear. On gross examination, there is a circumscribed mass, frequently with ulceration of the overlying skin (Fig. 2.72). On microscopic examination, the mass consists of sheets of epithelial cells with abundant, vacuolated cytoplasm, frequently with foci of necrosis and leukocytic infiltration (Figs. 2.73 and 2.74). Depending on their histological pattern, they are classified as adenomas or adenocarcinomas. The malignant tumors are locally invasive, but not metastatic.

———. 1985. Behavior of transplanted large granular lymphocytic leukemia in Fischer 344 rats. Lab. Invest. 53:200–207.

Ward, J.M., and Reynolds, C.W. 1983. Large granular lymphatic leukemia. A heterogeneous lymphocytic leukemia in F344 rats. Am. J. Pathol. III:1–10.

Mammary Tumors

Barsoum, N.J., et al. 1984. Morphologic features and incidence of spontaneous hyperplastic and neoplastic mammary gland lesions in Wistar rats. Toxicol. Pathol. 12:26–38.

Hotchkiss, C.E. 1995. Effect of surgical removal of subcutaneous tumors on survival of rats. J. Am. Vet. Med. Assoc. 206:1575–77

Ito, A., et al. 1984. Prolactin and aging: X-irradiated and estrogen-induced rat mammary tumorigenesis. J. Natl. Cancer Inst. 73:123–26.

MacKenzie, W.F., and Garner, F.M. 1973. Comparison of neoplasms from six sources of rats. J. Natl. Cancer Inst. 50:1243–57.

Okada, M., et al. 1981. Characteristics of 106 spontaneous mammary tumours appearing in Sprague-Dawley female rats. Br. J. Cancer 43:689–95.

Russo, J., et al. 1989. Classification of neoplastic and nonneoplastic lesions of the rat mammary gland. In *Monographs on Pathology of Laboratory Animals: Integument and Mammary Glands,* ed. T.C. Jones et al., pp. 275–304. New York: Springer-Verlag.

Tucker, M.J. 1979. The effects of long term food restriction on tumors in rodents. Br. J. Cancer 23:803–7.

Pituitary Gland Tumors

Carlton, W.W., and Gries, C.L. 1986a. Adenoma, pars intermedia, anterior pituitary, rat. In *Monographs on Pathology of Laboratory Animals: Endocrine System,* ed. T.C. Jones et al., pp. 145–49. New York: Springer-Verlag.

———. 1986b. Adenoma and carcinoma, pars distalis, rat. In *Monographs on Pathology of Laboratory Animals: Endocrine System,* ed. T.C. Jones et al., pp. 134–45. New York: Springer-Verlag.

McComb, D.J., et al. 1984. Pituitary adenomas in old Sprague-Dawley rats: A histologic, ultrastructural, and immunohistochemical study. J. Natl. Cancer Inst. 73:1143–66.

Nagatani, M., et al. 1987. Relationship between cellular morphology and immunocytological findings of spontaneous pituitary tumours in the aged rat. J. Comp. Pathol. 97:11– 20.

Pickering, C.E., and Pickering, R.G. 1984a. The effect of repeated reproduction on the incidence of pituitary tumours in Wistar rats. Lab. Anim. 18:371–78.

———. 1984b. The effect of diet on the incidence of pituitary tumours in female Wistar rats. Lab. Anim. 18:298–314.

Sandusky, G.E., et al. 1988. An immunocytochemical study of pituitary adenomas and focal hyperplasia

in old Sprague-Dawley and Fischer rats. Toxicol. Pathol. 16:376–80.

Tucker, M.J. 1979. The effects of long term food restriction on tumours in rodents. Br. J. Cancer 23:803–7.

Testicular Tumors

Goodman, D.G., et al. 1979. Neoplastic and nonneoplastic lesions in aging F344 rats. Toxicol. Appl. Pharmacol. 48:237–48.

Troyer, H., et al. 1982. Leydig cell tumor induced hypercalcemia in the Fischer rat. Am. J. Pathol. 108:284–90.

General Bibliography

Boorman, G.A., and DeLellis, R.A. 1983. C cell adenoma, thyroid, rat. In *Monographs on Pathology of Laboratory Animals: Endocrine System,* ed. T.C. Jones et al., pp. 197–200. New York: Springer-Verlag.

Boorman, G.A., et al. 1990. *Pathology of the Fischer Rat: Reference and Atlas.* New York: Academic.

Burek, J.D. 1978. *Pathology of Aging Rats.* Boca Raton, Fla.: CRC.

Goelz, M.F., et al. 1993. Pleural and peritoneal nodules in a Fischer 344 rat (Diagnostic exercise). Lab. Anim. Sci. 43: 616–18.

Goodman, D.G., et al. 1980. Neoplastic and nonneoplastic lesions in aging Osborne-Mendel rats. Toxicol. Appl. Pharmacol. 55:433–47.

———. 1979. Neoplastic and nonneoplastic lesions in aging F344 rats. Toxicol. Appl. Pharmacol. 48:237–48.

MacKenzie, W.F., and Garner, F.M. 1973. Comparison of neoplasms from six sources of rats. J. Natl. Cancer Inst. 50:1243–57.

McMartin, D.N., et al. 1992. Neoplasms and related proliferative lesions in control Sprague-Dawley rats from carcinogenicity studies. Historical data and diagnostic considerations. Tox. Path. 20: 212–25.

Schuh, J.C.L., and Wojcinski, Z.W. 1996. Kidney masses in Wistar rats (Diagnostic exercise). Lab. Anim. Sci. 46:98–100.

Squire, R.A., et al. 1978. Tumors. In *Pathology of Laboratory Animals,* ed. K. Benirschke et al., pp. 1052–1283. New York: Springer-Verlag.

Stewart, H.L., et al. 1980. Histologic typing of liver tumors of the rat. J. Natl. Cancer Inst. 64:180–206.

Turusov, V.S., et al., eds. 1976. *The Pathology of Tumours in Laboratory Animals. I. Tumours of the Rat.* Lyon, France: IARC Scientific Publications.

Zwicker, G.M., et al. 1992a. Spontaneous skin neoplasms in aged Sprague-Dawley rats. Tox. Path. 20:327–340.

———. 1992b. Spontaneous brain and spinal cord/nerve neoplasms in aged Sprague-Dawley rats. Tox. Path. 20:576–84.

———. 1992c. Spontaneous renal neoplasms in aged Crl:CD BR rats. Tox. Path. 20:125–30.

———. 1992d. Naturally occurring intestinal epithelial neoplasms in aged CRL:CD BR rats. Tox. Path. 20: 253-259.

A number of different genera and species of hamsters are used in the research laboratory: the Syrian or golden hamster (*Mesocricetus auratus*); Chinese or gray hamster (*Cricetulus griseus*); European or black-bellied hamster (*Cricetus cricetus*); Armenian or migratory hamster (*Cricetulus migratorius*); Dzungarian, Siberian, dwarf, striped hairy-footed hamster (*Phodopus sungorus*); South African hamster or white-tailed rat (*Mystromys albicaudatus*); and others. However, the majority of those used in research are the Syrian and Chinese hamsters. Most of the Syrian hamsters that are now so commonly used in the research laboratory and kept as pets appear to have originated from a litter captured in Syria in 1930. The original animals were bred in captivity at Hebrew University, and their offspring later served as the foundation stock for *Mesocricetus auratus* in other countries. Although often referred to as outbred, Syrian hamsters are understandably genetically homozygous. It has been claimed that Syrian hamsters are so inbred that they can accept tissue transplants among one another. *Cricetulus griseus* was first domesticated in Beijing, China, around 1920. Based on clinical assessment, Syrian hamsters are susceptible to a number of serious enteric microbial infections, are remarkably susceptible to a number of xenogeneic viruses, and are prone to induction of tumors with many such viruses. This is likely to be due to a limited major histocompatibility complex (MHC) repertoire resulting from their highly inbred nature. The life span of the Syrian hamster varies from 1–3 yr. Female Syrian hamsters are hyperactive during estrus and are capable of traveling a considerable distance during this period (Richards 1966). This chapter deals primarily with diseases of the Syrian hamster. Very little is known about diseases of other types of hamsters, and it must be kept in mind that generalizations cannot be made, since hamsters represent different, distantly related genera.

ANATOMIC FEATURES

The anatomy of the Syrian hamster has been thoroughly reviewed by Bivin et al. (1987) and Magalhaes (1968). Hamsters have a characteristic, compact body, short legs, and very short tails. They possess four digits on the front feet and five on the rear feet. Syrian hamsters have remarkably abundant and loose skin. Adult females are larger than males. The female urethra has a separate opening from the vagina. Both sexes possess paired flank organs, which are most prominent in males. These organs consist of sebaceous glands, pigment cells, and terminal hair. They are darkly pigmented in mature males and appear to play a role in conversion of testosterone to dihydrotestosterone. Hamsters have prominent depots of brown fat beneath and between the scapulae, in the axilla and neck, and around the adrenals and kidneys. The gastrointestinal tract has a number of significant features. As in mice and rats, the incisors (but not the molars) grow continuously. Many, although not all, genera of hamsters possess buccal pouches, which extend dorsolaterally from the oral cavity on either side of the shoulder region. These structures have been utilized as immunologically privileged sites, which allow xenograft transplants to survive. The utility of hamster cheek pouches as an experimental tool has been largely supplanted by the athymic nude mouse. The stomach is divided into nonglandular and glandular segments, which are divided by a muscular sphincter. Paneth cells are a normal constituent of small intestinal crypts. The cecum is divided into apical and basal portions separated by a semilunar valve. In fact, there are a series of four valves in the ileococolic region of the hamster. The liver is divided into four lobes, with a gallbladder. As in the mouse and rat, intranuclear cytoplasmic invagination (inclusions) and eosinophilic cytoplasmic inclusions in hepatocytes can be found, particularly in diseased livers. The respiratory tract is similar to that of mice, rats, and guinea pigs, with no respiratory bronchioles. Lungs have a single left lobe and five lobes on the right side (cranial, middle, caudal, intermediate, and accessory). As desert animals, Syrian hamsters have water-conserving kidneys with elongated single papillae that extend into the ureters. The female reproductive tract consists of a duplex uterus with two cervical canals that merge into a single external cervical os. There are seven pairs of mammary glands. The male testes and accessory glands, as with most rodents, are comparatively large and prominent. Adult males develop large adrenal glands, due to enlargement of the zona reticularis to three times the size of females. This enlargement is related to season and sexual maturity. The hamster placenta differs somewhat from the hemochorial placentation of other laboratory rodents and is termed "labyrinthine hemochorial." Trophoblastic giant cells of the fetal placenta are in direct contact with the maternal bloodstream and tend to migrate in the maternal tissues. They have a tropism for arterial, not venous, blood and can be found inside uterine vessels and arteries in the mesometrium (Fig. 3.1). They can persist for up to 3 wk postpartum.

Polychromasia is relatively common in hamster erythrocytes, with moderate anisocytosis. Erythrocyte life spans vary from 50 to 78 days. Life spans are increased during hibernation. Leukocyte counts are 5000–10,000 ml^3. Approximately 60–75% of the circulating leukocytes are lymphocytes. Neutrophils have densely staining eosinophilic granules and thus may be referred to as heterophils.

BIBLIOGRAPHY FOR INTRODUCTION AND ANATOMIC FEATURES

Bivin, W.S., et al. 1987. Morphophysiology. In *Laboratory Hamsters,* ed. G.L. Van Hoosier, Jr., and C.W. McPherson, pp. 9–41. New York: Academic.

Burek, J.R., et al. 1979. The pregnant hamster as a model to study intravascular trophoblasts and associated maternal blood vessel changes. Vet. Pathol. 16:553–66.

Clark, J.D. 1987. Historical perspectives and taxonomy. In *Laboratory Hamsters,* ed. G.L. Van Hoosier, Jr., and C.W. McPherson, pp. 3–7. New York: Academic.

Magalhaes, H. 1968. Gross Anatomy. In *The Golden Hamster: Its Biology and Use in Medical Research,* pp. 91–109. Ames: Iowa State University Press.

Richards, M.P.M. 1966. Activity measured by running wheels and observations during the oestrous cycle, pregnancy and pseudopregnancy in the golden hamster. Anim. Behav. 14:450–58.

Thomson, F.N., and Wardrop, K.J. 1987. Clinical chemistry and hematology. In *Laboratory Hamsters,* ed. G.L. Van Hoosier, Jr., and C.W. McPherson. pp. 43–59. New York: Academic.

VIRAL INFECTIONS

DNA VIRAL INFECTIONS

Adenoviral Infection. Adenoviral intranuclear inclusion bodies have been observed in ileal enterocytes in tissues collected from hamsters during the first few weeks of life. In addition, antibodies to the MAD-2 (K87) strain of mouse adenovirus are commonly present in hamsters from commercial suppliers in the United States.

PATHOLOGY. Large, amphophilic, intranuclear inclusions may be present in the enterocytes lining villi and goblet cells of the jejunum and ileum and, rarely, in the cryptal epithelial cells. In the typical case, animals are asymptomatic, and there is no evidence of intestinal tract damage or inflammatory response. To date, typical adenoviral inclusions have been observed only in hamsters less than 4 wk of age.

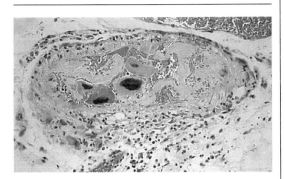

FIG. 3.1—Trophoblast epithelial cells present within mesometrial vessel in a pregnant hamster.

DIAGNOSIS. The presence of adenoviral infection may be confirmed by electron microscopy and serology.

SIGNIFICANCE. Infected hamsters are considered to be asymptomatic, and the significance of the infection in this species is currently unknown.

Cytomegaloviral Infection. Cytomegalovirus-like lesions have been observed in salivary glands of subclinically infected Chinese hamsters. Intranuclear and intracytoplasmic inclusions with cytomegaly occur in the acinar epithelium of the submaxillary salivary glands. Cytomegaloviruses are generally considered to be host-specific, but the relationship of the hamster agent to cytomegaloviruses of other species has not been defined.

Parvoviral Infection. An epizootic of high mortality with malformed and missing incisors has been observed among suckling and weaning pups in a breeding colony of Syrian hamsters. Necrosis and inflammation of the dental pulp with mononuclear leukocytic infiltration of the dental lamina and osteoclasis of alveolar bone was noted. This epizootic was associated with seroconversion to Toolan H-1 virus, a parvovirus of rats that has previously been shown to cause facial and dental deformities in experimentally infected neonatal hamsters. Seroconversion to both rat virus and H-1 virus occurs without disease in hamsters.

More recently, an outbreak of disease in a commercial breeding colony of Syrian hamsters was attributed to a newly recognized parvovirus. The epizootic was confined to suckling and weanling hamsters. Affected animals typically presented with domed calvaria, a pot-bellied appearance, marked discoloration and malformation of the incisor teeth, and high mortality. On microscopic examination, lesions associated with the infection included enamel hypoplasia of the incisor teeth, periodontitis, suppuration with mineralization of the dental pulp, multifocal hemorrhage, multifocal cerebral mineralization, and testicular atrophy with multifocal necrosis and mineralization of cells lining seminiferous tubules. A similar pattern of disease with mortality was observed in suckling SPF hamsters inoculated with this isolate. Based on polymerase chain reaction (PCR) assays, the hamster parvovirus is distinct from the rodent parvoviruses minute virus of mice (MVM), rat H-1 parvovirus (H-1), and Kilham rat virus (RV), but closely related to the mouse parvovirus MPV-1. Whether the Syrian hamster or another rodent is the natural host for this virus is currently not known. The proposed HaPV designation for the isolate will undoubtedly cause confusion, since the same term (HaPV) is currently in use for the hamster polyoma virus.

Polyoma Viral Infection: Transmissible Lymphoma. Hamster polyoma virus (HaPV) belongs to the polyoma virus subgroup of Papoviridae. It is structurally and biologically very similar to polyoma virus of mice but is a distinctly different virus (see Chap. 1). HaPV has suffered a longstanding history of misunderstanding. It is the cause of transmissible lymphoma, which can occur in epizootics among young hamsters, of keratinizing skin tumors of hair follicle origin, or of subclinical infections. This agent has erroneously been called hamster papillomavirus because of its ability to induce papilloma-like skin lesions. It clearly does not belong to the papillomavirus subgroup of Papoviridae, and thus the name should not be used.

EPIZOOTIOLOGY AND PATHOGENESIS. HaPV is not common, but infections of Syrian and European hamster colonies have been reported on several occasions in the United States and Europe. The origin of these infections has not been definitively determined. HaPV is probably one of few truly hamster-origin agents, but its atypical virulence in Syrian hamsters is due to xenogeneic infection among distantly related hamster genera. It was probably introduced to laboratory Syrian hamsters in Eastern Europe through acquisition of wild European hamster stocks and mixing with laboratory Syrian hamsters. The biology of HaPV closely parallels that of polyoma virus of mice, but there are unique features peculiar to the hamster, especially its sensitivity to the oncogenic effects of DNA viruses in general. HaPV is probably spread by environmental contamination with infected urine. Like polyoma virus of mice, it causes a multisystemic infection with persistence in the kidney and shedding in the urine. This behavior is typical of many viruses of the polyoma virus subgroup, which infect a number of different species. Like polyoma virus of mice,

HaPV is also oncogenic, but tumor formation is a side effect of infection and not critical to the virus life cycle. HaPV infection can result in the formation of lymphomas and hair follicle epitheliomas in hamsters. Other types of tumors have not been described. Typical of polyoma viruses, HaPV can infect cells lytically with virus replication or transform cells without virus replication. Thus, lymphomas do not have detectable infectious virus. On the other hand, HaPV epitheliomas have HaPV replication in keratinizing epithelium, similar to the behavior of papillomaviruses. Polyoma virus of mice can cause similar virus-replicating skin tumors in mice as well, but unlike mice, hamsters are susceptible to the oncogenic effects of this virus (and other DNA viruses) beyond the neonatal period and following natural exposure.

With the above brief synopsis, the epizootiology of HaPV can be understood. When first introduced to a naive population of breeding hamsters, HaPV can result in epizootics of lymphoma, with attack rates as high as 80% among young hamsters within 4–30 wk postexposure, which is a diagnostic phenomenon, since lymphomas normally occur in very low incidence and only among aged hamsters. Infected hamsters may also have a variable incidence of epitheliomas, usually around the face and feet. Although the epitheliomas contain infectious virus, they are not necessary for virus transmission, which occurs primarily through the urine. Lymphomas do not contain infectious HaPV, but HaPV nucleic acid can be detected in their genome. Hamster leukemia virus particles also occur in these tumors, as they do in other tumors and normal tissues as an incidental finding. Once enzootic, the incidence of lymphoma declines to much lower levels because young hamsters are presumably protected from infection and the virus infects only older hamsters, which tend to resist the oncogenic effects. Infection of older hamsters results in a clinically silent infection with persistent viruria, typical of polyoma viruses. Enzootically infected hamsters, however, tend to develop a higher incidence of HaPV skin tumors than do hamsters during the epizootic form. These complex features have led to considerable confusion as to the etiology of transmissible lymphoma, including claims that it is caused by a DNA viroid–like agent. These claims have been refuted and the etiological role of HaPV confirmed. Barthold (1991) presents a thorough review of HaPV biology.

PATHOLOGY. Affected hamsters appear thin, often with palpable masses in their abdomens. Lymphomas usually arise in the mesentery without involvement of the spleen, but they can arise in axillary and cervical lymph nodes. Infiltration of liver, kidney, thymus, and other organs can also occur (Fig. 3.2). Tumors vary cytologically. They are usually lymphoid, but erythroblastic, reticulosarcomatous, and myeloid types have been described. Lymphoid tumors are variably differentiated, usually immature, although sometimes they have plasmacytoid features. Lymphomas of the abdomen have been shown to possess B-cell markers, and those of the thymus T-cell markers. Mesenteric masses involve the intestinal wall and lymph nodes, with necrosis of the central region. Infiltration of hepatic sinusoids is also common

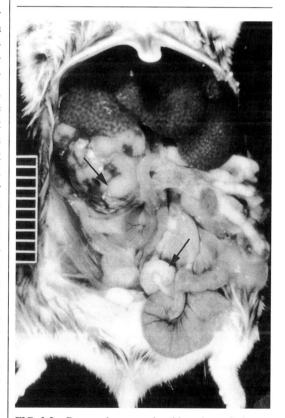

FIG. 3.2—Papovavirus-associated lymphoma in hamster. Note the marked enlargement of lymph nodes (*arrows*) in the abdominal cavity. (Courtesy Barthold et al. 1987, reprinted by permission)

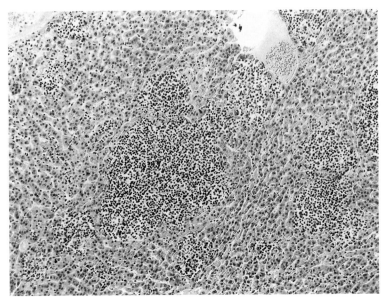

FIG. 3.3—Hepatic lesions associated with hamster papovavirus infection. Note the marked infiltration of neoplastic lymphoid cells in sinusoids.

(Fig. 3.3). Affected hamsters may also present few to many nodular masses involving nonglabrous skin. These lesions consist of keratinizing follicular structures reminiscent of trichoepitheliomas (Figs. 3.4 and 3.5).

DIAGNOSIS. Epizootic HaPV is unmistakable. Lymphoid tumors are otherwise rare in hamsters, and when they occur, it is usually in aged hamsters. As stated earlier, electron microscopy of lymphoid tumors in an effort to visualize HaPV is a vacuous exercise. Trichoepitheliomas have not been described in hamsters unless associated with HaPV. If present, they offer the opportunity to visualize HaPV crystalloids in the nucleus of keratinizing epithelial cells. A serological test for this virus is not available. *Differential diagnoses* must include transmissible ileal hyperplasia, which can cause palpable enlargement of the terminal ileum, spontaneous lymphoid tumors, and skin lesions such as *Demodex* folliculitis.

SIGNIFICANCE. HaPV can cause devastating epizootics, which have caused the total loss of some inbred strains of Syrian hamsters. Once enzootic, the virus cannot be effectively eliminated without slaughter of the entire population and thorough decontamination of the premises. Even under these circumstances, repeated outbreaks have been known to occur, possibly because of the resistance of the virus to environmental decontamination.

RNA VIRAL INFECTIONS

Arenaviral Infection: Lymphocytic Choriomeningitis (LCM). LCM virus is an arenavirus with a wide host range, including rodents and human and nonhuman primates. Its principal natural reservoir host is the wild mouse (see Chap. 1).

EPIZOOTIOLOGY AND PATHOGENESIS. Infection with LCM virus may occur by exposure to saliva or urine from animals shedding the virus. Portals of entry include the oronasal route and skin abrasions. Cage-to-cage transmission via aerosols does not appear to play an important role in spread. Congenital infections also occur in hamsters. Cell cultures or transplantable tumors contaminated with the virus are an important source of the virus in the laboratory. The patterns of disease that occur in hamsters postexposure will depend on the age of the animal, strain and dose of the virus, and route of administration. In one study, newborn hamsters were inoculated subcu-

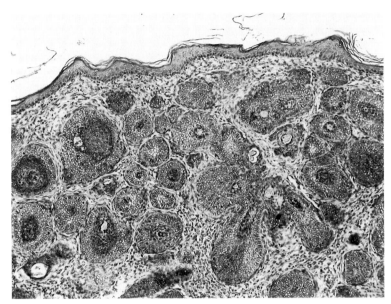

FIG. 3.4—Section of skin from hamster, illustrating trichoepithelioma associated with HaPV infection.

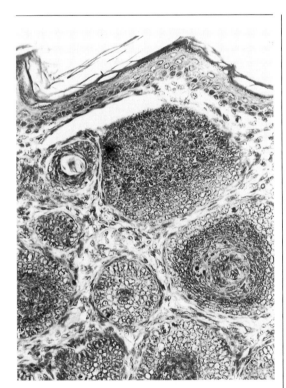

FIG. 3.5—Higher magnification of Figure 3.4. Note the prominent hair follicle formation.

taneously with LCM virus. Approximately half of the recipients cleared the virus, with minimal to moderate lymphocytic infiltration in the viscera. In the remaining inoculated animals, viremia and viruria persisted for approximately 3 and 6 mo, respectively. In addition, there was chronic wasting, and lymphocytic infiltration was observed in tissues such as liver, lung, spleen, meninges, and brain. Vasculitis and glomerulitis were present in hamsters examined histologically at 6 or more months postinoculation. Antigen-antibody complexes were demonstrated in arterioles and glomerular basement membranes.

SIGNIFICANCE. LCM virus–infected hamsters are recognized to be the primary source of the virus in human patients. Thus, the public health aspects are an important consideration. Epidemics of LCM have occurred in laboratory personnel exposed either to hamsters shedding virus or to infected cell lines. Pet hamsters are also the recognized source of virus in some human cases. In one outbreak reported in Europe, there were approximately 200 reported cases of LCM in humans after contact with subclinically infected pet hamsters. It was suggested that there may have been up to 4000 additional cases of exposure in pet owners after hamsters were distributed to homes nationwide from the supplier of infected animals. In human cases, sequelae postexposure may vary from subclinical infections to influenzalike symptoms. On rare occasions, viral meningitis or encephalomyelitis may occur.

DIAGNOSIS. Serology is the recognized method for confirming the diagnosis. Sera collected from hamsters infected early in life may have a high percentage of samples with anticomplementary activity, thus complicating interpretations if the complement fixation test is used. Hamsters that acquire LCM infections as adults usually seroconvert early in the disease and remain seropositive for a long period of time. The indirect fluorescent antibody test is one procedure recommended for serological testing.

Paramyxoviral Infections

PNEUMONIA VIRUS OF MICE (PVM). Laboratory hamsters, rats, and mice can be naturally infected with this paramyxovirus. In an early report, interstitial pneumonitis with consolidation was observed in hamsters inoculated with an infectious agent interpreted to be contaminated with PVM, but there are few details of the morphologic changes. Conventional colonies of hamsters may be seropositive, usually in the absence of clinical disease. Based on current information, it is evident that PVM infections in this species normally go unrecognized as a subclinical event. Thus the significance of PVM infection in hamsters is currently unknown; it does, however, represent a potential complicating factor, particularly in research related to respiratory function.

DIAGNOSIS. In suspected cases of pneumonitis due to Sendai virus or PVM, the demonstration of seroconversion is the most practical method to confirm the diagnosis. *Differential diagnoses* would include alveolar changes secondary to congestive heart failure.

SENDAI VIRUS. Based on serological surveys, Sendai virus infections are relatively widespread in some colonies of hamsters. However, there are few reports of confirmed clinical disease due to Sendai virus infections in this species. Seronegative hamsters introduced into a facility housing infected rodents may seroconvert, but it is unlikely that any clinical signs will be observed,

although there are reports of mortality in newborn Syrian and Chinese hamsters. Currently mice, rats, and hamsters are regarded as the natural hosts for Sendai virus.

Young adult Syrian hamsters inoculated intranasally with Sendai virus remained asymptomatic during the course of the study, although there were transient changes in the upper and lower respiratory tract evident by light microscopy, and virus was recoverable from the lung during the acute stages of the disease. Hamsters seroconverted by day 7 postinoculation. In general, most lesions had resolved by 12 days postinfection. In animals examined at 3–9 days postinoculation, lesions were very similar to those present in mice. There is a focal to segmental rhinitis progressing to necrotizing tracheitis, multifocal bronchitis, and bronchoalveolitis (Figs. 3.6 and 3.7). In the reparative stages, features include hyperplasia of epithelial cells lining affected airways and peribronchial lymphocytic infiltration.

Viral Infections of Uncertain Significance. Laboratory Syrian hamsters seroconvert to mouse encephalomyelitis virus, reovirus 3 and SV5 (a paramyxovirus), and parvoviruses of the rat (RV and H-1). Except for a single epizootic associated with H-1 virus (see Parvoviral Infection), disease has not been associated with these infections.

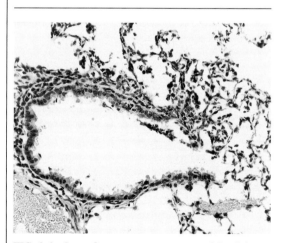

FIG. 3.6—Lung from spontaneous case of Sendai virus pneumonitis in Syrian hamster. There is a bronchoalveolitis with mobilization of alveolar macrophages.

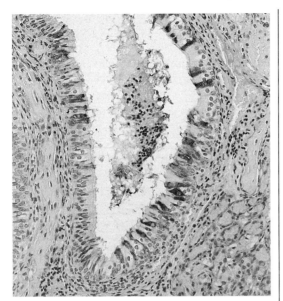

FIG. 3.7—Rhinitis in a Syrian hamster examined at 4 d postexposure to Sendai virus. Note the dark-staining viral antigen present in the cytoplasm of numerous ciliated epithelial cells. Immunoperoxidase stain.

Hamsters are also host to an endogenous retrovirus, which is expressed in tissues and cells as C-type particles without evidence of oncogenicity.

Virus-Associated Neoplasia. Newborn hamsters are recognized to be a sensitive in vivo test system to screen for potentially oncogenic viruses isolated from other mammalian species. A number of human adenoviruses have been shown to be oncogenic in young hamsters following experimental inoculation.

BIBLIOGRAPHY
FOR VIRAL INFECTIONS

DNA Viral Infections

Barthold, S.W. 1991. Hemolymphatic tumors. In *The Pathology of Tumours in Laboratory Animals, III. Tumours of the Hamster,* ed. U. Mohr et al. Lyon, France: IARC Scientific Publications.

Barthold, S.W., et al. 1987. Further evidence for papovavirus as the probable etiology of transmissible lymphoma of Syrian hamsters. Lab. Anim. Sci. 37:283–88.

Besselsen, D.G., et al. 1999. Natural and experimentally induced infection of Syrian hamsters with a newly recognized parvovirus. Lab. Anim. Sci. 49:308–12.

Gibson, S.V., et al. 1990. Naturally acquired enteric adenovirus infection in Syrian hamsters (*Mesocricetus auratus*). Am. J. Vet. Res. 51:143–47.

———. 1983. Mortality in weanling hamsters associated with tooth loss. Lab. Anim. Sci. 33:497.

Kuttner, A.G., and Wang, S. 1934. The problem of the significance of the inclusion bodies in the salivary glands of infants, and the occurrence of inclusion bodies in the submaxillary glands of hamsters, white mice and wild rats (Peiping). J. Exp. Med. 60:773–91.

Lussier, G. 1975. Murine cytomegalovirus (MCMV). Adv. Vet. Sci. Comp. Med. 19:223–47.

RNA Viral Infections
and General Bibliography

Bhatt, P.N., et al. 1986. Contamination of transplantable murine tumors with lymphocytic choriomeningitis virus. Lab. Anim. Sci. 36:136–39.

Biggar, R.J., et al. 1975. Lymphocytic choriomeningitis outbreak associated with pet hamsters: Fifty-seven cases from New York state. J. Am. Med. Assoc. 232:494–500.

Bowen, G.S., et al. 1975. Laboratory studies of a lymphocytic choriomeningitis virus outbreak in man and laboratory animals. J. Epidemiol. 102:233–40.

Carthew, P., et al. 1978. Incidence of natural virus infections of laboratory animals 1976–1977. Lab. Anim. 12:245–46.

Parker, J.C., and Richter, C.B. 1982. Viral diseases of the respiratory system. In *The Mouse in Biomedical Research, Vol. II. Diseases,* ed. H.L. Foster et al., pp. 107–55. New York: Academic.

Parker, J.C., et al. 1987. Viral diseases. In *Laboratory Hamsters,* ed. G.L. Van Hoosier, Jr., and C.W. McPherson, pp. 95–110. New York: Academic.

———. 1976. Lymphocytic choriomeningitis virus infection in fetal, newborn, and young adult Syrian hamsters (*Mesocricetus auratus*). Infect. Immun. 13:967–81.

Pearson, H.E., et al. 1940. A virus pneumonia of Syrian hamsters. Proc. Soc. Exp. Biol. Med. 45:677–79.

Percy, D.H., and Palmer, D. 1997. Experimental Sendai virus infection in the Syrian hamster. Lab. Anim Sci.47: 132–37.

Profeta, M.L., et al. 1969. Enzootic Sendai infection in laboratory hamsters. Am. J. Epidemiol. 89:316–24.

Reed, J.M., et al. 1974. Antibody levels to murine viruses in Syrian hamsters. Lab. Anim. Sci. 24:33–38.

Trentin, J.J. 1987. Experimental biology: Use in oncological research. In *Laboratory Hamsters,* ed. G.L. Van Hoosier, Jr., and C.W. McPherson. pp. 201–25. New York: Academic.

BACTERIAL AND MYCOTIC INFECTIONS

BACTERIAL ENTERIC INFECTIONS

Campylobacter jejuni **(***Lawsonia***) Infection.** *Campylobacter fetus* ssp. *jejuni* has been isolated on numerous occasions from clinically normal hamsters, as well as hamsters with enteritis. In one study, 24 of 30 hamsters acquired from pet stores were positive for *Campylobacter*. A few animals had watery diarrhea. Hamsters have been shown to be relatively resistant to experimental disease. Manipulations may be required in order to produce clinical disease consistently in inoculated animals. Subclinically infected hamsters may shed the organism in the feces for up to several months. An outbreak of enterocecocolitis with mortality in a breeding colony of Syrian hamsters was attributed to concomitant infections with *E. coli* and *Campylobacter*–like organisms. Adults were most frequently affected, and the cecum and colon were primarily involved.

SIGNIFICANCE. *Campylobacter*–infected hamsters represent a zoonotic threat to both pet owners and laboratory animal personnel. Confusion has reigned over *Campylobacter* and its role in proliferative ileitis (see *Lawsonia intracellularis* Infection, below). *Campylobacter* (*Lawsonia*) can be isolated in cell-free medium and does not cause proliferative ileitis, although it may be a co-infecting pathogen during proliferative ileitis.

Clostridium difficile Infections: Clostridial Enteropathies

ANTIBIOTIC-ASSOCIATED ENTEROCOLITIS. Antibiotics that have been associated with enterocolitis in hamsters include lincomycin, clindamycin, ampicillin, vancomycin, erythromycin, cephalosporins, gentamicin, and penicillin. In general, profuse diarrhea, with high mortality, occurs within 2–10 days following the oral or parenteral administration of certain narrow spectrum antibiotics.

PATHOGENESIS. The predominant bacterial flora in the hamster intestine are *Lactobacillus* and *Bacteroides*. Following therapy with certain narrow spectrum antibiotics, overgrowth with *Clostridium difficile* occurs, resulting in acute colitis, diarrhea, and death. In hamsters treated orally with vancomycin, the mortality rates may approach 100%. The oral administration of cecal contents from normal animals following vancomycin treatment has provided protection to the majority of recipients. Change may be precipi-

tated by the loss of gram-negative anaerobes or other clostridia following antibiotic treatment. This alteration of the "inhibitory barrier" may then allow colonization of *C. difficile* and elaboration of the toxin. Fatal typhlitis attributed to *C. difficile* has been observed in hamsters housed in the same room as antibiotic-treated hamsters. There is also some evidence that *C. difficile* may occur as an endogenous infection, and the organism has been isolated from the intestinal tract of normal hamsters. Deaths following antibiotic treatment have been attributed to the overgrowth of endogenous *C. difficile*.

PATHOLOGY. At necropsy, the cecum is distended with fluid contents, with extensive hemorrhage into the gut wall. Histopathology may reveal lesions varying from mild typhlitis to acute pseudomembranous typhlitis. Microscopic cecal changes include effacement of the mucosal epithelium, edema of the lamina propria, leukocytic infiltration, and mucosal hyperplasia. There may be some involvement of the terminal ileum and colon.

DIAGNOSIS. *C. difficile* should be recoverable on anaerobic culture. The cytotoxin may be demonstrated in intestinal contents by cell culture or mouse inoculation. The cytotoxin produced by this *Clostridium* may be neutralized by the homologous antitoxin or by *C. sordelli* antitoxin. For additional information, see Small (1987). *Differential diagnoses* include salmonellosis, enteropathogenic *Escherichia coli* infections, and Tyzzer's disease.

Non–Antibiotic-Associated Clostridial Enteropathy. Enteritis of acute onset with mortality has been associated with *Clostridium difficile* infection in hamsters with no previous history of antibiotic therapy. Necrotizing typhlitis with mucosal damage is the characteristic microscopic finding (Fig. 3.8). *C. difficile* cytotoxin may be demonstrated in cecal contents of affected hamsters. In another study, hamsters fed an atherogenic diet with a high fat content developed profuse diarrhea associated with a toxigenic strain of *C. difficile*. Enteritis with acute hemorrhagic typhlitis was evident at post mortem. In a subsequent study, the clostridial infection recurred in animals fed the

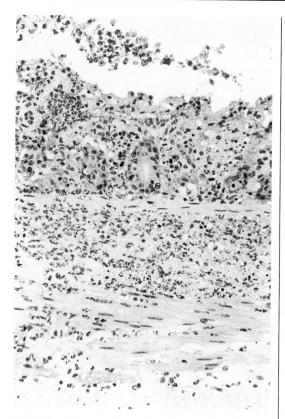

FIG. 3.8—Microscopic section of cecum from hamster with spontaneous clostridial enteropathy not associated with prior antibiotic treatment. There is a necrotizing typhlitis with mucosal effacement and leukocytic infiltration.

atherogenic diet, but not in control animals fed a normal diet. Whether the pathogenesis of this clostridial enteropathy was due to disruption of the gut flora and/or increased susceptibility of hamsters fed this abnormal diet is yet to be determined.

Cecal Mucosal Hyperplasia of Unknown Etiology. Spontaneous cases of cecal hyperplasia have been observed in suckling and weanling hamsters. Diarrhea, runting, and high mortality were associated with the disease. At necropsy, ceca are congested, contracted, and opaque. Microscopic changes observed in the cecum included increased mitotic activity and hyperplasia of enterocytes lining cecal crypts, as well as focal mucosal erosions. Bacterial cultures and ultrastructural studies failed to permit identification of a specific causative agent. The syndrome

probably represents the recovery phase of clostridial enteropathy.

***Clostridium piliforme* Infection: Tyzzer's Disease.** Epizootics of Tyzzer's disease have been observed in Syrian hamsters in various parts of the world. The causative agent, *Clostridium piliforme,* is a spore-forming bacillus that multiplies only within cells. The organism has a wide host range. (For additional details, see Tyzzer's disease in the rabbit, Chap. 6.)

EPIZOOTIOLOGY AND PATHOGENESIS. Hamsters may become infected by contact with affected animals or by contaminated bedding. Predisposing factors, such as poor sanitation, intestinal parasitism, and inappropriate feeding practices, may play a role in precipitating clinical outbreaks of the disease. Weanling hamsters are most often affected. In hamsters inoculated with infected liver homogenates, organisms and lesions are detectable in the mucosa of the small and large intestine by 3 days postinoculation, and multiple lesions and bacilli may be present in the liver by days 6–8 postexposure.

PATHOLOGY. At necropsy, there is a variable distribution of lesions. In some epizootics, lesions may be confined to either the liver or the intestinal tract. Multifocal hepatic necrosis is evident in some cases. Intestinal lesions, when evident grossly, usually involve the lower ileum, cecum, and colon and are associated with soiling of the perineum. Affected areas are edematous and dilated, with fluid contents. Microscopically, in the liver, there are foci of necrosis with leukocytic infiltration. Intracellular bundles of bacilli are usually best demonstrated at the periphery of hepatic lesions. When lesions are present in the intestinal tract, there is edema of the lamina propria, with polymorphonuclear cell infiltration and effacement of the mucosal architecture. There may be extension of the inflammatory process into the underlying muscular layers. Typical bacilli are usually demonstrable within enterocytes in the region (Fig. 3.9) and in hepatocytes adjacent to necrotic foci (Fig. 3.10). Focal granulomatous myocarditis, with conspicuous pale bulging nodules, has been associated with Tyzzer's disease in this species.

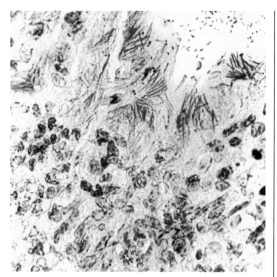

FIG. 3.9—Cecum from a spontaneous case of Tyzzer's disease in young hamster. There is an acute necrotizing typhlitis extending to the deeper layers. Bacilli are seen present in many enterocytes (Warthin-Starry stain). (Courtesy R.J. Hampson)

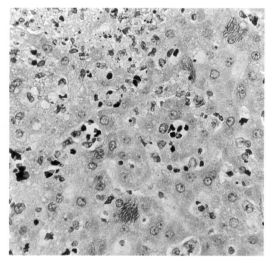

FIG. 3.10—Liver from a case of Tyzzer's disease in hamster (Warthin-Starry stain). Note the bundles of beaded bacilli in hepatocytes.

DIAGNOSIS. Confirmation of the diagnosis entails the demonstration of the typical intracellular bacilli in affected cells, using Warthin-Starry or Giemsa stains. *Differential diagnoses* include proliferative ileitis, salmonellosis, coliform enteritis, antibiotic-associated enterocolitis, and *Campylobacter* (*Lawsonia*) infections.

SIGNIFICANCE. Although documented cases of Tyzzer's disease are relatively rare, it does represent one cause of morbidity and mortality in hamsters. There is a possibility of interspecies transmission of the disease.

Escherichia coli Infection

EPIZOOTIOLOGY AND PATHOGENESIS. Isolates of *E. coli* from hamsters with enteritis have proven to be pathogenic when inoculated into susceptible recipient animals. Strains 1056, 1126, and 4165 have been isolated from naturally occurring cases of hamster enteritis. When inoculated into ligated intestinal loops to test for enteropathogenicity, the pathogenic strains produced changes in most of the inoculated weanling hamsters and in some of the adult animals.

One isolate of *E. coli,* strain 1056, has been recovered from ground ileal suspension prepared from a hamster with proliferative ileitis. Many of the weanling Syrian hamsters inoculated orally with this strain developed acute enteritis within 2 wk postinoculation. Animals inoculated with a nonenteropathogenic strain remained asymptomatic throughout the study.

PATHOLOGY. At necropsy, the small intestine may contain yellow to dark red fluid material. On microscopic examination, blunting and fusion of villi are frequently observed. Affected villi are lined by cuboidal epithelial cells. Degeneration and sloughing of enterocytes and polymorphonuclear cell infiltration in the lamina propria commonly occurs. In the mesenteric lymph nodes, changes may vary from lymphoid hyperplasia to diffuse polymorphonuclear cell infiltration. Focal coagulation necrosis in the liver, with polymorphonuclear cell infiltration, and gastric ulcers are other variable findings. Colitis and/or typhlitis may be present in some affected animals, sometimes with concomitant colonic intussusception. Ultrastructural studies of sections of ileum have revealed bacilli in the cytoplasm of enterocytes and blunting and irregularities in microvilli. *Differential diagnoses* include clostridial enterocolitis, *Lawsonia* proliferative ileitis, and salmonellosis.

SIGNIFICANCE. Enteropathogenic strains of *E. coli* may cause acute enteritis in weanling hamsters. It appears to be a different syndrome from proliferative ileitis, although concurrent *E. coli* infections may also play a role in this disease entity. Enterocecocolitis with mortality has been associated with infections with *E. coli* and *Campylobacter*–like organisms in adult hamsters.

***Helicobacter* sp. Infections.** A species of *Helicobacter* has been isolated from the gall bladders of Syrian hamsters with a high incidence of cholangiofibrosis. Based on sequence analysis of the 16S rDNA gene, the isolates were closely related to *H. pametensis,* and the name *H. cholecystis* has been proposed. Whether the organism plays a role in the development of the chronic biliary lesions in this species remains to be resolved. In another preliminary report, chronic gastritis and intestinal metaplasia of gastric mucosa in Syrian hamsters were associated with *Helicobacter sp.* infection.

***Lawsonia intracellularis* Infection: Proliferative Ileitis, Transmissible Ileal Hyperplasia.** Proliferative ileitis is among the most commonly recognized diseases in the Syrian hamster; it usually results in high morbidity and mortality. This specific condition has been referred to by a variety of names, including regional ileitis, hamster enteritis, terminal enteritis, atypical ileal hyperplasia, enzootic intestinal adenocarcinoma, proliferative bowel disease, and wet tail. It seems that each individual or group that has become involved in the study of this syndrome has endowed it with a unique epithet. The term "wet tail" should not be used because it includes virtually all the numerous conditions that may cause diarrhea in hamsters.

ETIOLOGY AND PATHOGENESIS. The etiology of proliferative enteritis is now considered to be *Lawsonia intracellularis.* The many past quests toward identifying the etiology of proliferative ileitis in hamsters have incriminated a number of apparently secondary and possibly contributory agents, including *Escherichia coli, Campylobacter,* and *Cryptosporidium. E. coli* isolates from cases of proliferative ileitis have been shown to be enteropathogenic in naive hamsters but did not induce proliferative disease. In another study, an organism was isolated and identified as a new species of *Chlamydia,* with close but distinctly different 16S ribosomal RNA homology to *C. trachomatis* and *C. psittaci.* Koch's postulates were fulfilled, but its true classification in the *Chlamydia* genus and importance in this disease remained controversial. In subsequent molecular studies, the organism was determined to be taxonomically related to the *C. trachomatis,* mouse pneumonitis strain. However, the intracellular organisms seen in enterocytes in typical cases of proliferative enteritis proved to be distinctly different from *C. trachomatis,* and it was concluded that chlamydial infections do not play a primary role in the disease. In typical cases of proliferative ileitis, intracellular bacterial forms are found abundantly in the apical cytoplasm of hyperplastic ileal enterocytes. In the past, these have been referred to as intracellular *Campylobacter*-like organisms (ICLOs). Based on 16S rDNA analysis, the ICLOs were found to be closely related to the genus *Disulfovibrio,* and the term "intracellular *Disulfovibrio*" (IDO) was proposed for a period of time. It is now recognized that *Lawsonia intracellularis* causes similar lesions, with similar intracytoplasmic bacteria, in a wide variety of species, including subjects of this text: hamsters, rats, guinea pigs, and rabbits. The organism seems to be genetically homogeneous, regardless of host species origin, and can be readily transmitted among vastly unrelated host species with ease. Experimental induction of proliferative ileitis requires inoculation of young, naive hamsters with homogenates of proliferative ileal lesions, because the agent cannot be grown on artificial medium.

CLINICAL SIGNS AND PATHOLOGY. Epizootics of the proliferative ileitis are usually confined to younger animals, particularly during the postweaning period. Hamsters are normally resistant to the experimental disease by 10–12 wk of age. Overcrowding, transport, diet, and experimental manipulations have also been identified as predisposing factors. In epizootics of the disease, there may be a morbidity rate of up to 60%, and mortality rates in affected animals may approach 90%. Clinical signs include lethargy; unkempt hair coat; anorexia; weight loss; foul-smelling,

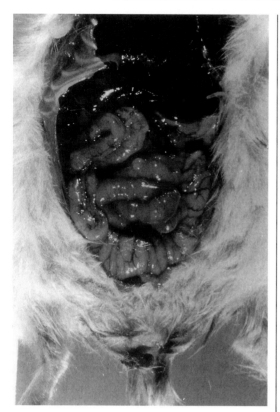

FIG. 3.11—Typical gross findings in a case of proliferative ileitis in young hamster. There is soiling of the perineal region and marked thickening and edema of the terminal small intestine.

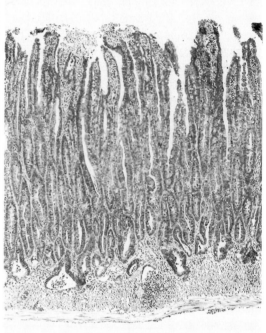

FIG. 3.12—Section of ileum from a spontaneous case of proliferative ileitis. There is marked hyperplasia of enterocytes lining crypts and villi, with extension into the submucosa. Some crypts are dilated and contain cellular debris.

watery diarrhea; and dehydration. Rectal prolapse or intussusceptions frequently occur.

Affected hamsters are runted and emaciated, with soiling of the perineum with diarrhea. The ileum is segmentally thickened, often with prominent serosal nodules and fibrinous peritoneal adhesions to adjacent structures (Fig. 3.11). The opened bowel reveals an abrupt transition of the craniad, normal ileum, and the caudal cecum with the affected, hyperplastic mucosa. Microscopic lesions, as noted, consist of marked crypt and villous epithelial hyperplasia, villous elongation, villous fusion, varying degrees of necrosis and hemorrhage, crypt invasion of underlying structures, crypt abscessation, and granulomatous inflammation (Figs. 3.12 and 3.13). With silver or PAS stains, numerous and characteristic small bacteria can be seen in the apical cytoplasm of proliferating enterocytes, and macrophages in the lamina propria and submucosa contain abundant granular PAS-positive material in their cytoplasm.

DIAGNOSIS. The demonstration of the typical lesions should be sufficient to confirm the diagnosis. *Differential diagnoses* would include Tyzzer's disease, salmonellosis, antibiotic-associated enterocolitis, coliform enteritis, and giardiasis. It is highly likely that co-infections are common and may even play an important role in the pathogenesis of ileal hyperplasia.

SIGNIFICANCE. Sporadic outbreaks of transmissible ileal hyperplasia are an important cause of disease and mortality in hamsters from pet stores and represent a potential complicating factor in hamsters used in research facilities.

Salmonellosis. Epizootics of salmonellosis are a rarity in the current era. However, Syrian hamsters are very susceptible to *Salmonella* infections. In one report from India, *Salmonella* was

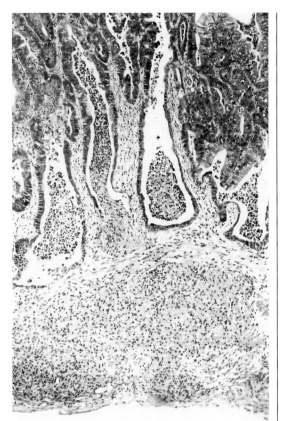

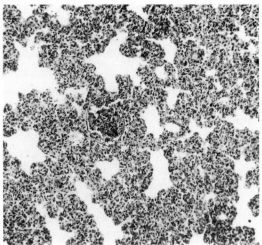

FIG. 3.14—Section of lung from a fatal case of salmonellosis in young hamster. There is marked interstitial pneumonitis, with hypercellularity of alveolar septa, leukocytosis, and sludging of blood in larger vessels.

FIG. 3.13—Higher magnification of Figure 3.12, illustrating the cryptal diverticula, with concurrent granulomatous inflammatory response in the submucosa and adjacent muscle.

isolated from close to 50% of diseased hamsters. *S. enteritidis* serotypes *typhimurium* and *enteritidis* are the most frequent isolates in this species. Transmission is probably primarily by the ingestion of contaminated food or bedding, and interspecies transmission is likely to occur. Explosive outbreaks of salmonellosis are characterized by depression, ruffled hair coat, anorexia, dyspnea, and high mortality.

PATHOLOGY. At necropsy, there may be multifocal, pinpoint-size, pale areas in the liver, with patchy pulmonary hemorrhage and reddened hilar lymph nodes. Microscopic changes in the lung are characterized by multifocal interstitial pneumonitis, with intraalveolar hemorrhage. In the pulmonary veins and venules, there may be a septic thrombophlebitis, with thrombi containing leukocytes, and erosion of venous walls (Fig. 3.14). Focal splenic necrosis and focal necrotizing hepatitis, with leukocytic infiltration, and venous thrombosis are typical lesions. Embolic glomerular lesions and focal splenitis may also occur.

DIAGNOSIS. In acute salmonellosis, the organism can usually be readily recovered from blood, lung, and other viscera. *Differential diagnoses* include Tyzzer's disease, pathogenic *Escherichia coli* infections, and other acute bacterial infections, such as pseudomoniasis.

SIGNIFICANCE. Although currently a rare occurrence in most areas of the world, salmonellosis can cause severe disease, with mortality, in a high percentage of infected hamsters. The public health aspects and dangers of interspecies spread should be emphasized.

Other Bacterial Infections

CORYNEBACTERIUM INFECTIONS. *Corynebacterium kutscheri* has been isolated from the oral cavities of clinically normal adult Syrian hamsters. In addition, the organism has been recovered from sites such as esophagus, cecal contents, submaxillary lymph nodes, and upper respiratory tract. In one study, Syrian hamsters were inoculated subcutaneously or intramuscularly with *C. kutscheri*. Localized granulomatous and suppurative lesions were the only changes observed. Another species, *C. paulometabulum,* was isolated from a hamster with respiratory signs.

SIGNIFICANCE. The Syrian hamster can serve as a reservoir host for *C. kutscheri* but appears to be relatively resistant to systemic corynebacterial infections. The importance of *C. paulometabulum* as a primary pathogen is this species is unknown.

FRANCISELLA TULARENSIS INFECTION: TULAREMIA. There is a single report of an outbreak of *Francisella tularensis* infection in a hamster breeding colony, resulting in 100% mortality. Hamsters were hunched, had ruffled fur, and died within 48 hr. Lungs were mottled with hemorrhage, livers were pale and swollen, and spleens were enlarged. Gut-associated lymphoid tissue was prominent and pale. Microscopic findings included lymphoid necrosis, focal hemorrhages, and bacteria.

LEPTOSPIRA BALLUM INFECTION: LEPTOSPIROSIS. Hamsters inadvertently infected with *Leptospira ballum* by inoculation with contaminated tissue from inapparently infected mice developed severe hemolytic disease, jaundice, hemoglobinuria, nephritis, and hepatitis within 4–6 days. Hamsters are highly susceptible to intentional experimental inoculation with a number of *Leptospira* spp., and thus they can be potentially susceptible to severe natural disease, although never reported.

YERSINIA INFECTION. Hamsters have been known to incur infections of *Yersinia pseudotuberculosis* via contaminated food or bedding. This organism produces chronic emaciation with intermittent diarrhea. Necropsy findings include necrotic caseous nodules in the intestine, mesenteric lymph nodes, liver, spleen, and lungs.

BACTERIAL RESPIRATORY INFECTIONS. Upper respiratory disease, otitis, and bronchopneumonia in hamsters have been associated with a number of bacteria, including *Pasteurella pneumotropica, Pasteurella* spp., *Streptococcus pneumoniae, S.*

agalactiae, and *Streptococcus* spp. The primary roles of these bacteria in respiratory disease in hamsters have not been definitively established. *Mycoplasma pulmonis* has been isolated from hamsters, but its pathogenic potential in hamsters is not known.

MASTITIS AND MISCELLANEOUS BACTERIAL INFECTIONS. Mastitis has been associated with beta-hemolytic *Streptococcus, P. pneumotropica,* and *Escherichia coli*. Cutaneous and cervical abscesses have been found to be colonized with a variety of organisms including *Actinomyces bovis, Staphylococcus aureus, Streptococcus* spp., and *P. pneumotropica. Pseudomonas aeruginosa* septicemia has also been observed in this species. Enteritis in postpartum dams has been attributed to *Pasteurella pneumotropica,* but a cause and effect relationship was not established.

MYCOTIC INFECTIONS. Spontaneous dermatophyte infections are rare in laboratory hamsters, and there are few reports of confirmed cases in the literature.

BIBLIOGRAPHY FOR BACTERIAL AND MYCOTIC INFECTIONS

Clostridial Infections and Antibiotic Toxicity

Barthold, S.W, and Jacoby, R.O. 1978. An outbreak of cecal mucosal hyperplasia in hamsters. Lab. Anim. Sci. 28:723–27.

Bartlett, J.G., et al. 1978. Antibiotic-induced enterocolitis in hamsters: Studies with eleven agents and evidence to support the pathogenic role of toxin-producing clostridia. Am. J. Vet. Res. 39:1525–30.

Blankenship-Paris, T.L., et al. 1995. In vivo and in vitro studies of *Clostridium difficile*–induced disease in hamsters fed an atherogenic, high-fat diet. Lab. Anim. Sci. 45:47–53.

Hawkins, C.C., et al. 1984. Epidemiology of colitis induced by *Clostridium difficile* in hamsters: Application of bacteriophage and bacteriocin typing system. J. Infect. Dis. 149:775–80.

Iaconis, J.P., and Rolfe, R.D. 1986. *Clostridium difficile*–associated ileocecitis in clindamycin-treated infant hamsters. Curr. Microbiol. 13:327–32.

Rehg, J.E. 1997. Clostridial enteropathies, hamster. In *Monographs on Pathology of Laboratory Animals: Digestive System,* ed. T.C. Jones et al., pp. 396–403. New York: Springer-Verlag.

Rehg, J.E., and Lu, Y.-S. 1982. *Clostridium difficile* typhlitis in hamsters not associated with antibiotic therapy. J. Am. Vet. Med. Assoc. 181:1422–23.

Ryden, E.B., et al. 1990. Non–antibiotic-associated *Clostridium difficile* enterotoxemia in Syrian hamsters. Lab. Anim. Sci. 40:544.

Small, J.D. 1987. Drugs used in hamsters with a review of antibiotic-associated colitis. In *Laboratory Hamsters,* ed. G.L. Van Hoosier, Jr., and C.W. McPherson, pp. 179–99. New York: Academic.

Wilson, K.H., et al. 1981. Suppression of *Clostridium difficile* by hamster cecal flora and prevention of antibiotic-associated cecitis. Infect. Immun. 34:626–28.

Clostridium piliforme Infection

Motzel, S.L., and Gibson, S.V. 1990. Tyzzer disease in hamsters and gerbils from a pet store supplier. J. Am. Vet. Med. Assoc. 197:1176–78.

Nakayama, M., et al. 1976. Typhylohepatitis in hamsters infected perorally with Tyzzer's organism. Jap. J. Exp. Med. 46:309–24.

Takasaki, Y., et al. 1974. Tyzzer's disease in hamsters. Jap. J. Exp. Med. 44:267–70.

Zook, B.C., et al. 1977. Tyzzer's disease in Syrian hamsters. J. Am. Vet. Assoc. 171:833–36.

Helicobacter Infections

Franklin, C.L., et al. 1996. Isolation of a novel *Helicobacter sp.* from the gallbladder of Syrian hamsters with cholangiofibrosis. Lab. Anim. Sci. 46:460.

Patterson, M.M., et al. 1998. *Helicobacter*–associated gastritis and intestinal metaplasia in Syrian hamsters. Contemp. Top. 37(4):90.

Proliferative Ileitis

Amend, N.K., et al. 1976. Transmission of enteritis in the Syrian hamster. Lab. Anim. Sci. 26:566–72.

Andrews, E.J. 1975. Alterations of selected intestinal enzymes in hamsters with hamster enteritis syndrome. Am. J. Vet. Res. 36:889–91.

Boothe, A.D., and Cheville, N.F. 1967. The pathology of proliferative ileitis in the golden hamster. Pathol. Vet. 4:31–44.

Cooper, D.M., and Gebhart, C.J. 1998. Comparative aspects of proliferative enteritis. J. Am. Vet. Med. Assoc. 212:1446–51.

Davis, A.J., and Jenkins, S.J. 1986. Cryptosporidiosis and proliferative ileitis in a hamster. Vet. Pathol. 23:632–33.

Dillehay, D.L., et al. 1994. Enterocolitis associated with *Escherichia coli* and *Campylobacter*–like organisms in a hamster (*Mesocricetus auratus)* colony. Lab. Anim. Sci. 44:12-16.

Fox, J.G., et al. 1994. The intracellular *Campylobacter*-like organism from ferrets and hamsters with proliferative bowel disease is a *Disulfovibrio* sp. J. Clin. Microbiol. 32:1229–37.

———. 1993. Antigenic specificity and morphologic characterization of *Chlamydia trachomatis,* strain SFPD, isolated from hamsters with proliferative ileitis. Lab. Anim. Sci. 43:405–10.

———. 1986. Colonization of Syrian hamsters with streptomycin resistant *Campylobacter jejuni.* Lab. Anim. Sci. 36:28–31.

———. 1983. The pet hamster as a potential reservoir of human campylobacteriosis. J. Infect. Dis. 147:784.

Frisk, C.S., and Wagner, J.E. 1977. Experimental hamster enteritis: An electron microscopic study. Am. J. Vet. Res. 38:1861–68.

Frisk, C.S., et al. 1981. Hamster (*Mesocricetus auratus*) enteritis caused by epithelial cell-invasive *Escherichia coli.* 31:1232–38.

———. 1978. Enteropathogenicity of *Escherichia coli* isolated from hamsters (*Mesocricetus auratus*) with hamster ileitis. Infect. Immun. 20:319–20.

Humphrey, C.D., et al. 1986. Morphologic observations of experimental *Campylobacter jejuni* infection in the hamster intestinal tract. Am. J. Pathol. 122:152–59.

Jacoby, R.O., and Johnson, E.A. 1981. Transmissible ileal hyperplasia. Adv. Exp. Med. Biol. 34:267–89.

Jasni, S., et al. 1994. Experimentally-induced proliferative enteritis in hamsters: An ultrastructural study. Res. Vet. Sci. 56:186–92.

Lentsch, R.H., et al. 1982. *Campylobacter fetus* ssp. *jejuni* isolated from Syrian hamsters with proliferative ileitis. Lab. Anim. Sci. 32:511–14.

Sheffield, F.W., and Beveridge, E. 1962. Prophylaxis of "wet-tail" in hamsters. Nature 196:294–95.

Stills, H.F. 1991. Isolation of an intracellular bacterium from hamsters (*Mesocricetus auratus*) with proliferative ileitis and reproduction of the disease with pure culture. Infect. Immun. 59:3227–36.

Salmonellosis

Innes, J.R.M., et al. 1956. Epizootic *Salmonella enteritidis* infection causing pulmonary phlebothrombosis in hamsters. J. Infect. Dis. 98:133–41.

Ray, J.P., and Mallick, B.B. 1970. Public health significance of *Salmonella* infections in laboratory animals. Indian Vet. J. 47:1033–37.

Other Bacterial Infections

Corynebacterium Infections

Amao, H. et al. 1995. Pathogenicity of *Corynebacterium kutscheri* in the Syrian hamster. J. Vet. Med. Sci. 57:715–19.

———. 1991. Isolation of *Corynebacterium kutscheri* from aged Syrian hamsters (*Mesocricetus auratus*). Lab. Anim. Sci. 41:265–68.

Tansey, G., et al. 1995. Acute pneumonia in a Syrian hamster: Isolation of a *Corynebacterium* species. Lab. Anim. Sci. 45:366–67.

Francisella Infection

Perman, V., and Bergeland, M.E. 1967. A tularemia enzootic in a closed hamster breeding colony. Lab. Anim. Care 17:563–68.

Leptospira Infection

Frenkel, J.K. 1972. Infection and immunity in hamsters. Prog. Exp. Tumor Res. 16:326–67.

Mastitis and Miscellaneous
Bacterial Infections

Huerkamp, M.J., and Dillehay, D.L. 1990. Coliform mastitis in a golden Syrian hamster. Lab. Anim. Sci. 40:325–27.

Lesher, R.J., et al. 1985. Enteritis caused by *Pasteurella pneumotropica* infection in hamsters. J. Clin. Microbiol. 22:448.

General Bibliography

Frisk, C.S. 1987. Bacterial and mycotic diseases. In *Laboratory Hamsters*, ed. G.L. Van Hoosier, Jr., and C.W. McPherson, pp. 111–33. New York: Academic.

Hagen, C.A., et al. 1965. Intestinal microflora of normal hamsters. Lab. Anim. Care 15:185–93.

Renshaw, H.W., et al. 1975. A survey of naturally occurring diseases of the Syrian hamster. Lab. Anim. 9:179–91.

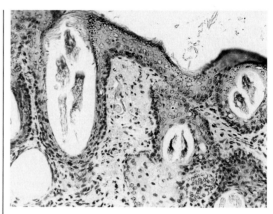

FIG. 3.15—Section of skin from case of acariasis in hamster with clinical manifestations. Mites and debris are present in dilated hair follicles

PARASITIC DISEASES

ECTOPARASITIC INFESTATIONS

Mite Infestations: Acariasis. Two species of the *Demodex* genus, *D. criceti* and *D. aurati,* occur as natural infestations in Syrian hamsters. These mites are relatively common in animal facilities. In one survey, the majority of animals in colonies surveyed were infected with *D. aurati* and/or *D. criceti,* and all colonies examined were positive. Hamsters born to infected dams normally acquire the parasite during the suckling period. Demodectic mange mites are normally of low pathogenicity, and clinical signs rarely occur in hamsters with demodicidosis. Lesions have been observed occasionally, particularly in older animals and hamsters under experimental manipulation. Hair loss may occur over the back, neck, and hindquarters. Denuded areas are nonpruritic, dry, and scaling, with multiple scabs. Microscopically, *D. criceti* are usually present in epidermal "pits," with sparing of the dermis. Mites of *D. aurati* are found in hair follicles and canals of the sebaceous glands. Hair follicles may be dilated with mites and debris, usually with minimal inflammatory response (Fig. 3.15).

Hamsters have also been found to be infested with *Notoedres notoedres,* a mite that burrows in the stratum corneum. Scabby lesions were found on the ears, nose, feet, and perianal areas, including large scabious masses around the anus. Numerous mites were present in skin scrapings and sections. Notoedric mange is rare but can be focally common in some hamster colonies. An outbreak of notoedric mange has also been described in which hamsters were infested with *N. cati.* In Europe, nasal mite (*Speleorodens clethrionomys*) infestations were observed in three separate hamster breeding colonies. Hamsters can also be host to *Ornithonyssus bacoti,* the tropical rat mite, and *O. sylvarium,* the northern fowl mite.

DIAGNOSIS. Specimens should be collected from males, since males usually have a larger mite parasite load than females. Mites can be demonstrated in skin scrapings cleared in 10% KOH or NaOH. *Differential diagnoses* include bacterial dermatitis, bite wounds, and dermatophyte infections.

SIGNIFICANCE. Demodex infestations are a common occurrence in Syrian hamsters. When skin lesions do occur, there are usually other identifiable predisposing factors, such as experimental manipulations and/or advanced age. The mites are species-specific, and there is no evidence of interspecies spread.

Myiasis. Rare cases of myiasis in hamsters can occur, due to *Wohlfahrtia vigil, Sarcophaga haemorrhoidalis,* and *Musca domestica.*

ENDOPARASITIC INFECTIONS

Protozoal Infections. Hamsters are host to many enteric protozoa, which are often listed and discussed in reviews of parasites, but very few protozoa have any pathogenic significance in the hamster. *Spironucleus muris,* of dubious pathogenic status in the mouse, is a common intestinal flagellate of hamsters. *Cryptosporidia* have also been found in hamsters with proliferative ileitis. *S. (Hexamita) muris* infections rarely are recognized to produce clinical disease in this species, although the organism has been identified frequently in stocks from commercial suppliers. The organisms normally feed on intestinal bacteria, and their presence is usually considered to be an incidental finding. However, under certain circumstances, mucosal damage and clinical signs may occasionally occur in infected laboratory rodents. Clinical signs attributable to spironucleosis have been recognized most frequently in laboratory mice, usually in animals that have been recently weaned or are immunocompromised. In the latter category, mice may be naturally immunodeficient, or they may have been subjected to experimental manipulation.

SIGNIFICANCE. The significance of *S. muris* infections in laboratory hamsters has not been determined. These flagellates have been found in the peripheral blood of hamsters with enteritis. In one study, transmission to rats was shown to occur. However, in another study, interspecies transmission occurred using clones of *S. muris* isolated from mice and hamsters, but not between these species and rats. Hexamitiasis may affect macrophage activity and the immune response in mice, but the significance of the infection in the Syrian hamster is yet to be determined.

GIARDIASIS. Naturally occurring giardiasis in hamsters has been attributed to *Giardia misocricetus* or *G. muris.* Based on morphologic similarities to *Giardia* in other small rodents and the ability to infect mice and rats with isolates from hamsters, *G. muris* appears to be the appropriate term. Infestations in hamsters are usually asymptomatic, although we have seen chronic emaciation and diarrhea in aged hamsters with concomitant advanced amyloidosis. These ham-

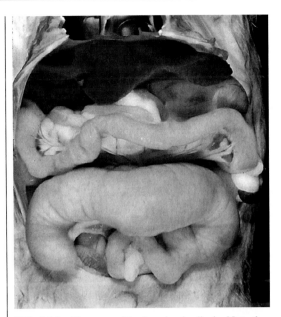

FIG. 3.16—Hamster with chronic giardiasis. Note the marked thickening of small intestine, cecum, and colon.

sters have the classic lesions of chronic giardiasis, with marked enterotyphlocolitis (Fig. 3.16), and diffuse infiltration of the intestinal lamina propria with plasma cells and lymphocytes and diffuse gross mural thickening of the small intestine and cecum (Figs. 3.17 and 3.18).

DIAGNOSIS. Wet mount preparations from the duodenal region should reveal the pear-shaped organisms that move with a characteristic rolling tumbling movement. The banded cyst forms can be visualized in wet mount preparations using phase contrast microscopy or with Giemsa-stained preparations. The typical thick-walled ellipsoidal cysts containing four nuclei can be visualized microscopically by the fecal flotation technique or in fecal smears stained with Lugol's iodine. In tissue sections of the small intestine collected from suspected cases, pear-shaped to ellipsoidal trophozoites are present along the brush borders of enterocytes. The protozoa normally congregate in the crypts of the duodenum, and in severe infestations they may be present in the intervillous regions, extending to the tips of the villi.

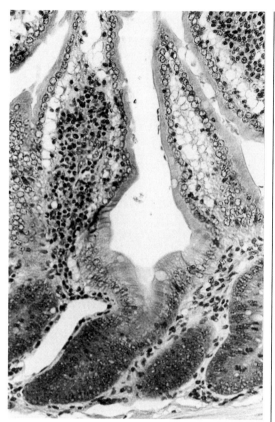

FIG. 3.17—Duodenum from hamster with enteritis associated with *Giardia* infestation. Note the pear-shaped organisms present in the intervillous regions and the mononuclear cell infiltration in the lamina propria.

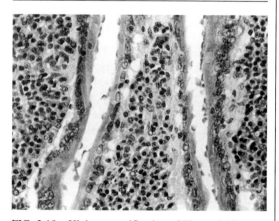

FIG. 3.18—Higher magnification of Figure 3.17. There is moderate flattening of enterocytes, with a prominent mononuclear cell infiltrate in the lamina propria.

SIGNIFICANCE. Although there have been numerous reports of *Giardia* infestations in hamsters, the significance of the organism, either as a primary or opportunistic pathogen in this species, has not been resolved. The possibility of interspecies transmission warrants consideration. Currently, there is no convincing evidence that infestations with *Giardia* in small rodents pose any direct threat to human contacts.

ENCEPHALITOZOONOSIS. There is relatively little information on *Encephalitozoon cuniculi* infections in hamsters. One report describes *Encephalitozoon* infection of a transplantable plasmacytoma of hamsters, but details of pathologic findings were not included. For additional information, see encephalitozoonosis in the rabbit (Chap. 6).

Helminth Infections: Pinworms. Hamsters can be infected with their own pinworm, *Syphacia mesocriceti*, but infection with the mouse pinworm, *S. obvelata*, is more common. These worms can be distinguished from each other on minor morphological criteria. Hamsters are also experimentally susceptible to the rat pinworm, *S. muris*.

DIAGNOSIS. Depending on the genus involved, diagnosis is made by demonstration of pinworm eggs either (1) by the microscopic examination of perianal cellophane tape impression smears or fecal flotations or (2) by the examination of the large intestine at necropsy for adult worms.

SIGNIFICANCE. In addition to the possibility that pinworm infections may have adverse effects on certain types of research, particularly those related to the alimentary tract, interspecies transmission is another consideration. Currently, there appears to be no documented evidence that hamsters are susceptible to *Aspicularis* spp. infections.

TRICHOSOMOIDES INFECTION. A number of reports have documented infection of the nasal cavity of hamsters with *Trichosomoides nasalis*. According to a review by Wagner (1987), other nematodes have been identified in wild-trapped hamsters.

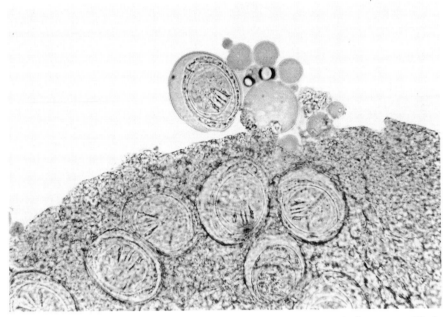

FIG. 3.19—Crush preparation of *Hymenolepis diminuta* collected from the intestinal contents of Syrian hamster. (Courtesy J.P. Lautenslager)

Helminth Infections: Tapeworms. Hamsters, like other rodents, have been found with liver cysts of *Cysticercus fasciolaris,* the intermediate stage of *Taenia taeniaformis,* a tapeworm of dogs and cats. Infection is incurred by contamination of food with feces from the definitive hosts. Infections with *Hymenolepis nana* and *H. diminuta* are relatively common in hamsters, compared with laboratory mice and rats. *H. nana* adults are found in the lower small intestine, whereas *H. diminuta* adults tend to be found in the upper small intestine (see Chap. 1). Unless there is a heavy infection, hamsters are usually asymptomatic. In view of the direct life cycle of *H. nana,* there is a danger of transmission to other rodents and to human contacts.

DIAGNOSIS. Diagnosis is made by identification of the eggs in fecal samples or in crush preparations (Fig. 3.19), or by demonstration of the adult worms at necropsy, or on histological examination. *H. nana* adults are relatively small, whereas *H. diminutia* adults are considerably larger (Figs. 3.20 and 3.21). Flynn (1973) and Wagner

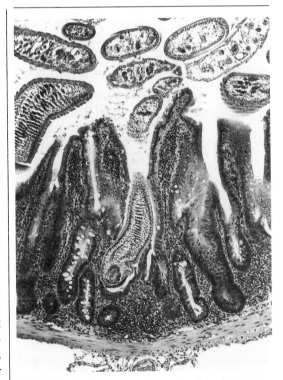

FIG. 3.20—Section of small intestine from hamster with *Hymenolepis nana* infestation.

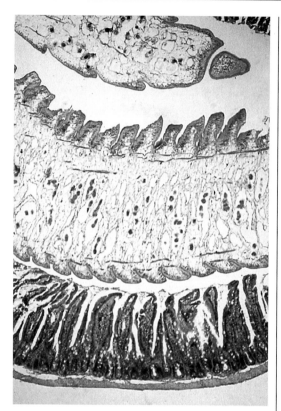

FIG. 3.21—Section of small intestine from another animal infected with *Hymenolepis diminuta*. Note the large size of the adult parasite with relation to the intestinal villi (vs. *H. nana*).

(1987) give additional information on parasites in Syrian hamsters.

BIBLIOGRAPHY
FOR PARASITIC DISEASES

Ectoparasitic Infections

Bornstein, S., and Iwarsson, K. 1980. Nasal mites in a colony of Syrian hamsters. Lab. Anim. 14:31–33.

Estes, P.C., et al. 1971. Demodectic mange in the golden hamster. Lab. Anim. Sci. 21:825–28.

Flatt, R.E., and Kerber, W.T. 1968. Demodectic mite infestation in golden hamsters. Lab. Anim. Dig. 4:6–7.

Owen, D., and Young, C. 1973. The occurrence of *Demodex aurati* and *Demodex criceti* in the Syrian hamster (*Mesocricetus auratus*) in the United Kingdom. Vet. Rec. 92:282–84.

Wagner, J.E. 1987. Parasitic diseases. In *Laboratory Hamsters*, ed. G.L. Van Hoosier, Jr., and C.W. McPherson, pp. 135–56. New York: Academic.

Endoparasitic Infections

Barthold, S.W. 1997a. *Giardia muris* infection, intestine, mouse, rat, and hamster. In *Monographs on Pathology of Laboratory Animals: Digestive System*, ed. T.C. Jones et al., pp. 422–26. New York: Springer-Verlag.

————. 1997b. *Spironucleus muris* infection, intestine, mouse, rat, and hamster. In *Monographs on Pathology of Laboratory Animals: Digestive System*, ed. T.C. Jones et al., pp. 419–22. New York: Springer-Verlag.

Davis, A.J., and Jenkins, S.J. 1986. Cryptosporidiosis and proliferative ileitis in a hamster. Vet. Pathol. 23:632–33.

Flynn, R.J. 1973. *Parasites of Laboratory Animals.* Ames: Iowa State University Press.

Grant, D.R., and Woo, P.T. 1978. Comparative studies of *Giardia* spp. in small mammals in southern Ontario. II. Host specificity and infectivity of stored cysts. Can. J. Zool. 56:1360–66.

Kunstyr, I., et al. 1992. Host specificity of *Giardia muris* isolates from mouse and golden hamster. Parasitol. Res. 78:621–22.

Meisser, J., et al. 1971. Nosematosis as an accompanying infection of plasmacytoma ascites in Syrian golden hamsters. Pathol. Microbiol. 37:249–60.

Roberts-Thomson, I.C., et al. 1976. Giardiasis in the mouse: An animal model. Gastroenterology 71:57–61.

Ross, C.R., et al. 1980. Experimental transmission of *Syphacia muris* among rats, mice, hamsters and gerbils. Lab. Anim. Sci. 30:35–37.

Ruitenberg, E.J., and Kruyt, B.C. 1975. Effect of intestinal flagellates on immune response of mice. Parasitology 71:R30.

Saxe, L.H. 1954. Transfaunation studies on the host specificity of the enteric protozoa of rodents. J. Protozool. 1:220–30.

Wagner, J.E. 1987. Parasitic diseases. In *Laboratory Hamsters*, ed. G.L. Van Hoosier, Jr., and C.W. McPherson, pp. 135–56. New York: Academic.

Wagner, J. E., et al. 1974. Hexamitiasis in laboratory mice, hamsters, and rats. Lab. Anim. Sci. 24:349–54.

General Bibliography

Flynn, R.J. 1973. *Parasites of Laboratory Animals.* Ames: Iowa State University Press.

Hsu, C.K. 1982. Parasitic diseases. In *The Mouse in Biomedical Research. II. Diseases,* ed. H.L. Foster et al., pp. 359–72. New York: Academic.

Kunstyr, I., and Friedhoff, K.T. 1980. Parasitic and mycotic infections of laboratory animals. In *Animal Quality and Models in Research,* ed. A. Spiegel et al., pp. 181–92. Stuttgart: Gustav Fischer Verlag.

Wagner, J.E. 1987. Parasitic diseases. In *Laboratory Hamsters,* ed. G.L. Van Hoosier, Jr., and C.W. McPherson, pp. 135–56. New York: Academic.

NUTRITIONAL AND METABOLIC DISORDERS

Spontaneous Hemorrhagic Necrosis (SHN) of the Central Nervous System of Fetal Hamsters. SHN has been recognized in fetal hamsters examined during the last trimester of pregnancy and in newborn hamsters. In affected litters, animals are stillborn or weak at birth and are frequently cannibalized by the dam. Microscopic changes are usually most extensive in the prosencephalon. Symmetrical, subependymal vascular degeneration occurs, with edema and hemorrhage in the adjacent neuropil (Fig. 3.22). Intraventricular hemorrhage has been observed, and lesions may extend down the neuroaxis. There appear to be strain-related variations in susceptibility to the disease. SHN has been reproduced by feeding dams a diet deficient in available vitamin E and alleviated by vitamin E supplementation.

Diabetes Mellitus. Scientists have capitalized upon this genetically recessive disorder of Chinese hamsters, which occurs in high incidence in some inbred lines. Hamsters display weight loss, glucose intolerance, mild to severe hyperglycemia, polyuria, polydipsia, glycosuria, hypoinsulinemia, ketonuria, and high levels of free fatty acids in the blood. Microscopic changes in the pancreas include islet involution with nuclear pyknosis; shrunken, eosinophilic cytoplasm; cytoplasmic vacuolation; and degranulation.

Other endocrine disorders are currently seldom recognized and poorly characterized in this species. They include adrenocortical disease resulting in a Cushings-like state (Fig. 3.23).

BIBLIOGRAPHY FOR NUTRITIONAL AND METABOLIC DISORDERS

Diani, A., and Gerritson, G. 1987. Use in research. In *Laboratory Hamsters,* ed. G.L. Van Hoosier, Jr., and C.W. McPherson, pp. 329–47. New York: Academic.

Hubbard, G.B., and Schmidt, R.E. 1987. Noninfectious diseases. In *Laboratory Hamsters,* ed. G.L. Van Hoosier, Jr., and C.W. McPherson, pp. 169–78. New York: Academic.

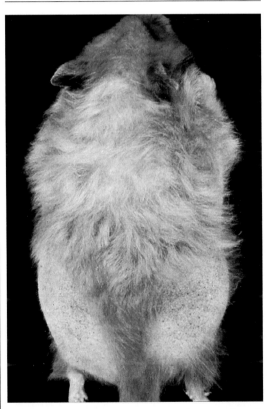

FIG. 3.23—Adult hamster demonstrating a confirmed case of Cushing's disease. Note the obesity and bilateral alopecia in the lumbosacral region.

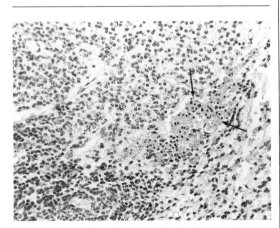

FIG. 3.22—Section of metencephalon from newborn Syrian hamster with hemorrhagic encephalopathy associated with vitamin E deficiency. There is marked extravasation of erythrocytes (*arrows*) and disruption of the neuropil. The marked cellularity in the adjacent nervous tissue is due to the large number of primordial cells present at this stage of development of the CNS.

Keeler, R.F., and Young, S. 1979. Role of vitamin E in the etiology of spontaneous hemorrhagic necrosis of the central nervous system of fetal hamsters. Teratology 20:127–32.

Margolis, G., and Kilham, L. 1976. Hemorrhagic necrosis of the central nervous system: A spontaneous disease of fetal hamsters. Vet. Pathol. 13:484–90.

Newberne, P.M. 1978. Nutritional and metabolic diseases. In *Pathology of Laboratory Animals,* ed. C.K. Benirschke et al., pp. 2065–2214. New York: Springer-Verlag.

ENVIRONMENTAL, GENETIC, AND OTHER DISORDERS

Bedding-Associated Dermatitis. Leg lesions have been associated with contact bedding in Chinese and Syrian hamsters. Lesions in animals housed on wood shavings are primarily on the footpads and are characterized by degeneration and atrophy of the digits, with granulomatous inflammatory response. Necrotic areas with ulceration may spread to the legs and shoulders. On histological examination, wood shavings and sawdust are frequently detectable in the dermis and subcutis, with leukocytic infiltration and multinucleate giant cell formation. The site of entry is likely the footpad, with subsequent subcutaneous migration to proximal areas. Rats and mice housed on the same bedding are not affected. *Differential diagnoses* include trauma and cannibalism.

Malocclusion. Like other rodents, hamsters can develop malocclusion or broken incisors, resulting in overgrowth of incisor teeth that are not in good opposition.

Periodontal Disease. Hamsters have served as experimental models of both periodontal disease and caries, which are induced by a combination of dietary and microbial factors. Spontaneous periodontal disease does occur but is apparently rare.

Behavioral Diseases. Syrian hamsters are desert-dwelling, solitary creatures that do not particularly enjoy each other's company except when breeding. They are easily disturbed and agitated. Females are very aggressive, particularly when pregnant or lactating, and prone to fight and kill other hamsters.

Cannibalism is common, especially when stressed, and primiparous females are renowned for their tendency to cannibalize their young. Sequelae may vary from limb amputation to death. Chinese hamsters are even more prone to pugilistic behavior. Hamsters are nocturnal, and their activity during darkness is high. Using exercise wheel revolutions as a measurement of activity, female Syrian hamsters have been shown to travel distances equal to several kilometers during a 24 hr period while in estrus. Olfactory cues play an essential role in mating behavior. They are active chewers and adept at escape. Although Syrian hamsters are of temperate desert origin, they carry the genetic baggage of a northern ancestry and are prone to hibernation and estivation. This occurs inconsistently, as they are regarded as permissive, rather than obligatory hibernators. **Hibernation** can be induced in some hamsters by a number of environmental stimuli, including low temperature, short days, solitude, nesting material, and adequate food stores. Likewise, high temperature, low water, and other factors may stimulate estivation. Under these and other less than optimal environmental conditions, the animals lose body weight while enlarging brown fat stores, and reproductive activity ceases with atrophy of reproductive organs. Even under stabilized conditions, hamsters enjoy a well-constructed and comfortable nest and endeavor to cache away impressive stores of food.

BIBLIOGRAPHY FOR ENVIRONMENTAL, GENETIC, AND OTHER DISORDERS

Griffin, H.E., et al. 1989. Hamster limb loss. Lab. Anim. 18(Sept.):19–20.

Hoffman, R.A. 1968. Hibernation and effects of low temperature. In *The Golden Hamster: Its Biology and Use in Medical Research,* ed. R.A. Hoffman et al., pp. 25–39. Ames: Iowa State University Press.

Meshorer, A. 1976. Leg lesions in hamsters caused by wood shavings. Lab. Anim. Sci. 26:827–29.

Murphy, M.R., and Schneider, G.E. 1970. Olfactory bulb removal eliminates mating behavior in the male golden hamster. Science 167:302–3.

Richards, M.P.M. 1966. Activity measured by running wheels and observations during the oestrus cycle, pregnancy and pseudopregnancy in the golden hamster. Anim. Behav. 14:450–58.

DISEASES ASSOCIATED WITH AGING

Hamster Glomerulonephropathy (Arteriolar Nephrosclerosis)

EPIZOOTIOLOGY AND PATHOGENESIS. Degenerative renal disease represents an important cause of morbidity and mortality in older hamsters. The disease occurs more frequently in females than in males. The etiology and pathogenesis of the disease is poorly understood. The disease in the hamster has been interpreted to be similar to progressive glomerulonephropathy in aged rats. It has been suggested that there is a direct relationship between the concentration of dietary protein and the severity of the renal lesions. Glomerular changes and arteriolar degeneration have been demonstrated in some experimental infections with lymphocytic choriomeningitis virus; therefore, a chronic viral infection has been proposed as another possible underlying cause. However, investigators have failed to demonstrate immunoglobulin deposits consistent with antigen-antibody complexes in such cases. Renovascular hypertension has also been implicated as a possible cause of the disease.

PATHOLOGY. Affected kidneys are pale and granular in appearance, with irregular cortical depressions (Fig. 3.24). There may be radiating cortical scarring evident on the cut surface. On micro-scopic examination, glomerular changes vary from segmental to diffuse thickening of basement membranes, with deposition of eosinophilic material. In severely affected animals, there may be complete obliteration of glomerular structures (Fig. 3.25). In advanced cases, frequently there is concurrent amyloid deposition on glomerular basement membranes and dilation and atrophy of degenerating tubules. Some tubules may be lined by poorly differentiated epithelial cells, and epithelial changes in other tubules vary from flattening to degeneration. There is a variable degree of interstitial fibrosis in a diffuse to segmental pattern, with thickening of basement membranes (Fig. 3.26). There is minimal inflammatory cell response. Proteinaceous, eosinophilic casts may be present in many tubules. Fibrinoid change may be present in the media of intrarenal vessels, but this is not a consistent finding.

DIAGNOSIS. *Differential diagnoses* include toxic nephropathy and uncomplicated amyloidosis.

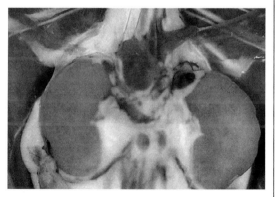

FIG. 3.24—Adult hamster with advanced glomerulonephropathy. Note the pale, irregular cortical surfaces.

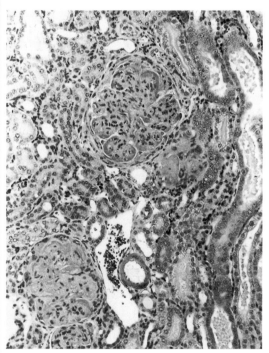

FIG. 3.25—Section of renal cortex from a spontaneous case of hamster nephropathy. Note the marked thickening of glomerular basement membranes, with obliteration of the normal architecture.

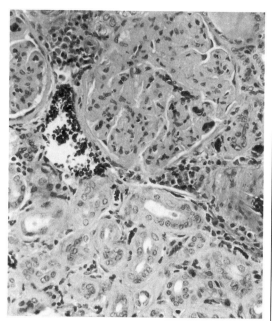

FIG. 3.26—Higher magnification of Figure 3.25, illustrating thickening of basement membranes of glomeruli and tubules.

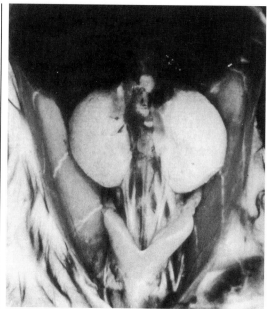

FIG. 3.27—Renal amyloidosis in aged hamster. The kidneys are pale and markedly swollen.

Amyloid deposition frequently occurs as a concurrent event, particularly in advanced cases of glomerulonephropathy.

SIGNIFICANCE. Progressive glomerulonephropathy is an important cause of disease and mortality in older hamsters. The etiopathogenesis requires further study.

Amyloidosis. Amyloidosis frequently occurs in older hamsters, and there is a marked variation in the incidence, depending on the colony under study. The disease is most common in females. Amyloid deposition may be detected as early as 5 mo, but it is much more common in hamsters examined at 15 or more months of age. There may be a drop in serum albumin and a rise in serum globulins. Amyloidosis may be produced experimentally in adult hamsters with regular injections of casein. Testosterone administration will inhibit the expression of amyloid in female hamsters.

PATHOLOGY. The kidneys can be pale and irregular (Fig. 3.27), and affected livers are swollen, with a prominent lobular pattern. On microscopic exami-

nation, the liver, kidneys, and adrenal glands are most frequently involved (Fig. 3.28). Other tissues that can be affected include spleen, stomach, testis, and intestine. In the liver, deposition of eosinophilic, homogeneous material is evident around portal triads and within vessel walls, with variable involvement of the sinusoidal regions. Amyloid deposition frequently occurs initially in the glomerular tufts. The early changes may be characterized by the appearance of PAS-positive hyalinlike deposits along the glomerular basement membranes. The early deposits may have the typical amyloid fibrils evident by electron microscopy but may be negative for amyloid (paramyloid), using the usual histochemical stains. In addition to deposition along glomerular basement membranes, the basement membranes of tubules are also frequently affected. In the adrenal glands, extensive cortical deposition may occur, with distortion of the normal architecture.

DIAGNOSIS. The presence of amyloid normally can be verified using techniques, such as Congo red or thioflavin T procedures. Deposits may be negative for amyloid using the alcian blue–PAS staining method. The primary *differential diagnosis* is hamster glomerulonephropathy.

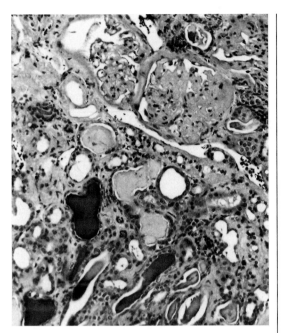

FIG. 3.28—Section of kidney from hamster with advanced renal amyloidosis. There is complete obliteration of the glomerular architecture.

SIGNIFICANCE. Amyloidosis is an important cause of renal insufficiency and mortality in older hamsters. In advanced cases, other organs with extensive amyloid deposition, such as the adrenal glands, may have severely compromised function.

Atrial Thrombosis

EPIZOOTIOLOGY AND PATHOGENESIS. The process, which usually involves the left auricle and atrium, is a common occurrence in older hamsters in some colonies. Females are usually affected earlier than males, and the syndrome is often associated with amyloidosis. Changes also occur in coagulation and fibrinolytic parameters consistent with consumptive coagulopathy. Atrial thrombosis may be due in part to local blood stasis secondary to cardiac insufficiency. Frequently there is concurrent myocardial degeneration and left-sided congestive heart failure.

PATHOLOGY. Hamsters with this disorder often present with severe dyspnea, due to congestive heart failure. The thrombus is usually present in the left auricle and atrium. A moderately firm to friable, pale thrombus is adherent to the adjacent endocardium (Fig. 3.29). Bilateral ventricular hypertrophy is a common finding. Lungs may be congested and edematous. Microscopically, there may be some degree of organization of the layered thrombus. Focal to diffuse myocardial degeneration, when present, is charac-

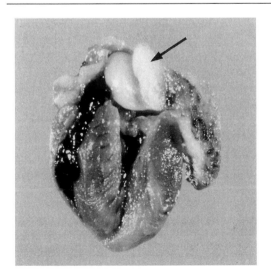
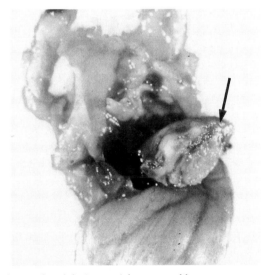

FIG. 3.29—Spontaneous thrombosis involving the left atrium and auricle (*arrows*) in two aged hamsters, one important cause of spontaneous deaths in older animals.

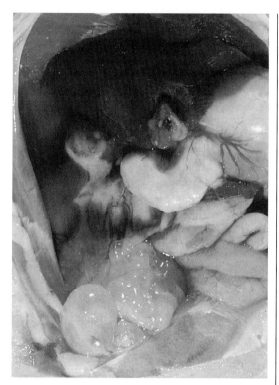

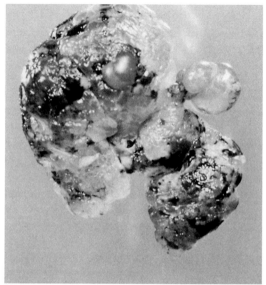

FIG. 3.31—Polycystic disease in an old hamster, advanced case. There are multiple cystic areas in the liver with compression and disruption of the adjacent parenchyma, as well as obliteration of the normal architecture.

FIG. 3.30—Polycystic disease in an old hamster, usually considered to be an incidental finding. Note the fluid-filled multiloculated cysts associated with the liver and peritesticular regions.

terized by nuclear hypertrophy, vacuolation of sarcoplasm, fiber atrophy, and interstitial fibrosis. There may be concurrent focal medial degeneration and calcification of coronary arteries. In the valves, fibrosis and myxomatous change can occur.

SIGNIFICANCE. In some facilities, atrial thrombosis is a common cause of mortality in older hamsters. Necropsy procedures in this species should always include a careful examination of the chambers of the heart for evidence of thrombotic change.

Polycystic Disease (Polycystic Liver Disease)

EPIZOOTIOLOGY AND PATHOGENESIS. Multiple hepatic cysts are occasionally seen in older hamsters at necropsy. They are considered to be of congenital origin and due to either failure of fusion of the intralobular and interlobular ducts or failure of superfluous bile ducts to disappear. Raised, cystic areas of variable size, up to 2 cm in diameter, are present on the capsule and within the parenchyma of the liver. True cysts may also be present in tissues such as epididymis, seminal vesicles, pancreas, and endometrium (Figs. 3.30 and 3.31). In one report, over 75% of hamsters studied had cystic lesions at necropsy and many had lesions at multiple sites. Cysts were most common in the liver and epididymis, followed by seminal vesicles and pancreas.

PATHOLOGY. The cysts are thin-walled, and contain clear, straw-colored fluid. On microscopic examination, there are multiple unilocular and multilocular cystic areas composed of a band of collagenous tissue and lined by flattened to cuboidal epithelial cells (Fig. 3.32). In the adjacent parenchyma of the liver, changes may include pressure atrophy of hepatic cords, hemosiderin deposition, proliferation of bile ducts, and periportal lymphocytic infiltration.

SIGNIFICANCE. Hepatic cysts occasionally occur as an incidental finding at necropsy in older

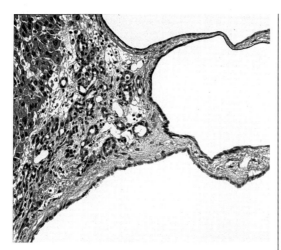

FIG. 3.32—Microscopic section of liver, illustrating the cystic areas lined by squamous to cuboidal epithelium (polycystic disease).

hamsters. They are interpreted to be of congenital origin.

Hepatic Cirrhosis. This spontaneous disorder occurs sporadically among laboratory hamsters, reaching an incidence of up to 20% in some colonies. It occurs in aged animals, particularly females. There is uniform nodularity to the capsular surface grossly, with microscopic evidence of periportal fibrosis and bile duct proliferation, analogous to the liver lesion encountered in aging rats. There is also nodular hepatocellular proliferation with concurrent degeneration, necrosis, and mixed leukocyte infiltration.

Other Changes Associated with Aging. Alveolar histiocytosis, fibrinoid degeneration of arterioles, and cerebral mineralization are examples of lesions that have been observed in older animals. Focal cerebral mineralization may be seen microscopically as an incidental finding at necropsy. There are foci of mineralization in the neuropil, with displacement of adjacent structures and minimal cellular response.

For additional information on age-related changes, see Schmidt et al. (1983), Hubbard and Schmidt (1987), Pour et al. (1976), and Pour et al. (1979).

BIBLIOGRAPHY FOR DISEASES ASSOCIATED WITH AGING

Chesterman, F.C., and Pomerance, A. 1965. Cirrhosis and liver tumours in a closed colony of golden hamsters. Br. J. Cancer 19:802–11.
Coe, J.E., and Ross, J.J. 1990. Amyloidosis and female protein in the Syrian hamster: Concurrent regulation by sex hormones. J. Exp. Med. 171:1257–66.
Doi, K., et al. 1987. Age-related non-neoplastic lesions in the heart and kidneys of Syrian hamsters of the APA strain. Lab. Anim. 21:241–48.
Gleiser, C.A., et al. 1971. Amyloidosis and renal paramyloid in a closed hamster colony. Lab. Anim. Sci. 21:197–202.
———. 1970. A polycystic disease of hamsters in a closed colony. Lab. Anim. Care 20:923–29.
Gruys, E., et al. 1979. Deposition of amyloid in the liver of hamsters: An enzyme-histochemical and electron-microscopical study. Lab. Anim. 13:1–9.
Hubbard, G.B., and Schmidt, R.E. 1987. Noninfectious diseases. In *Laboratory Hamsters,* ed. G.L. Van Hoosier, Jr., and C.W. McPherson, pp. 169–78. New York: Academic.
McMartin, D.N., and Dodds, W.J. 1982. Atrial thrombosis in aging Syrian hamsters: An animal model of human disease. Am. J. Pathol. 107:277–79.
Newberne, P.M. 1978. Nutritional and metabolic diseases. In *Pathology of Laboratory Animals,* ed. C.K. Benirschke et al., pp. 2065–2214. New York: Academic.
Pour, P., et al. 1979. Spontaneous tumors and common diseases in three types of hamsters. J. Natl. Cancer Inst. 63:797–811.
———. 1976. Spontaneous tumors and common diseases in two colonies of Syrian hamsters. 1. Incidence and sites. J. Natl. Cancer Inst. 56:931–35.
Schmidt, R.E., et al. 1983. *Pathology of Aging Syrian Hamsters.* Boca Raton, Fla.: CRC.
Slausen, D.O., et al. 1978. Arteriolar nephrosclerosis in the Syrian hamster. Vet. Pathol. 15:1–11.
Somvanshi, R., et al. 1987. Polycystic liver disease in golden hamsters. J. Comp. Pathol. 97:615–18.
Van Marck, E.A.E., et al. 1978. Spontaneous glomerular basement membrane changes in the golden hamster (*Mesocricetus auratus*): A light and electron microscopic study. Lab. Anim. 12:207–11.

NEOPLASMS

Although newborn hamsters are commonly used in vivo to screen for potentially oncogenic viruses, the incidence of spontaneous tumors in this species is relatively low. There is a marked variation in the incidence of neoplasms in different colonies. This probably reflects the influence of genetic factors, and possibly environmental conditions, on the occurrence of spontaneous tumors in this species. The spontaneous out-

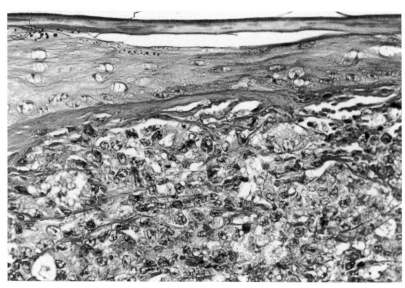

FIG. 3.33—Section of skin from adult hamster with spontaneous epidermotropic lymphoma. Note the infiltrate of poorly differentiated mononuclear cells in the dermis and excavation of the adjacent epidermis. (Courtesy B.M. Cross)

breaks of lymphomas and epithelial tumors associated with hamster papova virus have been discussed previously under Viral Infections. In addition, in aged Syrian hamsters there are spontaneous lymphomas that arise that are not associated with hamster papovirus. They are multicentric, often involving thymus, thoracic lymph nodes, mesenteric lymph nodes, superficial lymph nodes, spleen, liver, and other sites. Cell types are variable. *Cutaneous lymphoma* resembling mycosis fungoides, the epidermotropic lymphoma seen in humans, has been observed in adult hamsters. Lethargy, anorexia, weight loss, patchy alopecia, and exfoliative erythroderma have been observed in affected animals. Microscopic changes include dense infiltrates of neoplastic lymphocytes in the dermis, with extension into the epidermis (Fig. 3.33).

Of the other tumors that occur in this species, the majority are benign, and they frequently arise from the endocrine system or alimentary tract. *Adrenocortical adenomas* are one of the most frequently recorded tumors. For additional information on neoplasms see Pour et al. (1976), Pour et al. (1979), Strandberg (1987), Turusov et al. (1982), Van Hoosier and Trentin (1979), and Barthold (1992).

BIBLIOGRAPHY FOR NEOPLASMS

Barthold, S.W. 1992. Hemolymphatic tumors. In *The Pathology of Tumours in Laboratory Animals. III. Tumors of the Hamster,* ed. U. Mohr et al. Lyon, France: IARC Scientific Publications.

Harvey, R.G., et al. 1992. Epidermotropic cutaneous T-cell lymphoma (mycosis fungoides) in Syrian hamsters (*Mesocricetus auratus*). A report of six cases and the demonstration of T-cell specificity. Vet Dermatol. 3:13–19.

Pour, P., et al. 1979. Spontaneous tumors and common diseases in three types of hamsters. J. Natl. Cancer Inst. 63:797–811.

———. 1976. Spontaneous tumors and common diseases in two colonies of Syrian hamsters. 1. Incidence and sites. J. Natl. Cancer Inst. 56:931–35.

Saunders, G.K., and Scott, D.W. 1988. Cutaneous lymphoma resembling mycosis fungoides in the Syrian hamster (*Mesocricetus auratus*). Lab. Anim. Sci. 38:616–17.

Strandberg, J.D. 1987. Neoplastic diseases. In *Laboratory Hamsters,* ed. G.L. Van Hoosier, Jr., and C.W. McPherson, pp. 157–68. New York: Academic.

Trentin, J.J. 1987. Experimental biology: Use in oncological research. In *Laboratory Hamsters,* ed. G.L. Van Hoosier, Jr., and C.W. McPherson, pp. 95–110. New York: Academic.

Turusov, V.S., et al., ed. 1982. *Pathology of Tumours in Laboratory Animals. III. Tumours of the Hamster.* Lyon, France: IARC Scientific Publications.

Van Hoosier, G.L., Jr., and Trentin, J.J. 1979. Naturally occurring tumors of the Syrian hamster. Prog. Exp. Tumor Res. 23:1–12.

4 GERBIL

Gerbils are members of the subfamily Gerbillinae, family Muridae, with about 14 genera and 100 species. Most gerbils that are used for research are Mongolian gerbils (*Meriones unguiculatus*), also called jirds, clawed jirds, sand rats, and antelope rats. They are desert-dwelling, burrowing rodents with a high degree of resistance to heat stress and dehydration. A few other species of *Meriones* are used for research purposes, but most of the information available on pathology of gerbils relates to *M. unguiculatus,* as does this chapter. Most commercially available gerbils are outbred, although inbred strains exist.

ANATOMIC FEATURES

Hematology. The most conspicuous peculiarity of the gerbil is a high proportion of red cells with polychromasia, basophilic stippling, and reticulocytosis (Smith et al. 1976). This is particularly obvious in young gerbils up to 20 wk of age but occurs throughout life. This may be a reflection of the short half-life of erythrocytes (approximately 10 d), compared with other species. The predominant peripheral blood leukocyte is the lymphocyte, with a 3:1 or 4:1 ratio over granulocytes. Gerbils are normally lipemic (hypercholesterolemic) on standard diets, especially adult males.

Anatomy. The gross anatomy of the gerbil is quite similar to that of the mouse and rat. An obvious exception is its furred tail. Gerbils are utilized in stroke research because of their susceptibility to cerebral ischemia following common carotid artery ligation. This is because gerbils often have an incomplete circle of Willis, which is of no practical significance relative to spontaneous disease. Incisor teeth grow continuously, but molar teeth are rooted. Lung lobation is similar to that of mice and rats. Gerbils have a prominent gland on the midline of the ventral abdomen composed of sebaceous glands and specialized hair structures. It is inconspicuous in females but is prominent in sexually mature males. Gerbils do not have preputial glands. Auditory bullae are distinctively large, reflecting their highly adapted specialization for acute hearing. Microscopic adaptations in ear structure are also evident. The adrenal glands of the gerbil are quite large relative to other species of laboratory rodents. Renal function is adapted for urine concentration. The kidney has a very long papillus, and the ratio of papillus plus inner medulla to cortex is about twice that of a laboratory rat. This is a reflection of very long loops of Henle. Some Bowman's capsules in sexually mature male gerbils can be thickened due to the presence of cells that are morphologically intermediate between fibroblasts and smooth muscle cells (myofibroblasts). This lamina muscularis is unique to *Meriones.*

BIBLIOGRAPHY
FOR ANATOMIC FEATURES
Buchanan, J.G., and Stewart, A.D. 1974. Neurohypophysial storage of vasopressin in the normal and dehydrated gerbil (*Meriones unguiculatus*) with a note on kidney structure. J. Endocrinol. 60:381–82.

Bucher, O.M., and Kristic, R.V. 1979. Pericapsular smooth muscle cells in renal corpuscles of the Mongolian gerbil (*Meriones unguiculatus*). Cell Tissue Res. 199:75–82.

Dillon, W.G., and Glomski, C.A. 1975. The Mongolian gerbil: Qualitative and quantitative aspects of the cellular blood picture. Lab. Anim. 9:283–87.

Lay, D.M. 1972. The anatomy, physiology, functional significance and evolution of specialized hearing organs of gerbilline rodents. J. Morphol. 138:41–56.

Levine, S., and Sohn, D. 1969. Cerebral ischemia in infant and adult gerbils: Relation to incomplete circle of Willis. Arch. Pathol. 87:315–17.

Mays, A., Jr. 1969. Baseline hematological and blood biochemical parameters of the Mongolian gerbil. Lab. Anim. Care 19:838–42.

Ruhren, R. 1965. Normal values for hemoglobin concentration and cellular elements in the blood of Mongolian gerbils. Lab. Anim. Care 15:313–20.

Sales, N. 1973. The ventral gland of the male gerbil (*Meriones unguiculatus,* Gerbillidae): I. Histochemical features of the mucopolysaccharides. Ann. Histochem. 18:171–78.

Smith, R.A., et al. 1976. Erythrocyte basophilic stippling in the Mongolian gerbil. Lab. Anim. 10:379–83.

Williams, W.M. 1974. The anatomy of the Mongolian gerbil (*Meriones unguiculatus*). West Brookfield, Mass.: Tumblebrook Farms.

VIRAL INFECTIONS

There are no reported naturally occurring viral infections of gerbils, but this is probably a reflection of ignorance rather than reality. Certainly clinically significant viral infections are not currently recognized to be a problem.

BACTERIAL INFECTIONS

Clostridium piliforme Infection: Tyzzer's Disease

EPIZOOTIOLOGY AND PATHOGENESIS. There have been numerous documented cases of Tyzzer's disease in this species since the first reports of *Bacillus piliformis* (*C. piliforme*) infection in gerbils. The Mongolian gerbil is very susceptible to the disease. Frequently the successful reproduction of the disease in rodents requires treatment with immunosuppressive drugs, such as cortisone. However, Tyzzer's disease has been produced readily in gerbils without benefit of immunosuppression. Young gerbils have developed the typical disease following the oral inoculation of isolates from other species. Gerbils appear to be more susceptible to clinical disease following exposure to *C. piliforme* than do immunosuppressed mice. Housing sentinel gerbils on unautoclaved soiled bedding suspected to be contaminated with the organism has been used to detect carriers of the disease. Thus the Mongolian gerbil is recognized to be a useful sentinel animal to detect subclinical infections or environmental contamination with *B. piliformis.*

Typical lesions associated with Tyzzer's disease in gerbils include depression, ruffled hair coat, hunched posture, anorexia, and watery diarrhea. Following oral inoculation, severely affected animals usually die within 5–7 d postinoculation. In addition to focal hepatic necrosis, bacterial antigen has been observed in ileocecal enterocytes by 3 d postexposure. Extensive lesions and bacterial antigen has been demonstrated in the jejunum, ileum, and cecum by 5–6 d postinoculation. In affected gerbils, bacterial antigen may also be present in the muscle layers of the intestine and in Peyer's patches. Ileal enterocytes and Peyer's patches may be the initial sites for bacterial growth.

PATHOLOGY. At necropsy, pinpoint, pale foci up to 2 mm in diameter are usually present in the liver. Ecchymoses on the small intestine and cecum are variable findings. The walls of the small intestine and cecum are usually edematous. Intestinal contents are fluid and sometimes contain blood. The mesenteric lymph nodes may be enlarged and edematous. On microscopic examination, liver lesions frequently are concentrated in the periportal regions. In acute cases, there are foci of coagulation to caseation necrosis, with variable leukocytic infiltration, neutrophils predominating (Fig. 4.1). Intracytoplasmic bacilli are most numerous in hepatocytes adjacent to necrotic foci (Fig. 4.2). In hepatic lesions interpreted to be several days in duration, there may be focal fibrosis with mineralization. Intestinal lesions are usually most extensive in the ileum and cecum. Necrosis and sloughing of enterocytes, blunting of villi in affected areas, and transmural edema occur. Leukocytic infiltrates in the lamina propria consist of neutrophils and mononuclear cells. There may be necrosis of the adjacent intestinal smooth muscle, with leukocytic infiltration (Fig. 4.3). Frequently focal necrosis of Peyer's patches and mesenteric lymph nodes occurs. Intracytoplasmic bacilli are usually evident in enterocytes and sometimes in smooth muscle cells. Myocardial lesions, when present, consist of focal coagulation necrosis, with collapse of myofibers, and leukocytic infiltration (Fig. 4.4). There may be mineralization of cell debris. Bundles of bacilli may be evident in myofibers bordering necrotic foci using Warthin-

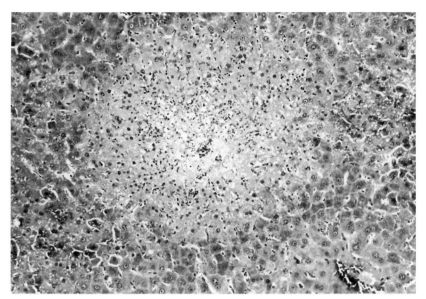

FIG. 4.1—Focal hepatitis with leukocytic infiltration in young Mongolian gerbil that died with acute Tyzzer's disease.

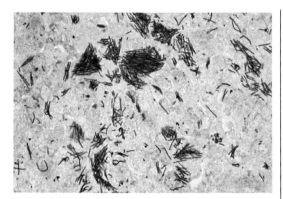

FIG. 4.2—Focal hepatic lesion stained with the Warthin-Starry method. Note the intracytoplasmic bacilli present in hepatocytes at the periphery of the lesion.

Starry or Giemsa stains. Diffuse suppurative encephalitis is another possible manifestation of Tyzzer's disease in this species.

DIAGNOSIS. The presence of the typical microscopic lesions and the demonstration of the intracellular bacilli are sufficient to confirm the diag-nosis. *Differential diagnoses* include acute bacterial infections, such as salmonellosis.

SIGNIFICANCE. The Mongolian gerbil is particularly susceptible to Tyzzer's disease. Aside from the complications due to morbidity and mortality, the gerbil is recognized to be a useful sentinel animal to detect the presence of *C. piliforme* in the research facility. The possibility of interspecies transmission is an important consideration.

***Salmonella* Infection: Salmonellosis.** Disease and mortality have been observed in young gerbils 3–10 wk of age that were naturally infected with *Salmonella typhimurium*. Clinical signs include moderate to severe diarrhea, dehydration, weight loss, and leukocytosis with neutrophilia. The mortality rate may be over 90%. In one report, animals also had a heavy infestation with *Hymenolepis nana*.

An outbreak of salmonellosis in a gerbil colony due to *Salmonella* group D has been reported. Dehydration, depression, testicular enlargement, and occasionally sudden death were observed.

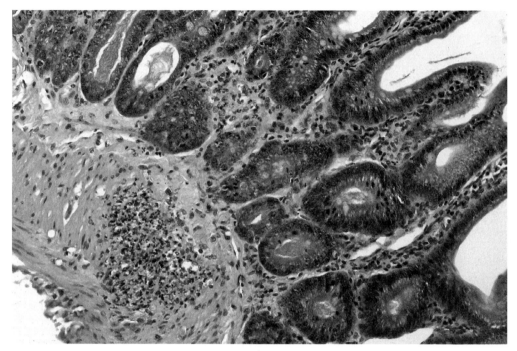

FIG. 4.3—Section of ileum from gerbil with Tyzzer's disease. Note the leukocytic infiltrate in the lamina propria, the scattered dilated intestinal crypts, and the focus of leukocytic infiltration in the adjacent smooth muscle.

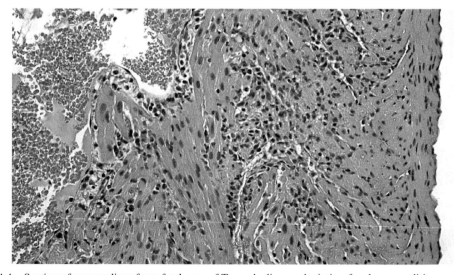

FIG. 4.4—Section of myocardium from fatal case of Tyzzer's disease depicting focal myocarditis.

Focal hepatitis, splenic necrosis, suppurative orchitis, interstitial pneumonitis, and purulent to pyogranulomatous leptomeningitis were lesions observed microscopically. *Salmonella*-infected cockroaches have been implicated as one possible source of the infection.

PATHOLOGY. At necropsy, the gastrointestinal tract is frequently distended with gas and fluid ingesta. Fibrinopurulent exudate may be present in the peritoneal cavity in some animals. Microscopic changes are characterized by multifocal hepatitis. Hepatic lesions may vary from foci of leukocytic infiltration to larger foci consisting of central caseation necrosis with variable mineralization and with epithelioid cells, lymphocytes, and neutrophils oriented around the periphery. Crypt abscesses are occasionally present in the intestine. *S. enteritidis* may be recovered from sites such as the small intestine, liver, spleen, and heart blood.

DIAGNOSIS. Isolation of the organism using the appropriate bacterial media, coupled with the typical lesions, will serve to confirm the diagnosis. *Differential diagnosis:* Tyzzer's disease is the primary one to rule out in this species.

SIGNIFICANCE. Although adult gerbils may be relatively resistant to experimental *Salmonella* infection, it is evident that younger animals may be very susceptible under certain circumstances. The dangers of interspecies transmission should be emphasized.

Staphylococcus Infection: Staphylococcal Dermatitis. Acute, diffuse dermatitis has been associated with beta-hemolytic *Staphylococcus aureus* infection. The disease appears to affect primarily young gerbils, and there may be a relatively high morbidity and mortality. The disease has been reproduced in gerbils inoculated in the nasal region with the staphylococcal isolate.

PATHOLOGY. On gross examination, there may be a diffuse moist dermatitis involving the face, nose, feet, legs, and ventral body surface. Alopecia, erythema, and moist brown exudate have been associated with the typical lesions. Micro-scopic changes are those of a suppurative dermatitis, with neutrophils infiltrating into the superficial and deep dermis and adnexae, with concurrent acanthosis and hyperkeratosis. Ulcerations may occur. Focal suppurative hepatitis may be present in some fatal cases of the disease.

DIAGNOSIS. Isolation and identification of the organism are necessary steps required to confirm the diagnosis.

SIGNIFICANCE. The isolation of a beta-hemolytic staphylococcus from the skin must be accompanied by the typical lesions.

Nasal Dermatitis. This is a frequently encountered problem in juvenile and adult Mongolian gerbils, appearing to be most common in postpuberal animals. Nasal dermatitis is characterized by dermatitis and alopecia around the external nares and upper labial region.

EPIZOOTIOLOGY AND PATHOGENESIS. The incidence of the disease in individual colonies may be over 15%, but an incidence of around 5% is more typical. The disease has been associated with infections with *Staphylococcus xylosus* (or *saprophyticus*) and *S. aureus.* However, staphylococci of identical type have been isolated from asymptomatic gerbils, and other factors have been implicated. Mechanical trauma may contribute to the disease in some circumstances, but porphyrin-containing lacrimal gland secretions have been shown to be an important contributing factor. Secretions from the Harderian gland normally bathe the eye and conjunctival sac and then are transported down to the external nares via the nasolacrimal duct. The secretions are mixed with saliva and spread widely over the pelage during the thermoregulatory grooming procedures. However, if these secretions are not removed routinely from the collection site at the external nares, chemical irritation and subsequent dermatitis may occur. Removal of the Harderian glands from affected animals has resulted in a marked improvement or recovery. Marked improvement was also seen in gerbils housed on sand. The failure to groom properly results in the accumulation of protoporphyrin-containing secretions around

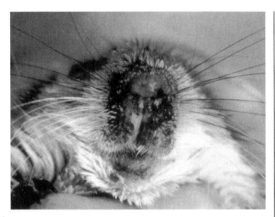

FIG. 4.5—Nasal dermatitis in mature Mongolian gerbil. There is marked reddening with encrustations around the external nares. (Courtesy M.E. Olson)

the external nares, which results in local irritation, scratching, hair loss, and dermatitis. Intact gerbils fitted with Elizabethan collars, which prevented self-grooming, develop nasal dermatitis, while those with bilateral Harderian gland adenectomy do not develop the disease. Synergism with a pathogenic bacterium such as *S. xylosus* or *S. aureus* may be necessary for the development of the moist, ulcerative form of the disease.

PATHOLOGY. On gross examination, there are varying degrees of dermatitis and alopecia involving the lateral and superior nasal area and the upper and lower lip (Fig. 4.5). Lesions may progress to a severe ulcerative dermatitis, with exudation and excoriation and crusting in the upper labial region. Dermatitis and hair loss may also be present on the forepaws and periocular regions. Histopathologically, there are hyperkeratosis and epidermal hyperplasia in active cases, with increased melanin deposition in the dermis. In acute, suppurative lesions, there are spongiosis, epidermal hyperplasia and necrosis, and infiltration with neutrophils. Other changes may include ulceration and epidermal abscessation.

DIAGNOSIS. The distribution and nature of the lesions are useful diagnostic criteria. The accumulated porphyrins will fluoresce under ultraviolet light. Routine bacteriology should be performed, since pathogenic staphylococci frequently play a role in the development of the lesions. *Differential diagnoses* include fighting injuries and nonspecific bacterial infections.

Other Bacterial Infections

BORDETELLA BRONCHISEPTICA INFECTION. This bacterium is a potential problem for gerbils but has not been reported as a natural disease. Young gerbils inoculated intranasally with *B. bronchiseptica* have developed severe disease with high mortality, while older gerbils appear to be more resistant. Both the *Meriones unguiculatus* and *M. shawi* species appear to be susceptible. Because of the frequency of *Bordetella* in laboratory guinea pigs and rabbits, contact with these species should be avoided.

CILIA-ASSOCIATED RESPIRATORY(CAR) BACILLUS INFECTION. Gerbils are susceptible to experimentally induced infections with the CAR bacillus. Young gerbils inoculated intranasally with a rat isolate remained asymptomatic during the study. However, at necropsy, there was colonization of the apices of epithelial cells lining the trachea and airways, with marked peritracheal and peribronchial lymphocytic infiltration. The relevance of these findings in the laboratory setting will require additional study.

LEPTOSPIRA INFECTION: LEPTOSPIROSIS. Leptospirosis has not been reported as a natural infection in gerbils, but they are quite susceptible to experimental infection. Acute disease is characterized by hemolytic icterus, with pale, mottled livers. Microscopically, there is degeneration of renal distal convoluted tubules and centrilobular hepatocytes with conspicuous erythrophagocytosis in the spleen. Spirochetes are present in kidney and liver in large numbers. Chronic infection occurs frequently, with chronic nonsuppurative inflammation, interstitial fibrosis, and development of progressively severe tubular degeneration and cyst formation. The infection may persist in the kidney for months to years.

BIBLIOGRAPHY
FOR BACTERIAL INFECTIONS

Carter, G.R., et al. 1969. Natural Tyzzer's disease in Mongolian gerbils (*Meriones unguiculatus*). Lab. Anim. Care 19:648–51.

Clark, J.D., et al. 1992. Salmonellosis in gerbils induced by a nonrelated experimental procedure. Lab. Anim. Sci. 42:161–63.

Fujiwara, K. 1978. Tyzzer's disease. Jap. J. Exp. Med. 48:467–77.

Gibson, S.V., et al. 1987. Diagnosis of subclinical *Bacillus piliformis* infection in a barrier-maintained mouse production colony. Lab. Anim. Sci. 37:786–91.

Harkness, J.E., and Wagner, J.E. 1995. Biology and Medicine of Rabbits and Rodents. Philadelphia: Lea and Febiger.

Lewis, C., and Grey, J.E. 1961. Experimental *Leptospira pomona* infection in the Mongolian gerbil (*Meriones unguiculatus*). J. Infect. Dis. 109:194–204.

Motzel, S.L., and Gibson, S.V. 1990. Tyzzer's disease in hamsters and gerbils from a pet store supplier. J. Am. Vet. Med. Assoc. 197:1176–78.

Olson, G.A., et al. 1977. Salmonellosis in a gerbil colony. J. Am. Vet. Med. Assoc. 171:970–72.

St. Claire, M.B., et al. 1999. Experimentally-induced infection of gerbils with cilia-associated respiratory bacillus. Lab. Anim. Sci. 49:421–23.

Veazy, R.S., et al. 1992. Encephalitis in gerbils due to naturally occurring infection with *Bacillus piliformis* (Tyzzer's disease). Lab. Anim. Sci. 42:516–18.

Waggie, K.S., et al. 1984. Experimentally induced Tyzzer's disease in Mongolian gerbils (*Meriones unguiculatus*). Lab. Anim. Sci. 34:53–57.

Winsser, J. 1960. A study of *Bordetella bronchiseptica*. Proc. Anim. Care Panel 10:87–104.

Yokomori, K., et al. 1989. Enterohepatitis in Mongolian gerbils (*Meriones unguiculatus*) inoculated perorally with Tyzzer's organism (*Bacillus piliformis*). Lab. Anim. Sci. 39:16–20.

Staphylococcal Infections and Nasal Dermatitis

Bresnahan, J.F., et al. 1983. Nasal dermatitis in the Mongolian gerbil. Lab. Anim. Sci. 33:258–63.

Donnelly, T.M. 1997. Nasal lesions in gerbils (What's your diagnosis?). Lab. Anim. 27(2):17–18.

Farrar, P.L., et al. 1988. Experimental nasal dermatitis in the Mongolian gerbil: Effect of bilateral Harderian gland adenectomy on development of facial lesions. Lab. Anim. Sci. 38:72–76.

Peckham, J.C., et al. 1974. Staphylococcal dermatitis in Mongolian gerbils (*Meriones unguiculatus*). Lab. Anim. Sci. 24:43–47.

Solomon, H.F. et al. 1990. A survey of staphylococci isolated from the laboratory gerbil. Lab. Anim. Sci. 40:316–18.

Theissen, D.D., and Kittrell, E.M.W. 1980. The Harderian gland and thermoregulation in the gerbil (*Meriones unguiculatus*). Physiol. Behav. 24:417–24.

Theissen, D.D., and Pendergrass, M. 1982. Harderian gland involvement in facial lesions in the Mongolian gerbil. J. Am. Vet. Med. Assoc. 181:1375–77.

Vincent, A.L., et al. 1979. The pathology of the Mongolian gerbil (*Meriones unguiculatus*): A review. Lab. Anim. Sci. 29:645–51.

PARASITIC DISEASES

ECTOPARASITIC INFESTATIONS

Mite Infestations (Acariasis). Gerbils can be infested with *Demodex*. The name *Demodex meriones* has been proposed, but it may represent *D. aurati* or *criceti* (hamster mites), since mites resembling both of these species have been found on the gerbil. *Demodex* mites have been demonstrated in skin scrapings from a 4-yr-old gerbil with diarrhea, cachexia, and rough hair coat. A lesion on the tail head was characterized by scaliness, hyperemia, and focal ulcerations. Old age and debilitation were considered to be important predisposing factors, and *Demodex* infections are not considered to be a problem in clinically healthy gerbils. The nature of the host-parasite relationship and the morphology of the mites are similar to the *Demodex* mite infections that occur in hamsters. Copra itch mites (*Tyrophagus castellani*), probably introduced through the food, have been found incidentally on gerbils. *Liponyssoides sanguineus,* an ectoparasite occasionally seen in house mice, has also been observed in Mongolian and Egyptian gerbils. Mites were also identified on laboratory mice and wild house mice on the same premises. No manifestations of disease were observed in affected animals. Mites were also present in the bedding in the cages.

ENDOPARASITIC INFECTIONS

Protozoal Infections: Giardiasis. Giardiasis has not been reported as a natural disease in gerbils, but they are highly susceptible to infection with *Giardia* cysts of human origin. Trophozoites can be found in the upper small intestine, and in heavy infestations they occur throughout the bowel.

Helminth Infections: Pinworms (Oxyuriasis) . Gerbils can become infected with several oxyurid nematodes, but none cause clinical problems. *Dentostomella translucida* has been reported in a variety of gerbils. It occurs in the anterior small intestine and has also been noted in the large intestine. Gerbils are susceptible to contact infection with the mouse and rat pinworms, *Syphacia obvelata* and *S. muris*.

Helminth Infections: Tapeworms. Severe infections with the "dwarf tapeworm" have been reported in pet gerbils. Dehydration and mucoid diarrhea are possible presenting signs. In another report describing an epizootic of salmonellosis in Mongolian gerbils, affected animals were also heavily parasitized with *Hymenolepis nana*. *H. diminuta* has also been identified at necropsy in gerbils.

At necropsy, small tapeworms are present in the small intestine. On microscopic examination of smears of intestinal mucosa, or of paraffin-embedded sections of small intestine, eggs and cysticercoids are readily identified. *H. nana* infections have been associated with debilitation and diarrhea in gerbils. In view of the direct life cycle, there is a possibility of transmission to human contacts.

BIBLIOGRAPHY
FOR PARASITIC DISEASES

Belosevic, M. 1983. *Giardia lamblia* infections in Mongolian gerbils: An animal model. J. Infect. Dis. 147:222–26.

Kellogg, H.S., and Wagner, J.E. 1982. Experimental transmission of *Syphacia obvelata* among mice, rats, hamsters and gerbils. Lab. Anim. Sci. 32:500–501.

Kunstyr, I., et al. 1993. Host specificity of cloned *Spironucleus* sp. originating from the European hamster. Lab. Anim. 27:77-80.

Levine, J.F., and Lage, A.L. 1984. House mouse mites infesting laboratory rodents. Lab. Anim. Sci. 34:393–94.

Lussier, G., and Loew, F.M. 1970. Natural *Hymenolepis nana* infection in Mongolian gerbils (*Meriones unguiculatus*). Can. Vet. J. 11:105–7.

Olson, G.A., et al. 1977. Salmonellosis in a gerbil colony. J. Am. Med. Assoc. 171:970–72.

Ross, C.R., et al. 1980. Experimental transmission of *Syphacia muris* among rats, mice, hamsters and gerbils. Lab. Anim. Sci. 30:35–37.

Schwartzbrott, S.S., et al. 1974. Demodicidosis in the Mongolian gerbil (*Meriones unguiculatus*): A case report. Lab. Anim. Sci. 24:666–68.

Vincent, A.L., et al. 1975. Spontaneous lesions and parasites of the Mongolian gerbil, *Meriones unguiculatus*. Lab. Anim. Sci. 25:711–22.

Wightman, S.R., et al. 1978a. *Dentostomella translucida* in the Mongolian gerbil (*Meriones unguiculatus*). Lab. Anim. Sci. 28:290–96.

———. 1978b. *Syphacia obvelata* in the Mongolian gerbil (*Meriones unguiculatus*): Natural occurrence and experimental transmission. Lab. Anim. Sci. 28:51–54.

GENETIC DISORDERS

Epilepsy. Epileptiform seizures are common among Mongolian gerbils that are subjected to stress, which may include cage changing. Susceptibility begins at around 2 mo of age and can reach an incidence of 40–80% within 6–10 mo and persist throughout life. The trait is inherited as a single autosomal locus with at least one dominant allele, with variable penetrance. The incidence therefore varies with different populations or lines of gerbils. Seizure-sensitive and -resistant strains have been selected for experimental purposes. Clinical signs include twitching of vibrissae and pinnae, motor arrest, myoclonic jerks, clonic-tonic seizures, vestibular aberrations, and occasionally death. Histopathologic lesions have not been found.

Periodontal Disease and Dental Caries. Gerbils that are maintained on a standard laboratory pelleted diet and water may develop progressively severe periodontal disease, which is first manifested at around 6 mo of age and is readily apparent by 1 yr. Advanced disease is present in gerbils over 2 yr of age, often with tooth loss. They are also prone to the development of dental caries, which can be enhanced with cariogenic diets.

Malocclusion. Lack of opposing occlusal contact results in tooth overgrowth in all species of rodents, including gerbils. Reported cases in gerbils are rare and have been due to loss of the upper incisors with overgrowth of the lower teeth. Molar teeth of gerbils do not grow continuously.

Behavioral Disease. Gerbils are usually relatively docile and easily handled. They are intermittently active day and night. Foot stomping is a common signal of startling, communication, and aggression. They tolerate each other very well if grouped before maturity, but mixing adult gerbils will usually provoke fighting, with death of the weaker animal.

BIBLIOGRAPHY FOR CONGENITAL/HEREDITARY DISORDERS

Afonsky, D. 1957. Dental caries in the Mongolian gerbil. NY State Dent. J. 23:315–16.

Fitzgerald, D.B., and Fitzgerald, R.J. 1965. Induction of dental caries in gerbils. Arch. Oral Biol. 11:139–40.

Loew, F.M. 1967. A case of overgrown mandibular incisors in a Mongolian gerbil. Lab. Anim. Care 17:137–39.

Loskota, W.J., et al. 1974. The gerbil as a model for the study of the epilepsies: Seizure patterns and ontogenesis. Epilepsia 15:109–19.

Moskow, B.S., et al. 1968. Spontaneous periodontal disease in the Mongolian gerbil. J. Periodont. Res. 3:69B83.

TOXIC AND METABOLIC DISORDERS

Streptomycin Toxicity. Members of the neomycin-streptomycin group of antibiotics can cause a direct neuromuscular blocking effect at excessive doses by inhibition of acetylcholine release. Although other rodents and rabbits are susceptible to this effect, they are less likely to be treated with these drugs and are, in addition, big enough to receive the proper dose. The margin of safety for streptomycin is low, and antibiotic preparations are seldom prepared so that an appropriate dose in a small volume can be administered to a rodent. Gerbils treated with these preparations have developed acute toxicity, characterized by depression, ascending flaccid paralysis, coma, and death within minutes of administration.

Lead Toxicity. Because of their urine-concentrating ability, gerbils are prone to accumulation of lead and chronic lead toxicity. They are used for this purpose experimentally, but the potential for natural toxicity in a laboratory environment is high because of their gnawing behavior. Chronically toxic animals become emaciated. Their livers become small and pigmented; their kidneys pale and pitted. Microscopic findings include acid-fast intranuclear inclusions in proximal convoluted tubular epithelium and chronic progressive nephropathy. Occasional intranuclear inclusions may be found in liver, but the predominant finding is lipofuscin pigment granules in hepatocytes and Kupffer's cells. Gerbils also develop a microcytic, hypochromic anemia with basophilic stippling. *Differential diagnoses* should include age-related renal disease, which is both mild and relatively rare in gerbils, and erythrocytic basophilic stippling, which should be differentiated from the condition that occurs normally in the gerbil, but to a lesser degree.

Amyloidosis. Amyloidosis has been reported in gerbils experimentally infected with a filariid worm. However, spontaneous cases occur, particularly in older animals. The liver, spleen, and lymph nodes are common sites of amyloid deposition. In one study, the majority of cases were secondary to chronic renal disease. Clinical signs, when present, include weight loss, dehydration, anorexia, and death.

Obesity and Diabetes. Approximately 10% of gerbils maintained on standard laboratory diet can become obese. This condition can be associated with reduced glucose tolerance, elevated insulin, and hyperplastic or degenerative changes in the endocrine pancreas.

Hyperadrenocortism/Cardiovascular Disease of Breeding Gerbils. A disease complex, attributed to hyperadrenocortism, has been described in repeatedly bred male and female, but not virgin, gerbils. Breeding females, and to a lesser extent males, develop mild to severe plaques of intimal and medial ground substance alterations with mineralization in the aorta and mesenteric, renal, and peripheral arteries. Breeders may have grossly visible plaques of the abdominal aorta, as well as aortic arch and the entire aorta in severe cases. Breeding animals have elevated serum triglycerides, enlarged pancreatic islets, fatty livers, thymic involution, adrenal hemorrhage, and adrenal lipid depletion, and some may have pheochromocytomas. Male breeders have been found to have a high incidence of focal myocardial necrosis and fibrosis. This phenomenon is also linked to diabetes and obesity. Cause and effect relationships have not been firmly established, but it is clear that these lesions occur frequently in gerbil populations and seem to occur in higher prevalence among breeders.

BIBLIOGRAPHY FOR TOXIC AND METABOLIC DISORDERS

Boquist, L. 1975. The Mongolian gerbil as a model for chronic lead toxicity. J. Comp. Pathol. 85:119–31.

————. 1972. Obesity and pancreatic islet hyperplasia in the Mongolian gerbil. Diabetologia 8:274–82.

Nakama, K. 1977. Studies on diabetic syndrome and influences of long-term tolbutamide administration in Mongolian gerbils (*Meriones unguiculatus*). Endocrinol. Jap. 24:421–33.

Port, C.D., et al. 1974. The Mongolian gerbil as a model for lead toxicity: I. Studies of acute poisoning. Am. J. Pathol. 76:79–94.

Vincent, A.L., et al. 1975. Spontaneous lesions and parasites of the Mongolian gerbil, *Meriones unguiculatus*. Lab. Anim. Sci. 25:711–22.

Wexler, B.C., et al. 1971. Spontaneous arteriosclerosis in male and female gerbils (*Meriones unguiculatus*). Atherosclerosis 14:107–19.

Wightman, S.R., et al. 1980. Dihydrostreptomycin toxicity in the Mongolian gerbil, *Meriones unguiculatus*. Lab. Anim. Sci. 30:71–75.

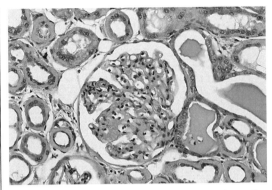

FIG. 4.7—Chronic progressive glomerulonephropathy in an aged Mongolian gerbil. Note the thickening of glomerular and peritubular basement membranes and the proteinaceous casts within tubules.

DISEASES ASSOCIATED WITH AGING

Focal Myocardial Degeneration. Focal myocardial degeneration and fibrosis are relatively common microscopic findings in older gerbils. In general, 50% or more of male breeders may be affected, and a smaller percentage of breeding females. Lesions are probably ischemic in origin, but the etiopathogenesis has not been adequately studied. On microscopic examination there are foci of degeneration of myofibers, with interstitial fibrosis (Fig. 4.6).

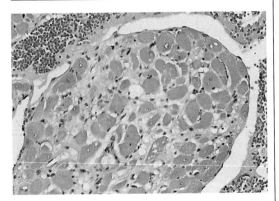

FIG. 4.6—Section of papillary muscle from a case of myocardial degeneration with interstitial fibrosis in an old Mongolian gerbil.

Chronic Nephropathy. Glomerular hypercellularity, tubular degeneration, and dilation and cast formation in tubules are changes seen in the kidneys of aging gerbils (Fig. 4.7) . Mononuclear cell infiltration consistent with chronic interstitial nephritis may be present in affected kidneys.

Aural Cholesteatoma. Spontaneous aural cholesteatomas occur in high frequency among adult gerbils, with an incidence of over 50% at 2 yr of age. These masses of keratinized epithelium arise from the outer surface of the tympanic membrane and external auditory canal. As keratin is accumulated, it displaces the tympanic membrane into the middle ear. Compression and secondary inflammation result in destruction of temporal bone and inner ear structures. Clinical signs include head tilt and accumulation of keratin plugs in the external ear canal. *Differential diagnosis* includes otitis media/interna, but this is rare in gerbils because of the vertical configuration of their eustachian tubes.

Cystic Ovaries. Female gerbils are prone to the development of ovarian cysts. Nearly 50% of gerbils over 400 d of age may be affected. Cysts range in size from 1 to 50 mm in diameter. Ovulation and corpus luteum formation continue to occur in the presence of cysts, but litter sizes are reduced, and severely affected females become infertile.

Ocular Proptosis. Aged gerbils can develop protrusion of the nictitating membrane and conjunctiva with bulbar proptosis. The underlying cause has not been characterized.

BIBLIOGRAPHY FOR DISEASES ASSOCIATED WITH AGING

Bingel, S.A. 1995. Pathologic findings in an aging Mongolian gerbil (*Meriones unguiculatus*) colony. Lab. Anim. Sci. 45:597–600.

Chole, R.A., et al. 1981. Cholesteatoma: Spontaneous occurrence in the Mongolian gerbil, *Meriones unguiculatus*. Am. J. Otol. 2:204—10.

Henry, K.R., et al. 1983. Age-related increase of spontaneous aural cholesteatoma in the Mongolian gerbil. Arch. Otolaryngol. 109:19–21.

Norris, M.L., and Adams, C.E. 1972. Incidence of cystic ovaries and reproductive performance in the Mongolian gerbil, *Meriones unguiculatus*. Lab. Anim. 6:337–42.

Rowe, S.E., et al. 1994. Spontaneous neoplasms in aging Gerbillinae. Vet. Pathol. 11:38–51.

NEOPLASMS

In general, the incidence of spontaneous tumors in this species is relatively low, with increasing incidence in gerbils over 2 yr of age. There is frequently a striking variation in the percentage of tumors that occur in different colonies of Mongolian gerbils. Ovarian, adrenocortical, and cutaneous tumors are the most commonly recognized neoplasms in this species. Of the ovarian tumors, granulosa cell tumors appear to be the most common in aged females. Granulosa cell tumors are frequently bilateral and vary from fleshy and lobulated to cystic masses (Fig. 4.8). Granulosa cells are the predominant cell type (Fig. 4.9). Dysgerminomas, luteal cell tumors, leiomyomas, and rarely thecal cell carcinoma have been identified. Adrenal cortical adenomas and carcinomas also occur. There is a relatively low incidence of tumors of the pituitary, mammary gland, and lung in the Mongolian gerbil. In a study involving other species of Gerbillinae, neoplasms included squamous carcinoma of the ear, thymoma, uterine adenocarcinoma, squamous cell carcinoma of the ventral marking gland (Figs. 4.10 and 11),

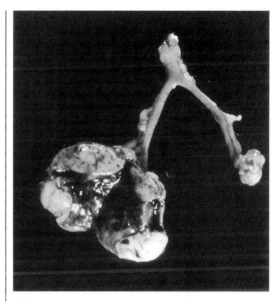

FIG. 4.8—Ovaries and uterine horns from an aged female Mongolian gerbil. The left ovary, which is markedly enlarged, fleshy, and lobulated, with variable dark red to pale tan areas, is a granulosa cell carcinoma. (Courtesy D. Schlafer)

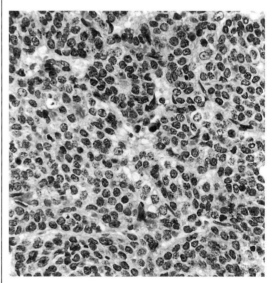

FIG. 4.9—Histological section from the granulosa cell tumor in Figure 4.8.

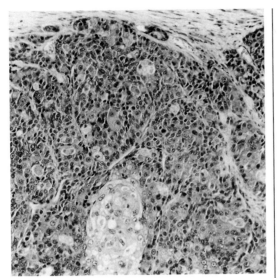

FIG. 4.10—Marking gland adenocarcinoma. Neoplasm was removed from the ventral midline (umbilical region) of a male Mongolian gerbil approximately 20 mo of age. Note the marked anisokaryosis, the variations in cytoplasmic volume and the staining properties, which vary from finely granular to vacuolated cytoplasm. (Courtesy B.M. Cross)

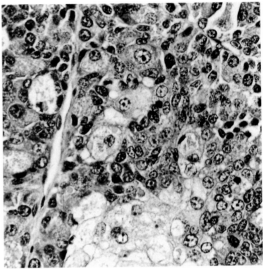

FIG. 4.11—Higher magnification of Figure 4.10. (Courtesy B.M. Cross)

adrenocortical tumors, and primary ovarian tumors.

BIBLIOGRAPHY FOR NEOPLASMS

Benitz, K.F., and Kramer, A.W. 1965. Spontaneous tumors in the Mongolian gerbil. Lab. Anim. Care 15:281–94.

Meckley, P.E., and Zwicker, G.M. 1979. Natur-ally-occurring neoplasms in the Mongolian gerbil (*Meriones unguiculatus*). Lab. Anim. 13:203–6.

Rowe, S.E., et al. 1974. Spontaneous neoplasms in aging Gerbillinae. Vet. Pathol. 11:38–51.

Vincent, A.L., et al. 1979. The pathology of the Mongolian gerbil (*Meriones unguiculatus*): A review. Lab. Anim. Sci. 29:645–61.

———. 1975. Spontaneous lesions and parasites of the Mongolian gerbil, *Meriones unguiculatus*. Lab. Anim. Sci. 25:711–22.

GUINEA PIG

There are relatively few strains of domesticated guinea pigs recognized in the world today; the so-called English shorthair or Hartley strain is most commonly used in the research facility. However, the long-haired Peruvian and Abyssinian breeds are popular in cavy club circles. Nervous in temperament, guinea pigs may refuse to eat or drink for some time following any significant change in location, feed, or management practices. Their long gestation period and relatively large offspring at full term may result in dystocia, particularly in sows that farrow with their first litter at 6 or more months of age. This has been attributed to failure of the iliosacral ligaments to relax sufficiently to permit passage of the fetuses at term. Unlike some of the smaller rodents, guinea pigs have relatively few viral infections recognized to be a significant cause of disease. In general, scurvy (either clinical or subclinical), respiratory tract infections, and enteric disease are the major diagnostic problems seen in this species.

Guinea pigs live in groups with a strong male-dominance hierarchy and a loose female hierarchy. They tend to live in family units centered around an alpha male. Mature boars, particularly strangers, will fight savagely, sometimes with fatal outcome. Females will also fight on occasion. Guinea pigs are active during daylight hours. They eat frequently, are coprophagic, and do not cache their food, as many rodents do. They require a constant source of water and tend to contaminate their water bowls with ingesta as they drink. They do not lick sipper tubes without training, a consideration that can lead to dehydration and death. They are indiscriminate defecators and renowned for their tendency to sit in and soil their food bowls. Breeding activity occurs year-round, and infants are highly precocious at birth. At parturition both males and females assist in grooming infants and eating placentas, and lactating sows will nurse other infants. Infants do not receive much maternal attention, other than anogenital grooming, which stimulates defecation and urination. They are normally weaned within 3 wk but can be weaned as early as 3–4 d if anogenital stimulation is provided. Vocalization is well developed and complex. They respond to sudden auditory stimulation and unfamiliar surroundings by freezing in place, whereas sudden movement often elicits a random stampede, which may result in injury to young animals.

ANATOMIC FEATURES

Hematology. Heterophils are the counterpart of the neutrophil in guinea pigs. These cells have distinct eosinophilic cytoplasmic granules. Lymphocytes are the predominant leukocyte in the peripheral blood, and both small and large forms are normally found.

Kurloff Cells (Foa-Kurloff Cells). These unique mononuclear leukocytes are found routinely in certain tissues in guinea pigs. In nonpregnant animals, Kurloff cells are located primarily in the sinusoids of the spleen and in stromal tissues of the bone marrow and thymus. They are not normally found in lymph nodes. Kurloff cells can be readily identified in impression smears of the spleen. They are usually present in the sinusoids of the spleen in tissue sections, particularly in females. The cells contain a finely fibrillar to granular structure (Kurloff body) 1–8 μm in diameter within a cytoplasmic vacuole, with displacement of the nucleus (Fig. 5.1). Theories regarding the origins of Kurloff cells have been varied and at times highly speculative. Interpretations have included intracellular parasites, phagocytic cells,

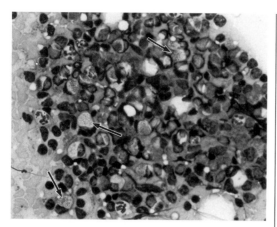

FIG. 5.1—Impression smear of spleen from adult female guinea pig, illustrating typical Kurloff cells (*arrows*). Note the large, finely granular Kurloff bodies within the cytoplasm of these mononuclear cells.

nuclear remnants, and secretory cells. It is now generally agreed that Kurloff cells are probably a member of the lymphoid series. The intracytoplasmic material is PAS-positive and stains positive for fibrinoid material with the Lendrum stain. It is interpreted to be mucopolysaccharide material secreted by the cell, and glycoprotein associated with a protein-polysaccharide material. On ultrastructural examination, inclusions are membrane-bound, and cytoplasmic organelles in these cells are consistent with secretory activity.

The possible function of these cells has been open to speculation. Kurloff cells, which are rarely seen in newborn guinea pigs, are present in relatively large numbers in adult female guinea pigs. Their numbers fluctuate with the stage of the estrous cycle. Treatment with estrogens produces a dramatic rise in the number of Kurloff cells in the viscera and circulation in both boars and sows. Increased numbers (e.g., more than 1–2%) are usually present in the peripheral blood during pregnancy. In addition, large numbers of these cells aggregate in the placental labyrinth in pregnant sows. Kurloff cells have been shown to release the material from the inclusion into the trophoblast and fetal endothelium of the placental labyrinth. In vitro studies have demonstrated that this material has a toxic effect on macrophages. It has been suggested that Kurloff cells may therefore play a role in preventing the maternal rejection of the fetal placenta during pregnancy.

There is evidence that Kurloff cells are the counterpart of natural killer (NK) cells in other species. As part of the internal monitoring system in mammals, NK cells are recognized to play an important role in the recognition and elimination of neoplastic cells. In vitro studies using Kurloff cells have demonstrated a cytotoxic effect on leukemic cells. In addition, Kurloff cells have been shown to reduce the incidence of leukemia in guinea pigs transplanted with lymphoblastic cells. Spontaneous neoplasms are relatively uncommon in guinea pigs. This may be due, at least in part, to the efficiency of the Kurloff cell in preventing the development of spontaneous tumors.

SIGNIFICANCE. It is important that pathologists be aware of these cells and not misinterpret the presence of Kurloff cells as a disease process. They have on occasion been interpreted as lupus erythematosus cells when found in blood samples collected from this species.

Respiratory Tract. Pulmonary arteries and arterioles have marked medial thickening in this species (Fig. 5.2). This should not be interpreted to be an abnormal finding. Larger airways are surrounded by prominent concentric bands of smooth muscle. The marked contraction of the peribronchial muscle may result in marked distortion and thickening and sloughing of the respiratory epithelium that lines affected airways. On occa-

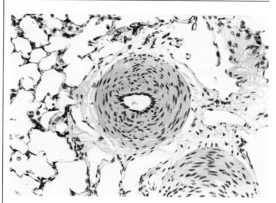

FIG. 5.2—Section of lung from guinea pig, illustrating typical medium-size pulmonary artery in this species. Note the medial thickness.

sion, such artifacts have been interpreted to be a bronchial tumor by the unwary pathologist. Clara cells are the prevalent cell type lining bronchioles, but they are absent in the trachea and larger bronchi.

PERIVASCULAR LYMPHOID NODULES. Aggregations of lymphocytes in the adventitia of pulmonary vessels are a frequent incidental finding in guinea pigs. A variety of strains may be affected. Microscopic foci have been observed in animals as young as 5 d of age, but nodules are more common in older animals. The incidence and extent of the involvement varies. Frequently animals of all ages are found to be free of these changes at necropsy. The perivascular changes are normally found only in the lung. At necropsy, close examination may reveal circumscribed, pale, pinpoint subpleural foci up to 0.5 mm in diameter. On microscopic examination, concentric to eccentric aggregations of small- to medium-size lymphocytes are oriented around small arteries and veins (Figs. 5.3 and 5.4). Nodules are focal to segmental in distribution in the perivascular regions. There may be focal to diffuse infiltrates of lymphocytes in alveolar septa in some animals, but the airways and alveoli are free of exudate in the typical cases. Ultrastructural studies have revealed morphologically normal

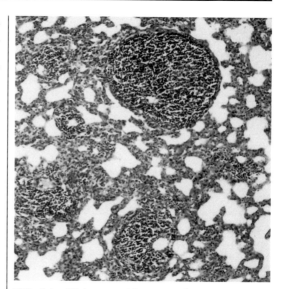

FIG. 5.4—Higher magnification of Figure 5.3. The infiltrates are present in the adventitia of arterioles and are composed of relatively well-differentiated lymphocytes. Note the thickening of alveolar septa, with mononuclear cell infiltration.

lymphocytes, and there was no evidence of viral agents associated with the cellular infiltrates. The lymphoid nodules have been ascribed to a variety of antigenic stimuli, but the pathogenesis and significance of these changes are currently not well understood.

SIGNIFICANCE. The presence of perivascular nodules, if present at necropsy, should be duly recorded. However, in the absence of other significant changes, undue importance should not be placed on this finding. They must be differentiated from the focal granulomatous pulmonary lesions seen in guinea pigs posttreatment with Freund's adjuvant.

OSSEOUS METAPLASIA (METAPLASTIC NODULES) IN THE LUNG. Bony spicules are occasionally observed in the lung in guinea pigs. Similar changes have been seen in other species, such as the rat and hamster. They are composed of dense, lamellar bone, with varying degrees of calcification. Usually there is no or minimal reaction in the adjacent alveolar septa. They have been interpreted to be inhaled fragments of bone of dietary origin, but there is evidence that in the guinea pig they are foci of osseous metaplasia.

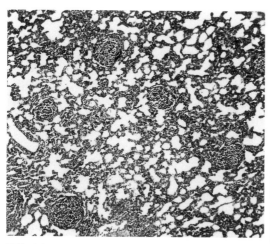

FIG. 5.3—Section of lung from adult guinea pig with prominent perivascular lymphoid nodules. These may be present as an incidental finding, particularly in adult animals.

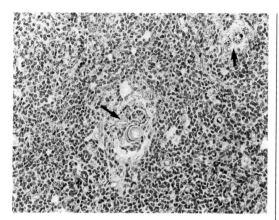

FIG. 5.5—Thymus from young guinea pig. Note the fragmentation of cells (*arrows*) associated with Hassall's corpuscles, a normal feature of the thymus in this species.

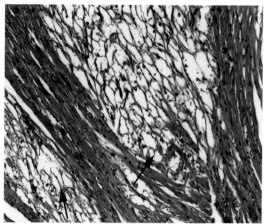

FIG. 5.6—Myocardium from adult guinea pig illustrating segmental rhabdomyomatosis, an incidental finding at necropsy. There is marked vacuolation of the sarcoplasm of affected myofibers (*arrows*).

Large numbers of metaplastic osseous foci, including well-differentiated bone marrow, have been observed in the lungs of guinea pigs following X-irradiation.

Hematopoietic System

THYMUS. Degenerate thymocytes are frequently observed in close association with Hassall's corpuscles, particularly in younger animals (Fig. 5.5). This should not be interpreted to be an abnormal change, as it is common in the guinea pig. These areas of degeneration may evolve into thymic cysts.

HEART: RHABDOMYOMATOSIS (NODULAR GLYCOGEN INFILTRATION). This condition is occasionally observed as an incidental finding in guinea pigs of various ages. It has been interpreted to be a degenerative condition and a congenital tissue malformation with "blastemoid" characteristics. It has been suggested that rhabdomyomatosis occurs more frequently in animals with scurvy, but this is speculation at this point. The current assessment is that rhabdomyomatosis is a congenital disease related to a disorder of glycogen metabolism.

PATHOLOGY. Smaller lesions are not visible on macroscopic examination. Occasionally larger areas appear as pale pink, poorly delineated foci or streaks. Rhabdomyomatosis has been observed in various regions of the heart, including ventricle, atria, interventricular septum, and papillary muscles. Lesions are most frequently found in the left ventricle. Microscopic examination reveals a spongy network of vacuolated myofibers composed of finely fibrillar to granular, eosinophilic cytoplasm (Fig. 5.6). Vacuoles are rounded to polygonal in shape and usually fill the sarcolemmal sheath. Vacuoles contain large quantities of glycogen, which is washed out in the fixation and processing procedures. Glycogen is readily demonstrated in PAS-stained, alcohol-fixed specimens. There may be displacement and flattening of myocyte nuclei in some affected fibers. In other fibers, there may be a cytoplasmic marginal rim with a round nucleus projecting into the vacuole (Fig. 5.7). Myofibers with centrally located nuclei and radiating fibrillar processes have been called "spider cells." Interspersed within the affected myofibers, there may be poorly differentiated fibers with identifiable cross-striations.

SIGNIFICANCE. Rhabdomyomatosis is considered to be an incidental finding in the guinea pig, and normally it does not significantly compromise cardiac function.

BIBLIOGRAPHY FOR ANATOMIC FEATURES

Hematology

Sanderson, J.H., and Phillips, C.E. 1981. *An Atlas of Laboratory Animal Haematology*. Oxford, Engl.: Clarendon.

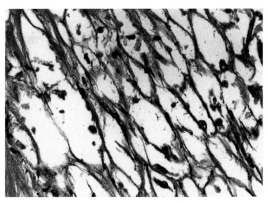

FIG. 5.7—Higher magnification of affected myocardium with rhabdomyomatosis. Note the cytoplasmic vacuolation, with fibrillar strands radiating from the nuclei.

Kurloff Cells
Christensen, H.E., et al. 1970. The cytology of the Foa-Kurloff reticular cells of the guinea pig. Acta. Pathol. Microbiol. Scand. (Suppl.) 212:15–24.
Debout, C., et al. 1995. Increase of a guinea pig natural killer cell (Kurloff cell) during leukemogenesis. Cancer Lett. 97:117–22.
———. 1993. In vitro cytotoxic effect of guinea pig natural killer cells (Kurloff cells) on homologous leukemic cells (L2C). Leukemia 7:733–35.
Ledingham, J.C.G. 1940. Sex hormones and the Foa-Kurloff cell. J. Pathol. Bacteriol. 50:201–19.
Marshall, A.H.E., et al. 1971. Studies on the function of the Kurloff cell. Int. Arch. Allergy 40:137–52.
Revell, P.A., et al. 1971. The distribution and ultrastructure of the Kurloff cell in the guinea pig. J. Anat. 109:187–99.

Respiratory Tract and Perivascular Lymphoid Nodules
Baskerville, A., et al. 1982. Ultrastructural studies of chronic pneumonia in guinea pigs. Lab. Anim. 16:351–55.
Brewer, N.R., and Cruise, L.J. 1997. The respiratory system of the guinea pig: Emphasis on species differences. Contemp. Top. 36(1):100–109.
Schiefer, B., and Stunzi, H. 1979. Pulmonary lesions in guinea pigs and rats after subcutaneous injection of complete Freund's adjuvant or homologous pulmonary tissue. Zentralbl. Vetinaermed. Med. (A) 26:1–10.
Thompson, S.W., et al. 1962. Perivascular nodules of lymphoid cells in the lungs of normal guinea pigs. Am. J. Pathol. 40:507–17.

Osseous Metaplasia in the Lung
Innes, J.R.M., et al. 1956. Note on the origin of some fragments of bone in the lungs of laboratory animals. Arch. Pathol. 61:401–6.

Knowles, J.F. 1984. Bone in the irradiated lung of the guinea pig. J. Comp. Pathol. 94:529–33.

Heart
Hueper, W.C. 1941. Rhabdomyomatosis of the heart in a guinea pig. Am. J. Pathol. 17:121–26.
Vink, H. 1969. Rhabdomyomatosis of the heart in guinea pigs. J. Pathol. 97:331–34.

General Bibliography
Breazile, J.E., and Brown, E.M. 1976. Anatomy. In *The Biology of the Guinea Pig,* ed. J.E. Wagner and P.J. Manning, pp. 54–62. New York: Academic.
Harper, L.V. 1976. Behavior. In *The Biology of the Guinea Pig,* ed. J.E. Wagner and P.J. Manning, pp. 31–51. New York: Academic.

VIRAL INFECTIONS

DNA VIRAL INFECTIONS

Adenoviral Infection: Adenoviral Pneumonitis. Outbreaks of respiratory disease attributed to an adenovirus have been recognized in Europe and North America. The disease is characterized by low morbidity and a mortality rate in clinically affected animals of up to 100%. In those cases described to date, frequently the animals have been subjected to experimental manipulations that may have resulted in impairment of the immune response.

PATHOLOGY. Consolidation of the cranial lobes of the lung and hilus is a characteristic finding at necropsy. Microscopic changes are those of a necrotizing bronchitis and bronchiolitis, with desquamation of lining epithelial cells and leukocytic infiltration, mononuclear cells predominating. Some airways may be obliterated by cell debris, leukocytes, and fibrinous exudate. Numerous necrotic foci may be scattered throughout the lung. The nuclei of affected epithelial cells often contain round to oval basophilic inclusion bodies 7–15 μm in diameter (Fig. 5.8). The virus has not been recovered and characterized to date, but electron microscopic examination has revealed typical adenovirus particles in affected nuclei. Using homogenates of lung prepared from a spontaneous case of the disease, typical lesions have been produced in intranasally inoculated newborn guinea pigs. The incubation period is 5–10 d. Older inoculated animals are relatively

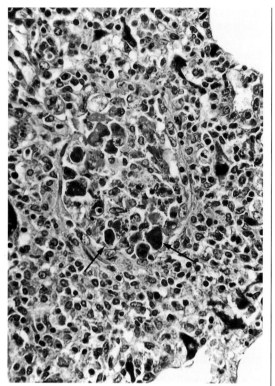

FIG. 5.8—Section of lung from spontaneous case of adenoviral bronchoalveolitis in young guinea pig. Prominent intranuclear inclusion bodies (*arrows*) are present in bronchial epithelial cells and in a few alveolar septal cells.

refractory to the disease. Typical adenoviral particles may be found in the nuclei of pulmonary epithelial cells of the lung.

DIAGNOSIS. The presence of nonsuppurative bronchitis and bronchiolitis in young guinea pigs with typical intranuclear basophilic inclusion bodies is consistent with adenoviral pneumonitis. The diagnosis may be confirmed by the demonstration of adenoviral particles in affected cells by electron microscopy. *Differential diagnoses* include cytomegalovirus infection and infections of the lower respiratory tract with bacteria, such as *Bordetella bronchiseptica.*

SIGNIFICANCE. Adenoviral infections in colonies of guinea pigs may be more prevalent than currently recognized. Clinical disease appears to occur primarily in young animals. Typical lesions have been observed in the airways of clinically

normal young adults, emphasizing that subclinical infections do occur. Other than the pulmonary lesions recognized to occur during the acute stages of the disease, the possible effects of adenoviral infections on other systems are currently unknown.

Herpesviral Infections

CYTOMEGALOVIRAL INFECTION. The cytomegalovirus (CMV) group are species-specific members of the family Herpesviridae. Natural infections occur in several mammals, including human and nonhuman primates, mice, rats, and guinea pigs. Members of the CMV group produce characteristic large, intranuclear and intracytoplasmic inclusion bodies and may persist in the host as an inapparent or latent infection for years. Under natural conditions, primary target tissues for CMV in the guinea pig are the salivary glands, kidney, and liver.

EPIZOOTIOLOGY AND PATHOGENESIS. Most guinea pigs housed under conventional conditions may seroconvert by a few months of age. A high percentage have been shown to have salivary gland lesions in some surveys. The virus may be transmitted by exposure to infected saliva or urine or as a transplacental infection. Systemic disease, with associated lesions, has been produced in weanling guinea pigs inoculated subcutaneously with CMV. In the experimental disease, focal lesions with intranuclear inclusion bodies may be present in salivary glands, liver, spleen, lung, and kidney. Pregnant guinea pigs have been shown to develop more extensive visceral lesions when inoculated with CMV than do nonpregnant animals. Lymphoproliferative disease, with mononucleosis-like syndrome and lymphadenopathy, has been observed in guinea pigs postinoculation with CMV. However, naturally occurring CMV infections rarely cause detectable clinical disease in the guinea pig, a pattern similar to that observed in human CMV infections. There is one report of systemic CMV infection with visceral lesions in two young guinea pigs introduced into a conventional facility. Focal destructive lesions with large intranuclear and cytoplasmic inclusion bodies were observed in various tissues including spleen, liver, kidney, and lung.

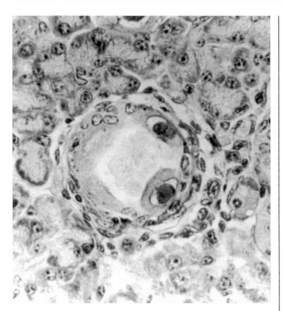

FIG. 5.9—Submandibular salivary gland from adult guinea pig with cytomegalovirus infection (an incidental finding). Note the karyomegaly of infected cells, the large intranuclear inclusion bodies, and the margination of nuclear chromatin. (Courtesy G.D. Hsiung)

PATHOLOGY. Lesions are usually regarded as an incidental finding at necropsy and are confined primarily to the ductal epithelial cells of the salivary glands. Large eosinophilic inclusion bodies are associated with marked karyomegaly and margination of the nuclear chromatin in affected cells (Fig. 5.9). Intracytoplasmic inclusions are occasionally present in ductal epithelial cells. There may be a concurrent mononuclear cell infiltration around infected ducts. In the acute systemic form of the disease, interstitial pneumonitis and multifocal areas of necrosis may be present in the lymph nodes, spleen, liver, kidney, lung, and other viscera. Intranuclear and intracytoplasmic inclusion bodies may be present in affected foci.

SIGNIFICANCE. Subclinical CMV infections are common in guinea pigs housed in conventional facilities. Spontaneous generalized cytomegalovirus infection with mortality seldom occurs, and there has been speculation that these cases may be associated with a compromised immune system. Lymphoid hyperplasia, lymphadenopathy, and mononucleosis have been observed in Hartley guinea pigs inoculated subcutaneously with guinea pig CMV. CMV infections in guinea pigs are considered to be a useful animal model for CMV infections in other species, including human patients.

OTHER CAVIAN HERPESVIRAL INFECTIONS. Guinea pig "herpeslike virus" (GPHLV) has been isolated from degenerating primary kidney cell cultures prepared from guinea pigs, but to date GPHLV has not been shown to be capable of producing disease in the natural host. Guinea pig "X virus" (GPXV) is a herpesvirus originally isolated from the leukocytes of strain 2 guinea pigs. Based on serological studies and DNA analyses, GPXV is different from either GPHLV or guinea pig CMV. Following experimental inoculation of GPXV into Hartley strain guinea pigs, viremia, focal hepatic necrosis, and mortality may occur.

SIGNIFICANCE. Current information suggests it is unlikely that GPHLV and GPXV will prove to be important primary pathogens in the guinea pig. However, they represent a possible complicating factor, should either occur as an inapparent infection in guinea pigs under experiment in the laboratory.

Viral Infections Associated with Cavian Leukemia. Cavian leukemia has been associated with a retroviral infection, and C-type viral particles have been visualized in transformed lymphocytes. GPHLV has also been associated with guinea pig leukemia. However, herpesviral particles interpreted to be GPHLV have been demonstrated in cells of leukemic guinea pigs that also were infected with a retrovirus. Based on current information, it seems unlikely that GPHLV plays an important role in leukemia in this species.

RNA VIRAL INFECTIONS

Arenaviral Infection: Lymphocytic Choriomeningitis (LCM)

EPIZOOTIOLOGY AND PATHOGENESIS. LCM is a relatively rare disease in guinea pigs, but it does represent an infection that can complicate research projects and is of public health significance. Lesions observed in guinea pigs with LCM have included lymphocytic infiltrates in the meninges, choroid plexi, and ependyma, and in liver, adrenals, and lungs. There is a wide host range, including wild mice, and exposure may occur by inhalation or ingestion, and apparently in guinea pigs through the intact skin.

DIAGNOSIS. Confirmation requires the demonstration of viral antigen in affected tissues and/or positive serological tests.

SIGNIFICANCE. LCM virus infection has been shown to prolong the life of guinea pigs carrying a leukemia agent, which emphasizes the potential for the virus to be an important complicating factor in certain types of research. Several species, including humans, are susceptible to LCM viral infection.

Coronavirus-like Infection. A syndrome characterized by wasting, anorexia, and diarrhea has been observed in young guinea pigs following their arrival at a research facility. The disease was characterized by a low morbidity and mortality.

PATHOLOGY. There is an acute to subacute necrotizing enteritis involving primarily the distal ileum, and copious amounts of mucoid material may be present throughout the gastrointestinal tract. On microscopic examination, lesions are particularly prominent in the terminal small intestine. There is blunting and fusion of affected villi, with necrosis and sloughing of enterocytes from the tips of villi and frequently syncytial giant cell formation in the intestinal mucosa. Viral particles consistent with the morphology of a coronavirus were demonstrated in fecal samples examined by electron microscopy. In another study, clinically normal guinea pigs of different ages were observed to shed coronavirus-like particles in the feces for long periods of time.

SIGNIFICANCE. The importance of suspected coronaviral infections in this species is currently unknown. However, until additional information is available, it should be considered in the differential diagnoses in cases of enteritis and/or wasting in young guinea pigs.

Paramyxoviral Infections. Serological surveys indicate that guinea pigs may occasionally seroconvert to pneumonia virus of mice (PVM) and Sendai virus. Guinea pigs inoculated intranasally with PVM develop antibodies within 2 wk postinoculation, but lesions attributable solely to PVM have not been observed. Natural seroconversion to PVM may be due to infection with an antigenically related paramyxovirus.

Picornaviral Infection. Antibodies to murine encephalomyelitis virus (TMEV strain GDVII) are occasionally observed when guinea pigs are tested for this virus. Lameness was observed in two guinea pigs that had high antibody titers to murine poliovirus. The clinical disease was attributed to the viral infection, although the animals recovered following treatment with vitamin C. The significance of the murine poliovirus infections in this species has not been resolved.

Other Viral Infections. Serology studies indicate that guinea pigs will develop antibody to other rodent viruses, including reovirus 3. The significance of these findings has not yet been determined.

BIBLIOGRAPHY FOR VIRAL INFECTIONS

Infections with DNA Viruses

Adenoviral Infection
Brennecke, L.H., et al. 1983. Naturally occurring virus-associated respiratory disease in two guinea pigs. Vet. Pathol. 20:488–91.
Crippa, L., et al. 1997. Asymptomatic adenoviral respiratory tract infection in guinea pigs. Lab. Anim. Sci. 47:197–99.
Feldman, S.H., et al. 1990. Necrotizing viral bronchopneumonia in guinea pigs. Lab. Anim. Sci. 40:82–83.
Kaup, F.-J., et al. 1984. Experimental viral pneumonia in guinea pigs: An ultrastructural study. Vet. Pathol. 21:521–27.
Kunstyr, I., et. al. 1984. Adenovirus pneumonia in guinea pigs: An experimental reproduction of the disease. Lab. Anim. 18:55–60.
Naumann, S., et al. 1981. Lethal pneumonia in guinea pigs associated with a virus. Lab. Anim. 15:255–42.

Herpesviral Infections

Bhatt, P.N., et al. 1971. Isolation and characterization of a herpes-like (Hsiung-Kaplow) virus from guinea pigs. J. Infect. Dis. 123:178–89.

Bia, F.J., et al. 1980. New endogenous herpesvirus of guinea pigs: Biological and molecular characterization. J. Virol. 36:245–53.

Connor, W.S., and Johnson, K.P. 1976. Cytomegalovirus infection in weanling guinea pigs. J. Infect. Dis. 134:442–49.

Cook, J.E. 1958. Salivary-gland virus disease of guinea pigs. J. Natl. Cancer Inst. 20:905–9.

Griffith, B.P., et al. 1983. Enhancement of cytomegalovirus infection during pregnancy in guinea pigs. J. Infect. Dis. 147:990–98.

———. 1976. Cytomegalovirus-induced mononucleosis in guinea pigs. Infect. Immunol. 13:926–33.

Jungeblut, C.W., and Opler, S.R. 1967. On the pathogenesis of cavian leukemia. Am. J. Pathol. 51:1153–60.

Lucia, H.L., et al. 1985. Lymphadenopathy during cytomegalovirus-induced mononucleosis in guinea pigs. Arch. Pathol. Lab. Med. 109:1019–23.

Ma, B.I., et al. 1969. Detection of virus-like particles in germinal centers of normal guinea pigs. Proc. Soc. Exp. Biol. Med. 130:586–90.

Nayak, D.P. 1971. Isolation and characterization of a herpesvirus from leukemic guinea pigs. J. Virol. 8:579–88.

Opler, S.R. 1968. New oncogenic virus producing acute lymphocytic leukemia in guinea pigs. Proc. 3rd Int. Symp. Comp. Leuk. Res. 31:81–88.

Van Hoosier, G.L., Jr., et al. 1985. Disseminated cytomegalovirus in the guinea pig. Lab. Anim. Sci. 35:81–84.

Weller, T.H. 1971. The cytomegaloviruses: Ubiquitous agents with protean manifestations. New Engl. J. Med. 285:203–14, 267–72.

Infections with RNA Viruses

Arenaviral Infection

Hotchin, J. 1971. The contamination of laboratory animals with lymphocytic choriomeningitis virus. Am. J. Pathol. 64:747–69.

Jungeblut, C. W., and Kodza, H. 1962. Interference between lymphocytic choriomeningitis virus and the leukemia transmitting agent of leukemia L2C in guinea pigs. Arch. Gesamte Virusforsch. 12:522–60.

Shaughnessy, H.J., and Zichis, J. 1940. Infection of guinea pigs by application of virus of lymphocytic choriomeningitis to their normal skins. J. Exp. Med. 72:331–43.

Coronavirus-like Infection

Jaax, G.P., et al. 1990. Coronavirus-like virions associated with a wasting syndrome in guinea pigs. Lab. Anim. Sci. 40:375–78.

Marshall, J.A., and Doultree, J.C. 1996. Chronic excretion of coronavirus-like particles in laboratory guinea pigs. Lab. Anim. Sci. 46:104–6.

General Bibliography

Griffith, J.W., et al. 1996. Experimental pneumonia virus of mice infection of guinea pigs spontaneously infected with *Bordetella bronchiseptica*. Lab. Anim. 31:52–57.

Hansen, A.K., et al. 1997. A serological indication of the existence of a guinea pig poliovirus. Lab. Anim. 31:212–18.

Van Hoosier, G.L., Jr., and Robinette, L.R. 1976. Viral and chlamydial diseases. In *The Biology of the Guinea Pig*, ed. J.E. Wagner and P.J. Manning, pp. 137–52. New York: Academic Press.

BACTERIAL INFECTIONS

BACTERIAL ENTERIC INFECTIONS

Clostridial Infections

ANTIBIOTIC-ASSOCIATED DYSBACTERIOSIS ("ANTIBIOTIC TOXICITY"). In guinea pigs, following treatment with certain antibiotics, within 1–5 d up to 50% or more may develop a profuse diarrhea, with high mortality. The antibiotics associated with this pattern of disease are those with an antibacterial action primarily against gram-positive organisms, including penicillin, bacitracin, and ampicillin.

PATHOGENESIS. In guinea pigs, gram-positive organisms such as streptococci and lactobacilli predominate in the small and large intestine. However, when a narrow spectrum antibiotic with antibacterial activity against gram-positive bacteria is administered per os or parenterally, striking changes occur in the gut flora. Following the administration of a single intramuscular dose of 50,000 units of penicillin, there was an estimated 100-fold decrease in cultivable gram-positive bacteria within 12 hr, followed by up to a 10,000,000-fold increase in gram-negative bacteria. A high incidence of bacteremia due to *Escherichia coli* has also been observed in treated animals. The problem can be prevented by treating with broader spectrum antibiotics. Antibiotics such as ampicillin and penicillin are excreted, at least in part, in the bile, which explains their profound effects on the bacterial flora of the gut, even after parenteral administration. Paradoxically, clostridial overgrowth has also been identified in antibiotic-associated diarrhea in guinea pigs. Following treatment with penicillin or ampicillin, large numbers of *Clostridium difficile* have been recovered from animals with diarrhea. In addition, *C. difficile* enterotoxin has been demonstrated in the intestinal contents posttreatment with penicillin. This organism is normally not present in intestinal contents of normal guinea pigs. Isolates of *C. difficile* tested to date have been sensitive to penicillin. This suggests that antibiotic treatment causes sufficient disruption of the gut flora to permit the proliferation of a pathogenic organism not normally recoverable from this species.

PATHOLOGY. At necropsy, the cecal mucosa is edematous and frequently hemorrhagic. Microscopically, in the terminal ileum, there is hyperplasia of the mucosa, with mononuclear cell infiltration in the lamina propria. In the cecum, there is degeneration and sloughing of enterocytes, edema of the lamina propria, and leukocytic infiltration.

DIAGNOSIS. The history of recent antibiotic treatment and the typical gross and microscopic changes should provide an accurate provisional diagnosis. Bacteriology, and the assay of cecal contents for *C. difficile* toxin, are recommended. *Differential diagnoses* include acute coccidiosis, idiopathic cecitis/typhlitis, cryptosporidiosis, and other bacterial enteritides.

SPONTANEOUS CLOSTRIDIAL TYPHLITIS/CECITIS. Acute, frequently fatal typhlitis occurs sporadically in guinea pigs of all ages. At necropsy, the cecum usually contains fluid ingesta and gas. Microscopic examination reveals degeneration and sloughing of enterocytes, with necrosis of the adjacent submucosa. *C. perfringens* has been isolated from cases of enterotoxemia in ex-germ-free guinea pigs, and spirochetes have been associated with some spontaneous cases of acute typhlitis in guinea pigs. Tyzzer's disease, *C. difficile* infection post–antibiotic treatment, and coccidiosis are other possible etiologic agents. Typhlitis due to *C. difficile* may also occur in the absence of prior antibiotic treatment. However, in some cases the etiology of the typhlitis complex has not been determined.

CLOSTRIDIUM PILIFORME INFECTION: TYZZER'S DISEASE. Spontaneous cases of Tyzzer's disease have been recognized in this species. In some reported cases in young guinea pigs, lesions were confined to the intestinal tract. Typical *C. piliforme* organisms were identified in enterocytes. The typical disease has been produced in young guinea pigs inoculated orally with *C. piliforme*. Lesions were observed in the ileum, large intestine, and liver by 4 d postinoculation. Typical bacilli were demonstrated in the gut lesions at 4–10 d and in the liver only at 8–10 d postinoculation. Vertical transmission has been reported to occur in a hysterectomy-derived, gnotobiotically reared guinea pig.

PATHOLOGY. Necrotizing ileitis and typhlitis, frequently with transmural involvement, are typical findings in cavian Tyzzer's disease. Hepatic lesions, when present, are characterized by focal coagulative necrosis in periportal regions, with variable polymorphonuclear cell infiltration. Intracellular bacilli are best demonstrated by the Warthin-Starry or Giemsa stains. The significance of the spirochetes seen in association with *C. piliforme* infections in guinea pigs in some outbreaks has not been determined.

***Lawsonia* Infection: Adenomatous Intestinal Hyperplasia.** Segmental epithelial hyperplasia of the duodenum attributed to *Campylobacter*-like organisms (now *Lawsonia intracellularis*) has been observed in guinea pigs on steroid treatment. A spontaneous outbreak of diarrhea, with weight loss and mortality, was reported from Asia. Adenomatous changes were observed in the jejunum and ileum, and intracellular organisms interpreted to be *Campylobacter* (*Lawsonia*) were observed in immature crypt epithelial cells by electron microscopy. The changes observed were very similar to those seen in *Lawsonia*-associated hamster ileitis.

***Salmonella* Infection: Salmonellosis.** Salmonella infections were a common occurrence in the first half of this century. However, with the current standards of husbandry and hygiene, improved wild rodent control, and the feeding of good-quality prepared feeds, the disease seldom occurs in well-managed facilities. *S. typhimurium* and *S. enteritidis* are the most common isolates from guinea pigs. *S. dublin* has also been isolated from fatal cases of salmonellosis in this species.

EPIZOOTIOLOGY AND PATHOGENESIS. Salmonellosis affects guinea pigs of all ages and strains, but young weanlings and sows around farrowing time are considered to be particularly at risk. Inapparent carriers may occur. Recovered animals may shed the organism intermittently in the feces, representing a possible source of reinfection. Ingestion of contaminated feces or feed is considered to be the usual source of the organism. Clinical signs observed include depression, conjunctivitis, and abortions. Diarrhea is a variable manifestation of the disease. The mortality rate may be 50% or higher.

PATHOLOGY. Gross lesions are similar to those observed in salmonellosis in other mammals. Pinpoint-size, pale foci may be present on the liver and spleen. Massive splenomegaly frequently occurs. Necrotic miliary foci may also be present in other viscera, including lymph nodes. Lesions may be absent in peracute cases. Frequently there is a multifocal granulomatous hepatitis, splenitis, and lymphadenitis, with infiltration by histiocytic cells and polymorphs. Focal suppurative lesions may also occur in lymphoid tissues of the intestinal tract.

DIAGNOSIS. Recovery of the organism from heart blood, spleen, and feces is best accomplished with media selective for *Salmonella*. In the absence of bacteriology, the characteristic paratyphoid nodules seen in organs such as liver and spleen are useful morphologic criteria. *Differential diagnoses* include clostridial enterotoxemia, yersiniosis, Tyzzer's disease, and pneumococcal septicemia.

SIGNIFICANCE. Aside from the dangers of interspecies spread in the animal facility, the zoonotic potential must be emphasized. Identical phage types have been recovered from guinea pigs and human contacts in epizootics of the disease. Slaughter is recommended. In one reported epizootic, shedders were identified by mass fecal sampling and culture, then removed. Strict hygienic measures and the culling of all contact animals have been used to eliminate the organism from an infected colony.

***Yersinia* Infection: Pseudotuberculosis.** Spontaneous outbreaks of disease and mortality due to *Yersinia pseudotuberculosis* are relatively rare. Inapparent carriers may also occur. Yersiniosis may be produced experimentally in guinea pigs inoculated orally or parenterally with *Y. pseudotuberculosis*. In the acute form of the disease, miliary, cream-colored nodules are present in the intestinal wall, with enteritis and mucosal ulceration, particularly in the terminal ileum and cecum. In the subacute and chronic forms of the disease, miliary to caseous lesions may be present in mesenteric lymph nodes, spleen and liver, and lung. Recovery and identification of the organism are necessary to confirm the diagnosis.

OTHER GRAM-NEGATIVE BACTERIA

***Bordetella bronchiseptica* Infection.** *Bordetella bronchiseptica* is a small, gram-negative rod that is an important cause of respiratory disease in the guinea pig.

EPIZOOTIOLOGY AND PATHOGENESIS. The organism is harbored in the upper respiratory tract in several other species, including dogs, cats, and rabbits, and it is likely that interspecies transmission can occur. To date, there is no evidence that there are variations in virulence of the isolates when tested in guinea pigs. Guinea pigs of all ages are susceptible and develop respiratory tract lesions following intranasal inoculation. However, disease and mortality occur most often in young guinea pigs, particularly during winter months. In some outbreaks, there may be other identifiable manipulations or environmental factors that could precipitate disease. Guinea pigs may harbor the organism in the upper respiratory tract and trachea as an inapparent infection. In enzootically infected colonies, the incidence of nasal shedders may be relatively high. Infection rates are usually highest in the winter months. Most animals appear to develop solid immunity and eventually eliminate the organism, but a small percentage may remain carriers. The organism is readily transmitted as an airborne infection. It has an affinity for ciliated respiratory epithelium and has been shown to cause ciliostasis in

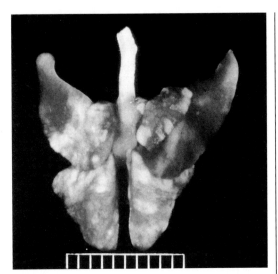

FIG. 5.10—Cranioventral bronchopneumonia from juvenile guinea pig with acute *Bordetella bronchiseptica* infection.

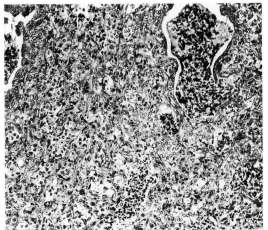

FIG. 5.11—Suppurative bronchopneumonia from spontaneous case of *Bordetella* infection. There is marked infiltration with heterophils and mononuclear cells, with obliteration of the normal architecture.

other species. During epizootics of bordetellosis, pregnant sows may die, abort, or produce still-born offspring. *Bordetella* has also been isolated from a case of pyosalpinx in the guinea pig.

PATHOLOGY. At necropsy the external nares, nasal passages, and trachea frequently contain mucopurulent or catarrhal exudate. Consolidated areas vary from dark red to gray, are anteroventral in distribution, and may involve entire lobes or individual lobules (Fig. 5.10). Mucopurulent exudate is present in affected airways, pleuritis occasionally occurs, and purulent exudate may be present in the tympanic bullae. Histologically, there is an acute to chronic suppurative bronchopneumonia, with marked infiltration by heterophils in airways and affected alveoli and obliteration of the normal architecture (Figs. 5.11 and 5.12). In some acute cases, there may be fibrinous exudation into terminal airways and alveoli.

DIAGNOSIS. The organism can usually be readily recovered on blood agar cultures from the respiratory tract, affected tympanic bullae, and in cases of metritis, the uterus. If the results of bacterial cultures are unrewarding, or not available, *differential diagnoses* include acute pneumococcal, *Klebsiella,* or staphylococcal infections, as well as a systemic form of *Streptococcus zooepi-*

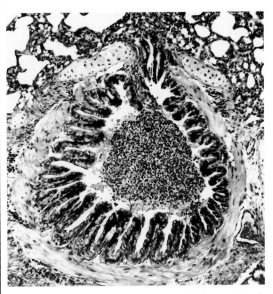

FIG. 5.12—Chronic suppurative bronchitis associated with *Bordetella* infection in mature guinea pig.

demicus infection. If there is a history of prior administration of Freund's adjuvant, chronic interstitial fibrosis and granulomatous pulmonary lesions may occur. These must be differentiated from resolving lesions due to other causes, including *B. bronchiseptica* infections.

SIGNIFICANCE. *B. bronchiseptica* infections are a major cause of respiratory disease in this species. Exacerbations of subclinical infections may occur. Attempts have been made to correlate cases of interstitial pneumonitis and perivascular lymphoid nodules with previous *Bordetella* infections, but without success. The dangers of interspecies transmission should be emphasized. Commercial and autogenous bacterins have been used to reduce the incidence of disease. However, immunization does not necessarily eliminate the carrier state.

Chlamydial Infection: Guinea Pig Inclusion Conjunctivitis (GPIC).

GPIC is a spontaneously occurring conjunctival infection due to *Chlamydia psittaci,* a member of the psittacosis-lymphogranuloma-trachoma group.

EPIZOOTIOLOGY AND PATHOGENESIS. Based on the available information, it appears likely that *C. psittaci* is relatively widespread in conventional colonies of guinea pigs. In enzootically infected colonies, animals are frequently asymptomatic, although the organism may be demonstrable in conjunctival smears. Guinea pigs 4–8 wk of age are most frequently actively infected with the organism in such herds, and most adults are likely to be seropositive under these circumstances. Young seronegative animals, when introduced into a conventional colony enzootically infected with the organism, may then develop the typical clinical disease. Transmission is probably primarily by direct contact. In addition to conjunctival lesions, rhinitis and genital tract infections may occur. Abortions and lower respiratory tract disease have been attributed to the organism, although lung lesions may be complicated by concurrent streptococcal or *Bordetella* infections. Sows cervically infected by *C. psittaci* have transmitted GPIC to offspring.

PATHOLOGY. The conjunctiva is reddened, with a serous to a purulent exudate. Conjunctival smears stained with the Giemsa method usually reveal sloughed epithelial cells and a scattering of heterophils and lymphocytes. Intracytoplasmic inclusions and bacteria may also be present in stained smears (Fig. 5.13).

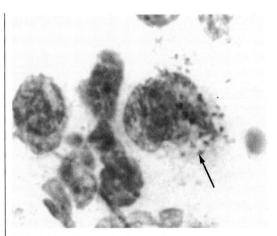

FIG. 5.13—Conjunctival swab from spontaneous case of inclusion conjunctivitis. Note the intracytoplasmic location of organisms in affected conjunctival cells (*arrow*).

DIAGNOSIS. The demonstration of the typical intracytoplasmic inclusion bodies in conjunctival epithelial cells is one recommended method for confirming the diagnosis. However, inclusions may be difficult to demonstrate, particularly if preparations are smudged and there are numerous bacteria in the smear. The demonstration of antigen in conjunctival smears using specific antibody and immunofluorescence microscopy is considered to be a more sensitive and reliable method. Serology using procedures such as the indirect fluorescent antibody technique has been used to demonstrate antibody to the organism. Bacterial culture of conjunctival swabs is recommended in an effort to differentiate GPIC from a primary bacterial conjunctivitis.

SIGNIFICANCE. GPIC is usually a self-limiting disease, and animals normally recover with no residual damage. The possibility of other complications, such as rhinitis and abortions, should be considered, particularly in animals with increased susceptibility due to immunosuppression or other predisposing factors.

***Citrobacter* Infection.** An epizootic of *Citrobacter* septicemia with high mortality was reported in guinea pigs. Pneumonia, pleuritis, and enteritis were observed, and *C. freundii* was isolated from lung, liver, spleen, and intestine at necropsy. No predisposing factors or possible sources of the infection were identified.

***Klebsiella* Infection.** Epizootics of acute infections due to *Klebsiella pneumoniae* have been reported on rare occasions. Patterns of disease vary from acute septicemia to acute necrotizing bronchopneumonia, with pleuritis, pericarditis, peritonitis, and splenic hyperplasia.

***Pseudomonas* Infection: Pulmonary Botryomycosis.** In one report, pulmonary botryomycosis was attributed to *Pseudomonas aeruginosa* infection. Sulfur granules were present within the focal suppurative pulmonary lesions.

***Streptobacillus moniliformis* Infection.** *S. moniliformis* has been isolated from a few cases of cervical lymphadenitis, from abscesses, and from a young guinea pig with pyogranulomatous bronchopneumonia. Suppurative lesions contain caseous to creamy exudate and are similar to those associated with streptococcal infections.

INFECTIONS WITH GRAM-POSITIVE BACTERIA

Staphylococcal Infections

Ulcerative pododermatitis. Bumblefoot is frequently associated with coagulase-positive staphylococcal infections. Predisposing factors include trauma due to defective or rusty cage wire and poor sanitation. The plantar surface of the forefeet typically is swollen, painful, and encrusted with necrotic tissue and clotted blood. In some advanced cases, amyloid deposition has been observed in the spleen, liver, adrenals, and islets. Staphylococcal infections have also been associated with isolated cases of suppurative pneumonia, purulent mastitis, and conjunctivitis.

Acute Staphylococcal Dermatitis (Exfoliative Dermatitis). This condition was reported to occur most frequently in strain 13 guinea pigs. In clinically affected animals, there was an age-related variation in mortality that was negligible in adults and relatively high in young animals, particularly those born to affected dams. Clinically, the disease was characterized by alopecia and erythema in the ventral abdominal region, with exfoliation of the epidermis. In survivors, skin lesions usually regressed within 2 wk, with subsequent new hair growth.

PATHOLOGY. At necropsy, there is erythema and hair loss, with dull red scabs and cracks in the epidermis, particularly along the ventral abdomen and the medial aspect of the extremities. On microscopic examination, there is marked epidermal cleavage, with parakeratotic hyperkeratosis and minimal inflammatory response. *Staphylococcus aureus* has been isolated from the lesions in the majority of affected animals, and the disease has been reproduced in young guinea pigs inoculated with a coagulase-positive strain of *S. aureus* isolated from an affected animal. The organism may also be isolated from the upper respiratory tract and pharynx of many of the affected animals and from clinically normal guinea pigs. Abrasions of the skin may have been an important predisposing factor, resulting in colonization with pathogenic staphylococci and invasion of the epidermis.

SIGNIFICANCE. Staphylococcal infections may occur as an inapparent infection in colonies of guinea pigs and may be recoverable from a relatively high percentage of clinically normal animals. The infection may persist in a colony for years. The possibility of interspecies transmission is an important consideration.

Streptococcal Infections

Streptococcal Lymphadenitis/Septicemia. *Streptococcus zooepidemicus* of Lancefield's group C is a gram-positive encapsulated coccus that produces beta hemolysis on blood agar plates. It is associated with suppurative lymphadenitis in this species.

EPIZOOTIOLOGY AND PATHOGENESIS. The organism may be carried in the nasopharynx and conjunctiva as an inapparent infection. Females have been shown to be more susceptible to the disease than are males, and there is a strain-related variation in susceptibility. Steroid treatment does not appear to increase susceptibility to the disease. Lymphadenitis has been produced consistently in guinea pigs inoculated sublingually with *S. zooepidemicus*. Lesions have been readily produced by inoculation of the organism on the abraided mucosa, but not in unabraided animals. The usual route of invasion appears to be via abrasions in the oral mucosa, but inhalation, skin abrasions, and invasion of the genital tract at farrowing are other possible portals of entry. The disease has also been produced in young guinea pigs by inoculation of the intact nasal and conjunctival mucous membranes. Following penetration of the oral mucosa and invasion of the underlying tissue, the organism is likely transported to the draining cervical lymph nodes via the lymphatics. The pyogenic organism then proliferates, producing a chronic suppurative inflammatory process.

PATHOLOGY. Affected adults usually have lesions confined to the regional lymph nodes. In the localized form of the disease, there is bilateral enlargement of the cervical lymph nodes. The nodes are freely movable, firm to soft, and frequently nonfluctuant, and they contain thick purulent exudate (Fig. 5.14). Localized abscessation involving other sites such as mesenteric

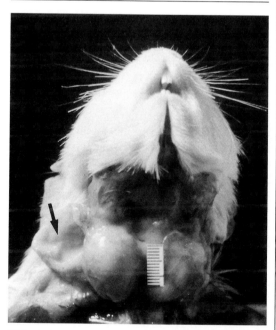

FIG. 5.14—Bilateral suppurative lymphadenitis associated with *Streptococcus zooepidemicus* infection. Note the purulent exudate (*arrow*) in the incised cervical lymph node.

lymph nodes is an infrequent finding. Retroorbital abscessation is another possible manifestation of the disease. Otitis media may also occur. Occasionally there is an acute systemic form of the disease, particularly in younger animals. In this case, fibrinopurulent bronchopneumonia, pleuritis, and pericarditis may be present at necropsy. On rare occasions, arthritis and abortions have been attributed to *S. zooepidemicus* infections. Microscopically, changes present in the cervical lymph nodes are those of a chronic suppurative lymphadenitis with central necrosis, peripheral fibrosis, and marked infiltration with heterophils. In the acute systemic form, fibrinopurulent pericarditis, focal myocardial degeneration, focal hepatitis, and acute lymphadenitis may be evident on histological examination. In one report, acute bronchopneumonia, hemopericardium, and hemothorax were associated with acute *S. pyogenes* infections.

DIAGNOSIS. The typical beta-hemolytic streptococci can usually be readily recovered from affected tissues, except in some cases of chronic lymphadenitis of some duration. *Differential diagnoses* in the acute systemic form of the disease include acute pneumococcal septicemia and acute *Bordetella* infection.

SIGNIFICANCE. Enzootic infections with *S. zooepidemicus* represent a potential complication in research. Culling the affected animals and thorough disinfection are required. Vaccination using a less virulent strain of the organism has provided a significant degree of protection against the disease.

DIPLOCOCCAL (PNEUMOCOCCAL) INFECTION. The organism *S. pneumoniae* is a lancet-shaped, gram-positive encapsulated coccus that occurs in pairs and short chains. Capsular polysaccharide type 19 is most frequently isolated from guinea pigs. Type 4 has also been identified.

EPIZOOTIOLOGY AND PATHOGENESIS. Pneumococcal infections have been recognized to occur in guinea pigs for decades, but the disease seldom occurs in well-managed facilities today. The organism may be carried as an inapparent infection in the upper respiratory tract. In affected colonies, up to 50% of the animals may be carriers of *S. pneumoniae.* Transmission is probably primarily by aerosols. Epizootics occur most often during winter months, and younger animals and pregnant sows are considered to be particularly at risk. Other predisposing factors include changes in environmental temperature, poor husbandry and experimental procedures, and inadequate nutrition. During epizootics, high mortality, abortions, and stillbirths may occur. The organisms do not produce toxins but are protected from phagocytosis primarily through their abundant polysaccharide capsules. Many pneumococci can activate the alternate complement pathway; thus complement activation may be the important stimulus for the early tissue changes.

PATHOLOGY. At necropsy, typical lesions include fibrinopurulent pleuritis, pericarditis, peritonitis, and marked consolidation of affected lobes of lung. Microscopic changes are those of an acute bronchopneumonia with fibrinous exudation and polymorphonuclear cell infiltration. Thrombosis of pulmonary vessels may occur in acute cases (Fig. 5.15). Infiltrating cells may be elongated and fusiform, forming pallisading patterns within affected airways and alveoli (Fig. 5.16). Fibrinopurulent pleuritis, pericarditis, and epicarditis fre-

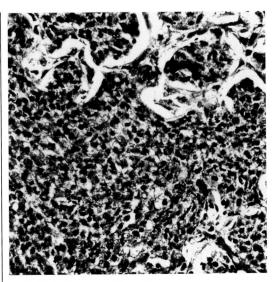

FIG. 5.16—Section of lung from young guinea pig with spontaneous diplococcal pneumonia (*Streptococcus pneumoniae*). There is necrotizing alveolitis with leukocytic infiltration and obliteration of the normal architecture.

quently occur. Splenitis, fibrinopurulent meningitis, metritis, focal hepatic necrosis, lymphadenitis, and ovarian abscessation have also been observed. *S. pneumoniae*–associated suppurative arthritis and osteomyelitis have been reported to occur in guinea pigs with borderline vitamin C deficiency.

DIAGNOSIS. Direct smears of Gram-stained inflammatory exudate should reveal the typical gram-positive diplococci. Using blood agar or enrichment media, the organism should be recoverable from affected tissues. (*S. pneumoniae* is more fastidious in growth requirements than are most other streptococci.) *Differential diagnoses* include acute septicemia due to *S. zooepidemicus* and acute *Bordetella* infections.

SIGNIFICANCE. Pneumococcal infections may be an important cause of disease and mortality in enzootically infected colonies and represent a potential complicating factor in research. Serotypes isolated from guinea pigs are identical to human isolates. The possibility of inter-

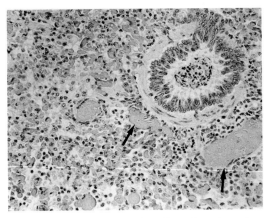

FIG. 5.15—Section of lung from juvenile guinea pig with peracute infection with *Streptococcus pneumoniae.* There is alveolar flooding, and thrombi (*arrows*) are present in small pulmonary vessels.

species transmission is feasible but not proven to date.

MISCELLANEOUS BACTERIAL SYNDROMES

Otitis Media. Middle ear infections frequently go undetected clinically in the guinea pig. Careful examination of the tympanic bullae should be performed at necropsy in order to detect subclinical cases. The otosclerosis associated with chronic middle ear infection may be detected antemortem by radiographic examination. Otitis media appears to be more common in colonies harboring pathogens in their upper respiratory tract. Organisms isolated from these cases include *S. pneumoniae, S. zooepidemicus, Bordetella,* and *Pseudomonas.*

Bacterial Mastitis. Mastitis occurs sporadically in colonies of guinea pigs, particularly in sows during early lactation. Cases usually are sporadic and may not be particularly contagious. The offspring may be unaffected.

PATHOLOGY. On gross examination, affected glands are red to purple, enlarged and firm, and congested and edematous on the cut surface. In sows with acute mastitis, lesions are characterized microscopically by mild degeneration to necrosis of ductal epithelium, with marked polymorphonuclear cell infiltration in ducts and alveoli, with a scattering of inflammatory cells in the interstitium. In chronic cases, there may be marked interstitial fibrosis, with mononuclear cell infiltration and obliteration of the normal architecture in severely affected areas. In one study, bacteria most frequently isolated (in decreasing order of frequency) were *Escherichia coli, Klebsiella pneumoniae,* and *Streptococcus zooepidemicus.*

BACTERIAL CONJUNCTIVITIS. Organisms isolated from cases of bacterial conjunctivitis include *S. zooepidemicus,* coliforms, *Staphylococcus aureus,* and *Pasteurella multocida.* Conjunctival smears should be examined to ensure that there is not a concurrent chlamydial infection.

BIBLIOGRAPHY FOR BACTERIAL INFECTIONS

Bacterial Enteric Infections

Clostridial Infections

Boot, R., et al. 1989. *Clostridium difficile*–associated typhlitis in specific pathogen free guinea pigs in the absence of antimicrobial treatment. Lab. Anim. 23:203–7.

Eyssen, H., et al. 1957. Further studies on antibiotic toxicity of guinea pigs. Antibiot. Chemother. 7:55–64.

Farrar, W.E., and Kent, T.H. 1965. Enteritis and coliform bacteremia in guinea pigs given penicillin. Am. J. Pathol. 47:629–42.

Lowe, B.R., et al. 1980. *Clostridium difficile*–associated cecitis in guinea pigs exposed to penicillin. Am. J. Vet. Res. 41:1277–79.

Maddon, D.L., et al. 1970. Spontaneous infection in ex-germ-free guinea pigs due to *Clostridium perfringens.* Lab. Anim. Care 20:454–55.

Rehg, J., and Pakes, S.P. 1981. *Clostridium difficile* antitoxin neutralization and penicillin-associated colitis. Lab. Anim. Sci. 31:156–60.

Young, J.D., et al. 1987. An evaluation of ampicillin pharmacokinetics and toxicity in guinea pigs. Lab. Anim. Sci. 37:652–56.

Clostridium piliforme Infection

Boot, R., and Walvoort, H.C. 1984. Vertical transmission of *Bacillus piliformis* infection in a guinea pig: Case report. Lab. Anim. 18:195–99.

McLeod, C.G., et al. 1977. Intestinal Tyzzer's disease and spirochetosis in a guinea pig. Vet. Pathol. 14:229–35.

Waggie, K.S., et al. 1987. Lesions of experimentally induced Tyzzer's disease in Syrian hamsters, guinea pigs, mice and rats. Lab. Anim. 21:155–60.

Zwicker, G.M., et al. 1978. Naturally occurring Tyzzer's disease and spirochetosis in guinea pigs. Lab. Anim. Sci. 28:193–98.

Lawsonia Infection

Elwell, M.R., et al. 1981. Duodenal hyperplasia in a guinea pig. Vet. Pathol. 18:136–39.

Muto, T., et al. 1983. Adenomatous intestinal hyperplasia in guinea pigs associated with *Campylobacter*-like bacteria. Jap. J. Med. Sci. Biol. 36:337–42.

Salmonella Infection

Fish, N.A., et al. 1968. Family outbreak of salmonellosis due to contact with guinea pigs. Can. Med. Assoc. J. 99:418–20.

John, P.C., et al. 1988. Natural course of salmonellosis in a guinea pig colony. Indian Vet. J. 65:200–204.

Nelson, J.B. 1928. Studies on a paratyphoid infection in guinea pigs. V. The incidence of carriers during the endemic stage. J. Exp. Med. 48:647–58.

Olfert, E.D., et al. 1976. *Salmonella typhimurium* infection in guinea pigs: Observations on monitoring and control. Lab. Anim. Sci. 26:78–80.

Onyekaba, C.O. 1983. Clinical salmonellosis in a guinea pig colony caused by a new *Salmonella* serotype *S. ochiogu*. Lab. Anim. 17:213–16.

Yersinia Infection

Ganaway, J.R. 1976. Bacterial, mycoplasma, and rickettsial diseases. In *The Biology of the Guinea Pig*, ed. J.E. Wagner and P.J. Manning, pp. 121–35. New York: Academic.

Obwolo, M.J. 1977. The pathology of experimental yersiniosis in guinea pigs. J. Comp. Pathol. 87:213–21.

Rigby, C. 1976. Natural infections of guinea pigs. Lab. Anim. 10:119–42.

Other Gram-negative Bacterial Infections

Bordetella bronchiseptica Infection

Baskerville, M., et al. 1982. A study of chronic pneumonia in a guinea pig colony with enzootic *Bordetella bronchiseptica* infection. Lab. Anim. 16:290–96.

Bemis, D.A., and Wilson, S.A. 1985. Influence of potential virulence determinants on *Bordetella bronchiseptica*-induced ciliostasis. Infect. Immunol. 50:35–42.

Ganaway, J.R. 1976. Bacterial, mycoplasma, and rickettsial diseases. In *The Biology of the Guinea Pig*, ed. J.E. Wagner and P.J. Manning, pp. 121–35. New York: Academic.

Ganaway, J.R., et al. 1965. Prevention of acute *Bordetella bronchiseptica* pneumonia in a guinea pig colony. Lab. Anim. Care 15:156–62.

Nakagawa, M., et al. 1971. Experimental *Bordetella bronchiseptica* infection in guinea pigs. Jap. J. Vet. Sci. 33:53–60.

Sinka, D.P., and Sleight, S.D. 1968. Bilateral pyosalpinx in guinea pig. J. Am. Vet. Med. Assoc. 153:830–31.

Traham, C.J. 1987. Airborne-induced experimental *Bordetella bronchiseptica* pneumonia in strain 13 guinea pigs. Lab. Anim. 21:226–32.

Yoda, H., et al. 1972. Development of resistance to reinfection of *Bordetella bronchiseptica* in guinea pigs recovered from natural infection. Jap. J. Vet. Sci. 34:191–96.

Chlamydial Infection

Deeb, B.J., et al. 1989. Guinea pig inclusion conjunctivitis (GPIC) in a commercial colony. Lab. Anim. 23:103–6.

Mount, D.T., et al. 1972. Infection of genital tract and transmission of ocular infection to newborn by the agent of guinea pig inclusion conjunctivitis. Infect. Immunol. 5:921–26.

Murray, E.S. 1964. Guinea pig inclusion conjunctivitis virus. J. Infect. Dis. 114:1–12.

Citrobacter freundii Infection

Ocholi, R.A., et al. 1988. An epizootic of *Citrobacter freundii* in a guinea pig colony: Short communication. Lab. Anim. 10:119–42.

Klebsiella Infection

Ganaway, J.R. 1976. Bacterial, mycoplasma, and rickettsial diseases. In *The Biology of the Guinea Pig*, ed. J.E. Wagner and P.J. Manning, pp. 121–35. New York: Academic.

Pseudomonas Infection

Bostrum, R.E., et al. 1969. Atypical fatal pulmonary botryomycosis in two guinea pigs due to *Pseudomonas aeruginosa*. J. Am. Vet. Med. Assoc. 115:1195–99.

Streptobacillus moniliformis Infection

Aldred, P., et al. 1974. The isolation of *Streptobacillus moniliformis* from cervical abscesses of guinea pigs. Lab. Anim. 8:275–77.

Kirchner, B.K., et al. 1992. Isolation of *Streptobacillus moniliformis* from a guinea pig with granulomatous pneumonia. Lab. Anim. Sci. 42:519–21.

Infections with Gram-Positive Bacteria

Staphylococcal Infections

Blackmore, D.K., and Francis, R.A. 1970. The apparent transmission of staphylococci of human origin to laboratory animals. J. Comp. Pathol. 80:645–51.

Ishihara, C. 1980. An exfoliative skin disease in guinea pigs due to *Staphylococcus aureus*. Lab. Anim. Sci. 30:552–57.

Markham, N.P., and Markham, J.G. 1966. Staphylococci in man and animals: Distribution and characteristics of strains. J. Comp. Pathol. 76:49–56.

Taylor, J.L., et al. 1971. Chronic pododermatitis in guinea pigs: A case report. Lab. Anim. Sci. 21:944–45.

Streptococcal Infections

Fraunfelter, F.C., et al. 1971. Lancefield type C streptococcal infections in strain 2 guinea pigs. Lab. Anim. 5:1–13.

Mayora, J., et al. 1978. Prevention of cervical lymphadenitis in guinea pigs by vaccination. Lab. Anim. Sci. 28:686–90.

Murphy, J.C., et al. 1991. Cervical lymphadenitis in guinea pigs: Infection via intact ocular and nasal mucosa by *Streptococcus zooepidemicus*. Lab. Anim. Sci. 41:251–54.

Okewole, P.A., et al. 1991. An outbreak of *Streptococcus pyogenes* infection associated with calcium oxalate urolithiasis in guinea pigs (*Cavia porcellus*). Lab. Anim. 25:184–86.

Olson, L.D., et al. 1976. Experimental induction of cervical lymphadenitis in guinea pigs with group C streptococci. Lab. Anim. 10:223–31.

Rae, V. 1936. Epizootic streptococcal myocarditis in guinea pigs. J. Infect. Dis. 59:236–41.

Diplococcal (Pneumococcal) Infections

Branch, A. 1927. Spontaneous infection in guinea pigs: Pneumococcus, Friedlander bacillus and pseudotuberculosis. J. Infect. Dis. 40:533–48.

Homburger, F., et al. 1945. An epizootic of *Pneumococcus* type 19 infections in guinea pigs. Science 102:449–50.

Keyhani, M., and Naghshineh, R. 1974. Spontaneous epizootic of pneumococcus infection in guinea pigs. Lab. Anim. 8:47–49.

Parker, G.A., et al. 1977. Extrapulmonary lesions of *Streptococcus pneumoniae* infection in guinea pigs. Vet. Pathol. 14:332–37.

Petrie, G.F. 1933. The pneumococcal disease of the guinea pig. Vet. J. 89:25–30.

Witt, W.M., et al. 1988. *Streptococcus pneumoniae* arthritis and osteomyelitis with vitamin C deficiency in guinea pigs. Lab. Anim. Sci. 38:192–94.

Yoneda, K., and Coonrod, J.D. 1980. Experimental type 25 pneumococcal pneumonia in rats. Am. J. Pathol. 99:231–42.

Otitis Media

Boot, R., and Walvoort, H.C. 1986. Otitis media in guinea pigs: Pathology and bacteriology. Lab. Anim. 20:242–48

Kohn, D.F. 1974. Bacterial otitis media in the guinea pig. Lab. Anim. 24:823–25.

Wagner, J.E., et al. 1976. Otitis media in guinea pigs. Lab. Anim. Sci. 26:902–7.

Bacterial Mastitis

Kinkler, R.J., et al. 1976. Bacterial mastitis in guinea pigs. Lab. Anim. Sci. 26:214–17.

General Bibliography

Ganaway, J.R. 1976. Bacterial, mycoplasma, and rickettsial diseases. In *The Biology of the Guinea Pig,* ed. J.E. Wagner and P.J. Manning, pp. 121–35. New York: Academic.

Rigby, C. 1976. Natural infections of guinea pigs. Lab. Anim. 10:119–42.

Smith, H. 1965. Observations on the flora of the alimentary tract of animals and factors affecting its composition. J. Pathol. Bacteriol. 89:95–122.

MYCOTIC INFECTIONS

Dermatophyte Infection: Dermatophytosis

EPIZOOTIOLOGY. Epizootics of "ringworm" in guinea pigs are usually due to *Trichophyton mentagrophytes*. In one survey of laboratory animals in Europe, over half of the guinea pigs sampled were positive for either *T. mentagrophytes* or *Microsporum canis*. The majority of the guinea pigs were asymptomatic. There appears to be a strain-related variation in susceptibility to the disease. In one recorded outbreak, the mortality rate in animals that developed the disease during the first week after birth was up to 50%. Spontaneous regression of lesions may occur, particularly in adults. However, in sows where skin lesions had disappeared, the clinical signs frequently recurred at parturition. High environmental temperatures and humidity may be other important predisposing factors in outbreaks of the disease. Cutaneous lesions may first appear on the nose, but other regions of the head, as well as neck, sides, and back areas, are frequently involved.

PATHOLOGY. On gross examination, there are circumscribed, scaly, pruritic lesions with a raised, erythematous border and localized alopecia (Fig. 5.17). Frequently there are pustule formations due to secondary bacterial infections. On microscopic examination, there is hyperkeratosis, epidermal hyperplasia, and polymorphonuclear cell infiltration. Pustules may be present in the superficial epidermis and hair follicles. Arthrospores can usually be readily demonstrated microscopically in H & E–stained, paraffin-embedded sections, particularly in hair follicles. PAS or methenamine silver staining procedures are best for the visualization of the fungi in section. Hyphae and arthrospores usually are readily demonstrated in wet mount

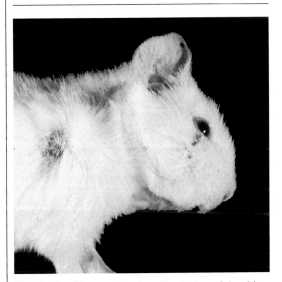

FIG. 5.17—Circumscribed, scaling lesion of the skin in spontaneous case of dermatophytosis.

preparations of hair shafts collected from lesions that are cleared in 10% KOH. Culture of skin scrapings or hair shafts on appropriate media, such as Sabouraud's dextrose, is recommended for positive identification.

SIGNIFICANCE. The dangers of transmission to human contacts should be emphasized. Depending on the circumstances, identification of affected animals, culling, and slaughter may be advisable. Systemic antifungal agents (griseofulvin) or topical ointments may be used. The teratogenic effects of griseofulvin have been demonstrated in some species; thus the treatment of pregnant guinea pigs with griseofulvin is counterindicated.

Other Mycotic Infections. There have been isolated reports of histoplasmosis, and candidiasis in the guinea pig. For additional information see Sprouse (1976).

BIBLIOGRAPHY
FOR MYCOTIC INFECTIONS

Correa, W.M., and Pacheco, A.C. 1967. Naturally occurring histoplasmosis in guinea pigs. Can. J. Comp. Med. 31:203–6.
Papini, R., et al. 1997. Survey of dermatophytes isolated from the coats of laboratory animals in Italy. Lab. Anim. Sci. 47:75–77.
Pombier, E.C., and Kim, J.C.S. 1975. An epizootic outbreak of ringworm in a guinea pig colony caused by *Trichophyton mentagrophytes*. Lab. Anim. 9:215–21.
Sprouse, R.F. 1976. Mycoses. In *The Biology of the Guinea Pig,* ed. J.E. Wagner and P.J. Manning, pp. 153–61. New York: Academic Press.

PARASITIC DISEASES

ECTOPARASITIC INFESTATIONS

Mite Infestations (Acariasis)

TRIXACARUS CAVIAE INFESTATION. Sarcoptic mange is associated with *T. caviae* infection. This pathogenic sarcoptid mite appears to be widespread in some conventional colonies of guinea pigs. Lesions are usually distributed over the neck, shoulders, inner thighs, and abdomen. Changes in the skin seen grossly are keratosis with scaling and crusting and alopecia. Marked pruritis may occur, and in severe cases, animals become thin and lethargic. Hematological changes include heterophilia, monocytosis, eosinophilia, and basophilia. Vigorous scratching may precipitate convulsive seizures. Some affected animals have exhibited flaccid paralysis. Untreated animals with extensive lesions may die. On microscopic examination of the typical lesions, there is epidermal hyperplasia, with orthokeratotic and parakeratotic hyperkeratosis. Irregular burrows in the stratum corneum contain mites and eggs. There may be spongiosis, with leukocytic infiltration in the underlying dermis. Hair follicles are normally not invaded by the parasite.

DIAGNOSIS. Skin scrapings of hair and scale cleared with 10% KOH and examined microscopically should reveal the typical mites and eggs. The parasites can also be demonstrated in paraffin-embedded sections of affected skin. *Differential diagnoses* include pediculosis, dermatophytosis, trauma, and idiopathic alopecia, a condition that is seen occasionally in guinea pigs.

SIGNIFICANCE. Urticaria may occur in human contacts. *T. caviae* infestations are an important cause of dermatitis in this species.

CHIRODISCOIDES CAVIAE INFESTATION. These mites have been identified in guinea pigs from commercial suppliers, in laboratory facilities, and in pet animals. The parasite tends to be concentrated in the lumbar region and lateral aspect of the hindquarters. Even parasite loads of up to 200/cm^2 appear to evoke minimal or no clinical evidence of pruritis or damage to the skin. Other predisposing factors, including concurrent disease, may have a significant influence on the incidence of acariasis in this species. Microscopic examination of the adult mite is necessary for positive identification.

DEMODEX CAVIAE INFESTATION. Although *D. caviae* has been recovered from guinea pigs in the absence of clinical signs, the incidence and significance of these infections in the laboratory guinea pigs is currently unknown. Infestations with ectoparasites such as *Myocoptes musculinus* and *Notoedres muris* are rare and may be due to interspecies infections.

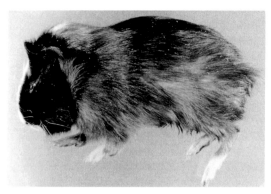

FIG. 5.18—Pediculosis due to *Gliricola porcelli.* Lice are attached to many hair shafts.

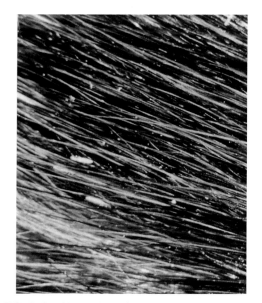

FIG. 5.19—Closer view of pellage in Figure 5.18.

Louse Infestation (Pediculosis). *Gliricola porcelli* and *Gyropus ovalis* are large biting lice that are associated with pediculosis in guinea pigs. Frequently, moderate infections are not accompanied by clinical signs. Pruritus, rough hair coat, and alopecia are seen in heavy infections (Figs. 5.18 and 5.19).

ENDOPARASITIC INFESTATIONS

Protozoal Infections

CRYPTOSPORIDIUM INFECTION: CRYPTOSPORIDIOSIS. *Cryptosporidium wrairi* is a recognized pro-tozoal pathogen in the guinea pig. Clinical infections occur most frequently in juvenile animals. Infection rates of 30–40% are considered to be typical in conventional colonies. Clinical signs include diarrhea, weight loss, and emaciation. In outbreaks of the disease, morbidity and mortality rates in young animals range from negligible to up to 50%.

PATHOLOGY. At necropsy, animals may be thin and pot-bellied, with fecal staining of the perineum. The small and large intestine usually contain watery material. Microscopically, acute lesions are usually concentrated in the jejunum, ileum, and cecum. There is hyperplasia of the crypt epithelium, edema of the lamina propria, and leukocytic infiltration. Necrosis and sloughing of enterocytes occur at the tips of the villi. In chronic lesions, villus atrophy and flattening of enterocytes commonly occur. Cryptosporidia are most numerous in acute cases. They are present within the brush border along the apices of enterocytes (Figs. 5.20 and 5.21). *Escherichia coli* has been associated with clinical cases of cryptosporidiosis.

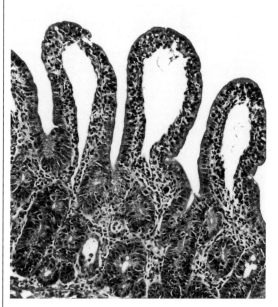

FIG. 5.20—Ileum from young guinea pig with cryptosporidiosis. There is marked dilation of lacteals and flattening of enterocytes.

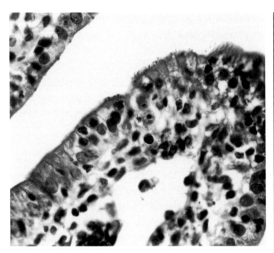

FIG. 5.21—Higher magnification of Figure 5.22, illustrating the organisms on the mucosal surface, with mononuclear cell infiltration in the lamina propria.

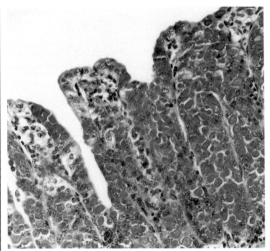

FIG. 5.22—Section of large intestine from a naturally occurring case of coccidiosis in a young guinea pig due to *Eimeria caviae.* Note the large numbers of macro- and microgametocytes.

DIAGNOSIS. Identification of the parasite by mucosal scrapings and examination by phase contrast microscopy is recommended. The organism may also be demonstrated in embedded sections of affected gut prepared for light or electron microscopy.

SIGNIFICANCE. Cryptosporidiosis is one recognized cause of enteritis in this species. Improved sanitation, and if necessary, sulfonamide treatment are recommended. The significance of the concurrent *E. coli* infections seen in some outbreaks has not been determined.

EIMERIA INFECTION: COCCIDIOSIS. In the guinea pig, intestinal coccidiosis is associated with *Eimeria caviae* infections. Following ingestion of the sporulated oocysts, sporozoites penetrate the intestinal mucosa, and schizogony is detectable by 7–8 d postinfection. Endogenous stages occur primarily in the cryptal cells of the anterior colon, although the cecum may also be involved. Diarrhea usually occurs at 10–13 d postexposure. The prepatent period is around 11 d, but severely affected animals may succumb with profuse diarrhea before oocysts are evident on fecal flotation. The time required for sporulation of oocysts to occur is from 2 to 3 d to up to 10 d. Clinical outbreaks of diarrhea occur predomi-

nantly in weanling animals. Seasonal fluctuations may occur. Mortality rates are variable but usually are relatively low.

PATHOLOGY. At necropsy, the large intestine usually contains fluid, fetid material, sometimes with brown flecks of blood. The mucosa is congested and edematous, with variable petechial hemorrhages. Microscopic changes are characterized by colonic hyperplasia and progress to sloughing of enterocytes, edema of the lamina propria, and infiltration with polymorphonuclear and mononuclear cells. Micro- and macrogametocytes are usually present in large numbers in the cecal and colonic mucosa (Fig. 5.22).

DIAGNOSIS. The demonstration of the organisms by mucosal scrapings, histopathology, and fecal flotation will confirm the diagnosis. Deaths may occur before oocysts are evident on fecal flotation. *Differential diagnoses* include cryptosporidiosis, clostridial enteropathies, and antibiotic-induced intestinal dysbacteriosis.

SIGNIFICANCE. *E. caviae* infections are relatively common in breeding colonies of guinea pigs. The organism is regarded as moderately pathogenic, and clinical disease usually indicates a heavy infection. Improved sanitation and husbandry are essential steps in the control of the disease.

RENAL COCCIDIOSIS (*KLOSSIELLA COBAYAE*). Sporadic cases of renal coccidiosis apparently occurred on a global basis in the early to mid–twentieth century. However, it is a rare occurrence under current laboratory conditions. The organism is shed in the urine, and following ingestion, the sporozoites of *K. cobayae* invade the intestinal mucosa and enter adjacent capillaries or lymphatics. Sporozoites reaching the kidney undergo schizogony in endothelial cells of the glomerular capillaries. Infected endothelial cells rupture, releasing merozoites, and schizogony is repeated in epithelial cells lining convoluted tubules. Gametogony occurs in epithelial cells of Henle's loop, and sporulated sporocysts are eventually released in the urine, to repeat the cycle. Clinical signs are normally absent, and the diagnosis is usually based on the demonstration of the schizogonous stage in glomerular capillaries or, more commonly, schizonts or the gametogenous stages in the cytoplasm of epithelial cells lining renal tubules.

ENCEPHALITOZOON INFECTION: ENCEPHALITOZOONOSIS. Spontaneous cases of *Encephalitozoon cuniculi* infection have been recognized in the guinea pig. Multifocal granulomatous encephalitis and interstitial nephritis occur. Lesions are similar to those seen in encephalitozoonosis in other species. The presence of lesions seen histologically as an incidental finding may represent an important complication when infected animals are used in certain types of research.

TOXOPLASMA INFECTION: TOXOPLASMOSIS. Naturally occurring infections have been reported in this species, but they rarely occur, particularly under current housing practices. Infections are frequently asymptomatic, although multifocal hepatitis and pneumonitis are possible manifestations in active infections. Cysts may be present in tissues such as myocardium and central nervous system in asymptomatic chronic infections. Animals may become infected through the ingestion of material contaminated with oocysts from *Feli-*

dae or via the accidental injection of contaminated biological material.

Helminth Infection

BAYLISASCARIS PROCYONIS. *B. procyonis* larval migrans has been reported in a colony of guinea pigs. Affected guinea pigs manifested cachexia, stupor, hyperexcitability, lateral recumbency and opisthotonos. They had multifocal malacia and eosinophilic granulomatous inflammation in the brain associated with the presence of nematode larvae. Eosinophilic granulomata containing nematode larvae were also found in the lungs of some animals. The source of the *Baylisascaris* eggs was wood shavings bedding that was contaminated with raccoon feces.

PARASPIDODERA UNCINATA. P. uncinata are small cecal worms up to approximately 25 mm in length that are located in the cecal and colonic mucosa. The life cycle is direct and is complete in around 65 d. No migration beyond the intestinal mucosa occurs, and infections are normally asymptomatic.

BIBLIOGRAPHY
FOR PARASITIC DISEASES

Ectoparasitic Infestations

Dorrestein, G.M., and Van Bronswijk, J.E.M.H. 1979. *Trixacarus caviae* as a cause of mange in guinea pigs and papular urticaria in man. Vet. Parasitol. 5:389–98.

Flynn, R.J. 1973. *Parasites of Laboratory Animals.* Ames: Iowa State University Press.

Fuentealbea, C., and Hanna, P. 1996. Mange induced by *Trixacarus caviae* in the guinea pig. Can. Vet. J. 37:749–50.

Henderson, J.D. 1973. Treatment of cutaneous acariasis in the guinea pig. J. Am. Vet. Med. Assoc. 163:591–92.

Hirsjarvi, P., and Phyala, L. 1994. Ivermectin treatment of a colony of guinea pigs infested with fur mite (*Chirodiscoides caviae*). Lab. Anim. 29:200–203.

Kummel, B.A., et al. 1980. *Trixacarus caviae* infestation of guinea pigs. J. Am. Vet. Med. Assoc. 177:903–8.

Ronald, N.C., and Wagner, J.E. 1976. The arthropod parasites of the genus *Caviae*. In *The Biology of the Guinea Pig*, ed. J.E. Wagner and P.J. Manning, pp. 201–25. New York: Academic.

Rothwell, T.L.W., et al. 1991. Haematological and pathological responses to experimental *Trixacarus caviae* infection in guinea pigs. J. Comp. Pathol. 104:179–85.

Wagner, J.E., et al. 1972. *Chirodiscoides caviae* infestation in guinea pigs. Lab. Anim. Sci. 22:750–52.

Protozoal Infections

Gibson, S.V., and Wagner, J.E. 1986. Cryptosporidiosis in guinea pigs: A retrospective study. J. Am. Vet. Med. Assoc. 189:1033–34.

Henry, L., and Beverly, J.K.A. 1976. Toxoplasmosis in rats and guinea pigs. J. Comp. Pathol. 87:97–102.

Markham, F.S. 1937. Spontaneous toxoplasma encephalitis in the guinea pig. Am. J. Hyg. 26:193–96.

Moffat, R.E., and Schiefer, B. 1973. Microsporidiosis (encephalitozoonosis) in the guinea pig. Lab. Anim. Sci. 23:282–83.

Muto, T., et al. 1985a. Studies on coccidiosis in guinea pigs. 1. Clinico-pathological observation. Exp. Anim. 34:23–30.

———. 1985b. Studies on coccidiosis in guinea pigs. 2. Epizootiological survey. Exp. Anim. 34:31–39.

Vetterling, J.M. 1976. Protozoan parasites. In *The Biology of the Guinea Pig,* ed. J.E. Wagner and P.J. Manning, pp. 163–96. New York: Academic.

Wan, C-H., et al. 1996. Diagnostic exercise: Granulomatous encephalitis in guinea pigs. Lab. Anim. Sci. 46:228–30.

Nematodes

Van Andel, R.A., et al. 1995. Cerebrospinal larva migrans due to *Baylisascaris procynonis* in a guinea pig colony. Lab. Anim. Sci. 45:27–30.

NUTRITIONAL, METABOLIC, AND OTHER DISORDERS

Scurvy (Hypovitaminosis C). One of the major scourges of explorers for centuries, scurvy also occurred in other populations, particularly in children up to the late nineteenth century. Frequently scurvy was complicated by concurrent ricketts in growing children.

PATHOGENESIS. Most species synthesize ascorbic acid by the glucuronic pathway. Ascorbic acid–dependent species are genetically deficient in the enzyme L-gulonolactone oxidase, which is involved in the conversion of L-gulonolac-tone to L-ascorbic acid. The lack of L-gulono-lactone oxidase is believed to be a genetic defect in species that normally have access to ascorbic acid in their natural diet. This biosynthetic activity occurs in the liver in mammals, but the synthesis of vitamin C occurs in the kidney in amphibians and reptiles. In addition to the inability of simian and human primates and guinea pigs to synthesize endogenous vitamin C, certain bats (e.g., Indian fruit bat), some birds (e.g., red-vented bulbul bird, northern shrike), some fish (e.g., channel catfish), and cetaceans also require supplemental vitamin C. Ascorbic acid is essential in the hydroxylase reactions necessary for the formation of hydroxyproline and hydroxylysine in the collagen molecule. Thus connective tissue cells are unable to synthesize collagen at a normal rate, resulting in deficient and defective production of interstitial osseous matrix. Vitamin C is also necessary for the catabolism of cholesterol to bile acids. In scurvy, cartilage produced in the epiphysis persists, while bone formation is suppressed. The cartilaginous lattice persists and lengthens, but it is not replaced by bone. This calcified cartilage scaffolding is relatively susceptible to mechanical forces; thus multiple microfractures occur in the epiphyseal region. Immobilization of the limb in a plaster cast will prevent the occurrence of microfractures, emphasizing the effect of the normal stresses and strains of limb movement on the development of the typical lesions. There is also increased capillary fragility. There is widening of intercellular spaces between endothelial cells, vacuolar degeneration of endothelium, and depletion of subendothelial collagenous tissue. There is also increased prothrombin time in animals with scurvy. The increased susceptibility of scorbutic guinea pigs to bacterial infections such as *Streptococcus pneumoniae* is probably due, at least in part, to impaired macrophage migration and depressed phagocytic activity of heterophils.

PATHOLOGY. At necropsy, there may be enlargement of the costochondral junctions, with hemorrhages into the regional soft tissues. Hemorrhages are present in the periarticular regions, particu-

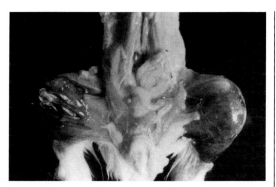

FIG. 5.23—Spontaneous scurvy in young guinea pig. Note the extensive periarticular hemorrhages.

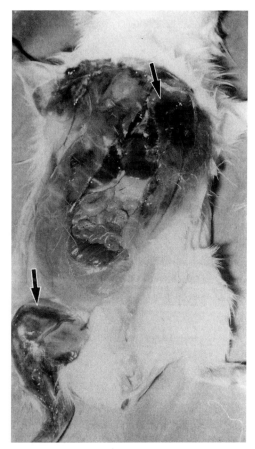

FIG. 5.24—Carcass of guinea pig with scurvy. There are prominent hemorrhages, particularly at the costochondral junctions and periarticular regions (*arrows*).

larly the hindlimbs (Figs. 5.23 and 5.24). Animals may be thin and appear unkempt. Evidence of diarrhea is a variable finding. Occasionally blood-tinged gut contents are observed, and there may by ecchymoses in the urinary bladder. Adrenal glands are frequently markedly enlarged. Microscopically, persistence and irregularities of the epiphyseal cartilage is evident in young growing animals. Microfractures of the cartilaginous spicules and hemorrhage are common findings. There is marked proliferation of poorly differentiated fusiform mesenchymal cells in the periosteal regions and medullary cavity, with displacement of normal hematopoietic cells. Frequently there are aggregations of eosinophilic material interspersed between the mesenchymal cells (Figs. 5.25, 5.26, and 5.27). Dental abnormalities also occur. Fibrosis of the pulp and derangement of odontoblasts have been observed during the early stages of the disease. In cases of subclinical scurvy, large numbers of hemosiderin-laden macrophages may be present in the lamina propria of the intestine. For a more complete description of microscopic changes, see Woodard (1978).

SIGNIFICANCE. Aside from the severe skeletal abnormalities and locomotor problems seen in scurvy, the disease may have significant effects on other processes, including cholesterol metabolism and resistance to bacterial infections. Prolonged clotting times and aberrations in amino acid metabolism may occur. Subclinical scurvy is identified as one important cause of diarrhea in guinea pigs. Recent pet store acquisitions may be particularly at risk. Regular dietary intake of vitamin C is essential, since animals have a limited ability to store vitamin C. Requirements are particularly high in young growing guinea pigs and in sows during pregnancy. Congenital scurvy may also occur. Commercial ration prepared for guinea pigs should be properly stored and fed within 3 mo of the milling date to ensure that vitamin C levels are adequate, because vitamin C levels drop at a relatively rapid rate in prepared rations.

Myopathies

MYOPATHY/MYOSITIS. Necrotizing myopathy, with necrosis of myofibers and leukocytic infiltration, has been reported in guinea pigs. Loss of

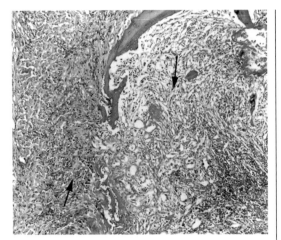

FIG. 5.25—Section of rib from a case of scurvy in guinea pig. There is marked proliferation of fusiform mesenchymal cells in the periosteal and medullary regions (*arrows*).

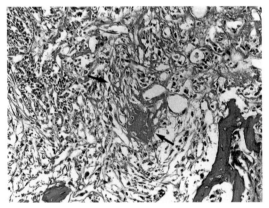

FIG. 5.26—Higher magnification of Figure 5.25, illustrating the amorphous eosinophilic material and the typical fusiform mesenchymal cells (*arrows*).

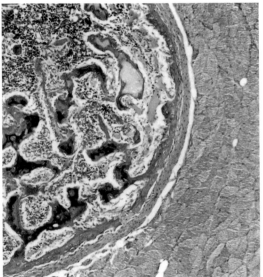

FIG. 5.27—Adjacent rib from animal in Figures 5.25 and 5.26. The cortical architecture and adjacent soft tissue is relatively normal, emphasizing the marked variation in the degree of involvement of bony structures in one animal.

cross-striations, multinucleated muscle bud formation, and variable mononuclear cell infiltration were features of the disease. The etiology was not determined, although a viral infection was suggested as a likely possibility. *Differential diagnoses* include nutritional muscular dystrophy and spontaneous muscular mineralization with degeneration.

NUTRITIONAL MUSCULAR DYSTROPHY. Myopathy has been reported to be associated with vitamin E/selenium deficiency. Depression and conjunctivitis may be present on clinical examination. In one report, spontaneous hindlimb weakness was a prominent clinical feature of the disease. There may be marked reduction in reproductive performance in affected sows. Severely affected animals may die within 1 wk of the onset of clinical signs. Elevated serum creatine phosphokinase (CPK) is a feature of the disease. Animals may respond to alpha tocopherol therapy.

PATHOLOGY. At necropsy, there is a marked pallor of the affected muscles. Microscopic changes are characterized by coagulative necrosis and hyalinization of myofibers, fragmentation of sarcoplasm, increased basophilia of the sarcoplasm, and rowing of nuclei in regenerating myofibers. Multinucleated muscle fibers may be present in regenerating myofibers. Mineralization of myofibers is apparently not an important feature of the disease. Testicular degeneration is a later development seen in vitamin E–deficient guinea pigs.

MYOCARDIAL AND SKELETAL MUSCLE DEGENERATION WITH MINERALIZATION. This is a poorly understood syndrome, and the contributing factors have not been clearly identified. Mul-

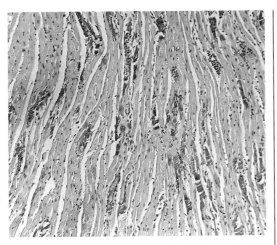

FIG. 5.28—Section of myocardium from adult guinea pig with spontaneous focal muscular degeneration and mineralization.

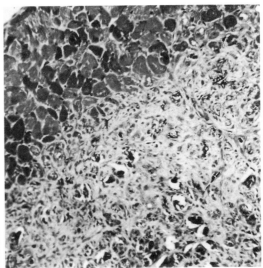

FIG. 5.29—Myocardial degeneration with extensive fibrosis and mineralization in aged guinea pig.

tifocal mineralization of individual muscle fibers may be seen as an incidental finding, particularly in the major muscles of the hindlimbs. Affected animals frequently are asymptomatic. On microscopic examination, there may be multifocal mineralization of skeletal muscle fibers, frequently with minimal cellular response. Myocardial degeneration with mineralization occasionally occurs. Changes are characterized by degeneration of myofibers, with variable mineralization and minimal mononuclear cell infiltration (Fig. 5.28). In chronic lesions of longer duration, there may be concurrent mineralization with fibrosis (Fig. 5.29). In one report, myocardial lesions were observed in crossbred Abyssinian/ Hartley guinea pigs. Vitamin E and selenium levels were within normal limits, and genetic factors were implicated in the disease.

"Metastatic Calcification." Metastatic calcification occurs most often in guinea pigs over 1 yr of age. Muscle stiffness and unthriftiness are variable findings. In some cases, mineral deposition may be confined to soft tissues around the elbows and ribs. There may be more widespread mineralization of tissues, such as lung, trachea, heart, aorta, liver, kidney, stomach, uterus, and sclera (Figs. 5.30 and 5.31). Dietary factors such as a low magnesium and a high phosphorus intake have been implicated in this syndrome. High-

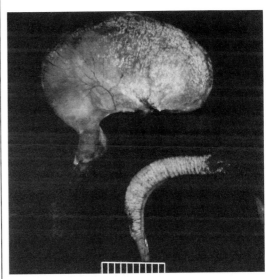

FIG. 5.30—Metastatic calcification in aged guinea pig. There are multiple linear chalky deposits on the serosal surface of the stomach and intestine.

calcium or high-phosphorus diets appear to interfere with magnesium absorption and metabolism. Therefore, this syndrome may not be the result of a deficiency of a single component but rather may be due to a dietary imbalance of two or more nutrients. However, the actual mechanisms

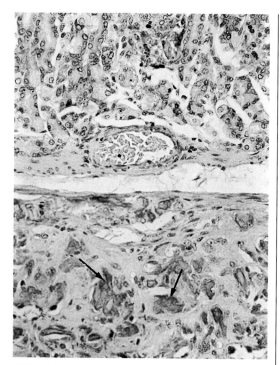

FIG. 5.31—Section of stomach from spontaneous case of calcification. There are prominent depositions of calcium in the gastric mucosa and underlying smooth muscle (*arrows*).

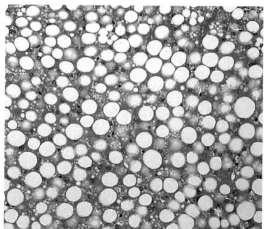

FIG. 5.32—Typical fatty change present in the liver of sow with the metabolic form of pregnancy toxemia.

involved, including possible constitutional and dietary factors, are yet to be determined.

Pregnancy Toxemia. Although the clinical signs are similar in many respects, there are now recognized to be two different patterns of disease associated with pregnancy toxemia in the guinea pig: the fasting or metabolic form and the circulatory or toxic form. Both forms normally occur in advanced pregnancy. Depression, acidosis, ketosis, proteinuria, ketonuria, and a lowered urinary pH from around 9 to 5–6 are frequent manifestations of the disease in both forms of pregnancy toxemia.

PREGNANCY TOXEMIA: METABOLIC/NUTRITIONAL FORM. This form occurs in obese sows during the last 2–3 wk of pregnancy, particularly in sows during their first or second pregnancy. The uterine contents of guinea pigs in advanced pregnancy may represent up to 50% of the weight of the nonpregnant dam, "a parasitism of stagger-

ing proportions," according to Ganaway and Allen (1971). Stress factors such as shipping or changes in feeding routines may be sufficient to precipitate the disease. In one study, withholding the usual supplemental cabbage ration resulted in a mortality rate of approximately 5% in obese dams. The syndrome has also been produced in obese, nonpregnant animals subjected to the stress of cabbage deprivation. Lowered blood glucose, ketosis, and hyperlipidemia are typical findings. Animals usually become comatose and die within 5–6 d after the onset of the disease. Presumably the disease is precipitated by reduced carbohydrate intake and the mobilization of fat as a source of energy, with disastrous results.

At necropsy, animals usually have abundant fat reserves, with marked fatty infiltration in the liver. Microscopically, fatty change is evident in the liver (Fig. 5.32), kidney, and adrenals, and lipid may be demonstrable in vessels with fat stains.

PREGNANCY TOXEMIA: CIRCULATORY FORM (PREECLAMPSIA). In this form, uteroplacental ischemia occurs due to compression of the aorta caudal to the renal vessels by the gravid uterus. This results in a significant reduction in blood pressure in the uterine vessels, with subsequent placental necrosis and hemorrhage, thrombocytopenia, ketosis, and death. On microscopic examination, there is uterine and placental hemorrhage, necrosis, and leukocytic infiltration. Multifocal periportal liver necrosis, nephrosis, and adrenocortical hemorrhage are typical findings. The disease has been reproduced in female guinea pigs by the banding and transection of uterine and ovarian vessels.

SIGNIFICANCE. Pregnancy toxemia is one cause of mortality during pregnancy in some facilities, particularly in obese animals. The circulatory form of the disease has been identified as a possible animal model for preeclampsia in pregnant women. The hypertension seen in human patients with pregnancy toxemia is a variable finding in guinea pigs with this form of the disease.

Diabetes Mellitus. Spontaneous diabetes mellitus has been reported in guinea pigs. Affected animals frequently show no clinical signs during the early stages of the disease. In one documented report, animals were usually affected by 6 mo of age, and the average age of onset was 3 mo. Both sexes were affected. Changes evident by clinical chemistry were hyperglycemia, glycosuria, and rarely ketonuria. There was a marked reduction in fertility in affected sows. Frequently animals introduced into the colony subsequently became diabetic; an infectious agent, currently not identified, appears to be involved.

PATHOLOGY. On microscopic examination, there is vacuolation of and degranulation of the beta islet cells with fatty infiltration of the exocrine cells and fibrosis of the vascular stroma. In advanced cases, there is thickening of basement membranes of the glomerular tufts, sometimes with sclerosis and scarring of Bowman's capsule.

SIGNIFICANCE. Diabetes in the guinea pig is identified as one animal model for juvenile diabetes. Based on current information, diabetes represents a possible cause of infertility in sows.

Alopecia. Bilateral alopecia commonly occurs in sows in advanced pregnancy and during lactation, particularly in older animals. Nutritional and genetic factors may be involved. In pregnant animals, hair loss may be due to reduced anabolism of maternal skin during fetal growth. The hair loss frequently occurs over the back and rump, and the pelage will return to normal in due course in the typical case. *Differential diagnoses* include barbering, pediculosis, and dermatophyte infections. Alopecia can also be associated with cystic rete ovarii.

Malocclusion. This condition most commonly involves the molar and premolar teeth in guinea pigs. The open-rooted cheek teeth grow continuously throughout life, and good opposition is required to prevent overgrowth. If the alignment is defective, the usual result is that the maxillary teeth overgrow labially and the mandibular teeth medially. Excessive salivation, inanition, and wasting occur in severely affected animals. Nutritional factors have been implicated, and fluorosis has been identified as one cause of "slobbers." However, there is evidence that genetic factors play an important role in this disease. There may be a single gene involved, or more than one gene with incomplete penetrance. The incidence is higher in some inbred strains. Anorexia and salivation are the usual clinical signs. At necropsy, food particles are frequently trapped around the cheek teeth. Cheek teeth have irregular contours and sharp edges on the occlusal surfaces (Fig. 5.33). In tooth abnormalities attributed to fluorosis, lesions were characterized by impair-

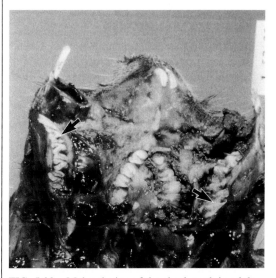

FIG. 5.33—Malocclusion of the cheek teeth in adult guinea pig. The mandibles have been separated. Note the irregular contours of the labial and lingual surfaces of the maxillary and mandibular molar teeth (*arrows*).

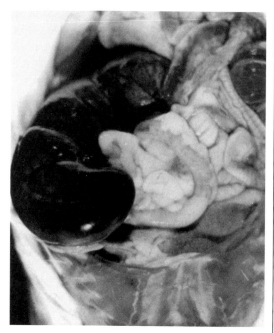

FIG. 5.34—Spontaneous cecal torsion in adult guinea pig. Note the hemorrhagic appearance of cecum associated with impaired circulation and infarction.

ment of dentin and enamel formation and by excessive wear. Abnormalities of this type are not evident in typical cases of malocclusion.

Gastric Dilatation. Multiple cases of acute gastric dilatation associated with gastric volvulus have been recognized in one colony of guinea pigs, and it occurs sporadically in other facilities. Frequently, affected animals were found dead, with no previous indication of disease. Typical cases have a 180-degree rotation along the mesenteric axis, and stomachs are distended with fluid and gas. Death has been attributed to respiratory impairment and possibly vascular shock. Contributing and/or predisposing factors have not been identified.

Cecal Torsion. Deaths due to cecal torsion are occasionally observed in this species. At necropsy, the displaced cecum is distended with fluid and gas and is edematous and hemorrhagic (Fig. 5.34).

Intestinal Hemosiderosis. Accumulations of hemosiderin-laden macrophages in the lamina propria of the intestine, particularly large bowel, is a common finding in the guinea pig. There is speculation that this is due to subclinical scurvy, whereas others believe that it is due to the normally zealous iron-binding of herbivores, with uptake of excessive dietary iron.

Focal Hepatic Necrosis. Multifocal coagulation necrosis of the liver is occasionally seen at necropsy. Affected areas are frequently subcapsular in distribution, with minimal or no inflammatory response. They are frequently interpreted to be a terminal event and may be due to hypoxic change secondary to impaired blood flow in the region. *Differential diagnoses* include bacterial hepatitis (e.g., Tyzzer's disease) and toxic change.

Chronic Idiopathic Cholangiofibrosis. Periportal fibrosis is occasionally seen in adult guinea pigs as an enzootic problem in individual facilities. Lesions, which are usually concentrated around portal triads, are characterized by hepatocyte degeneration, proliferation of cholangioles, and interstitial fibrosis (Fig. 5.35). The changes are suggestive of a toxin-induced change, but to date the etiopathogenesis has not been resolved. There is one report of chronic cholangiofibrosis in Syrian hamsters associated with infection with a *Helicobacter* sp. Whether this has any relevance for a similar pattern of disease in the guinea pig is unknown.

Liver Contusions. Fractures of the capsule of the liver, with hemorrhage into the peritoneal cav-

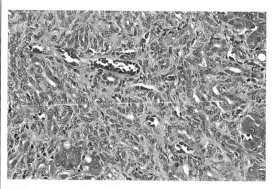

FIG. 5.35—Section of liver from adult guinea pig with spontaneous case of biliary cirrhosis of unknown etiopathogenesis. There is marked proliferation of bile ducts, with periportal fibrosis.

ity, are occasionally observed at necropsy. Traumatic lesions of this type may be caused by events such as mishandling or falls.

Foreign Body Pneumonitis (Pneumoconiosis).
Focal pulmonary lesions associated with aspirated food or bedding occur as an incidental finding, particularly in young guinea pigs. This has been observed in guinea pigs on various bedding materials, including wood products and rice straw.

PATHOLOGY. At necropsy, there may be foci of atelectasis or circumscribed nodules in the parenchyma of the lung, but frequently lesions are not detected on gross examination. On microscopic examination, in lesions of recent onset, plant fibers are lodged within small airways, with polymorphonuclear and mononuclear cell infiltration. In lesions of some duration frequently there is a focal granulomatous bronchiolitis and/or interstitial alveolitis, with mononuclear cell infiltration and foreign body multinucleated giant cell formation. Plant fibers may be identified in these areas. *Differential diagnoses* include osseous metaplasia, lesions of primary bacterial or viral origin, focal mycotic lesions (e.g., *Aspergillus* spp.), and granulomatous pulmonary lesions associated with the subcutaneous administration of Freund's adjuvant.

SIGNIFICANCE. Pneumoconiosis is usually regarded as an incidental finding, particularly if lesions are circumscribed and solitary. Aspirated plant fibers can serve as a nidus for opportunistic bacterial invaders. Pneumoconiosis could complicate research data, particularly if assessment of pulmonary changes is a component of the protocol.

Adjuvant-Associated Pulmonary Granulomas. Pulmonary granulomas may occur in guinea pigs and rats following subcutaneous injection with complete Freund's adjuvant. Microscopic changes are characterized by multifocal granulomatous inflammatory response (Fig. 5.36). *Differential diagnoses* include perivascular lymphoid nodules, pneumoconiosis, and focal pneumonitis due to infectious agents.

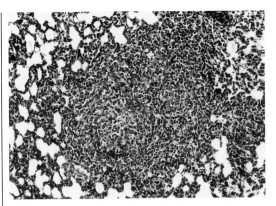

FIG. 5.36—Lung from guinea pig illustrating focal granulomas that may occur in animals treated with complete Freund's adjuvant. Note the granulomatous inflammatory response, with fibrosis and mononuclear cell infiltration.

Behavioral Diseases. Hair pulling is a common behavior pattern among guinea pigs in a group and can become an excessive activity once it is in vogue. An extension of this behavior is ear chewing, which can result in severe trauma and amputation of the ear pinnae. Frequently, sexually mature boars fight when placed together, and severe lacerations or death may be the end result. Very young guinea pigs in communal housing may be trampled by older animals in group stampedes.

BIBLIOGRAPHY FOR NUTRITIONAL, METABOLIC, AND OTHER DISORDERS

Scurvy
Clarke, G.L., et al. 1980. Subclinical scurvy in the guinea pig. Vet. Pathol. 17:40–44.
Eva, J.K., et al. 1976. Decomposition of supplementary vitamin C in diets compounded for laboratory animals. Lab. Anim. 10:157–59.
Follis, R.H. 1943. Effect of mechanical force on the skeletal lesions in acute scurvy in guinea pigs. Arch. Pathol. 35:579–82.
Gangulay, R., et al. 1976. Macrophage function in vitamin C–deficient guinea pigs. Am. J. Clin. Nutr. 29:762–65.
Gillespie, D.S. 1980. An overview of species needing vitamin C. J. Zoo. Anim. Med. 11:88–91.
Gore, I., et al. 1965. Endothelial changes produced by ascorbic acid deficiency in guinea pigs. Arch. Pathol. 80:371–76.
Kim, J.C.S. 1977. Ultrastructural studies of vascular and muscular changes in ascorbic acid–deficient guinea pigs. Lab. Anim. 11:113–17.

Nungester, W.J., and Ames, A.M. 1948. The relationship between ascorbic acid and phagocytic activity. J. Infect. Dis. 83:50–54.

Woodard, J.C. 1978. Bones. In *Pathology of Laboratory Animals,* ed. K. Benirschke et al., pp. 664–820. New York: Springer-Verlag.

Myopathies

Griffith, J.W., and Lang, C.M. 1987. Vitamin E and selenium status of guinea pigs with myocardial necrosis. Lab. Anim. Sci. 37:776–79.

Howell, J.M., and Buxton, P.H. 1975. Alpha tocopherol responsive muscular dystrophy in guinea pigs. Neuropathol. App. Neurobiol. 1:49–58.

Navia, J.M., and Hunt, C.E. 1976. Nutrition, nutritional diseases and nutrition research applications. In *The Biology of the Guinea Pig,* ed. J.E. Wagner and P.J. Manning, pp. 235–67. New York: Academic.

Pappenheimer, A.M., and Schogoleff, C. 1944. The testis in vitamin E deficiency in guinea pigs. Am. J. Pathol. 20:239–44.

Saunders, L.Z. 1958. Myositis in guinea pigs. J. Natl. Cancer Inst. 20:899–903.

Ward, G.S., et al. 1977. Myopathy in guinea pigs. J. Am. Vet. Med. Assoc. 171:837–38.

Webb, J.N. 1970. Naturally occurring myopathy in guinea pigs. J. Pathol. 100:155–62.

"Metastatic Calcification"

Galloway, J.H., et al. 1964. Relationship to diet and age to metastatic calcification in guinea pigs. Lab. Anim. Care 14:6–12.

Sparschu, G.L., and Christie, R.J. 1968. Metastatic calcification in a guinea pig colony: A pathological survey. Lab. Anim. Care 18:520–26.

Pregnancy Toxemia

Bergman, E.N., and Sellers, E.F. 1960. Comparison of fasting ketosis in pregnant and nonpregnant guinea pigs. Am. J. Physiol. 198:1083–86.

Ganaway, J.R., and Allen, A.M. 1971. Obesity predisposes to pregnancy toxemia (ketosis) of guinea pigs. Lab. Anim. Sci. 21: 40–44.

Golden, J.G., et al. 1980. Experimental toxemia in the pregnant guinea pig (*Cavia porcellus*). Lab. Anim. Sci. 30:174–79.

Seidl, D.C., et al. 1979. True pregnancy toxemia (preeclampsia) in the guinea pig (*Cavia porcellus*). Lab. Anim. Sci. 29:472–78.

Diabetes Mellitus

Lang, C.M., et al. 1977. The guinea pig as a model of diabetes mellitus. Lab. Anim. Sci. 27:789–805.

Other Disorders

Franklin, C.L., et al. 1996. Isolation of a novel *Helicobacter* sp. from the gall bladder of Syrian hamsters with cholangiofibrosis. Lab. Anim. Sci. 46:460.

Franks, L.M., and Chesterman, F.C. 1962. The pathology of tumours and other lesions of the guinea pig lung. Br. J. Cancer 16:696–700.

Hard, G.C., and Atkinson, F.F.V. 1967. "Slobbers" in laboratory guinea pigs as a form of chronic fluorosis. J. Pathol. Bacteriol. 94:95–104.

Lee, K.J., et al. 1977. Acute gastric dilatation associated with gastric volvulus in the guinea pig. Lab. Anim. Sci. 27:685–86.

Muto, T. 1984. Spontaneous organic dust pneumoconiosis in guinea pigs. Jap. J. Vet. Sci. 46:925–27.

O'Dell, B.L., et al. 1957. Diet composition and mineral imbalance in guinea pigs. J. Nutr. 63:65–67.

Rest, J.R., et al. 1982. Malocclusion in inbred strain-2 weanling guinea pigs. Lab. Anim. 16:84–87.

Schiefer, B., and Stunzi, H. 1979. Pulmonary lesions in guinea pigs and rats after subcutaneous injection of complete Freund's adjuvant or homologous pulmonary tissue. Zentrabl. Veterinaermed. (A) 26:1–10.

Wagner, J.E. 1976. Miscellaneous disease conditions of guinea pigs. In *The Biology of the Guinea Pig,* ed. J.E. Wagner and P.J. Manning, pp. 227–34. New York: Academic.

DISEASES ASSOCIATED WITH AGING

Segmental Nephrosclerosis. Irregularly pitted, granular renal cortices are a common finding at necropsy, particularly in guinea pigs that are at least 1 yr of age. It is frequently considered to be an incidental finding, but lesions may be extensive enough to result in renal insufficiency.

PATHOGENESIS. The pathogenesis of the segmental interstitial renal scarring has not been resolved, but theories proposed have included autoimmune disease, infectious agents, and vascular disease. In one study, treatment with immunosuppressants failed to prevent the development of the disease, and gamma globulin was not demonstrated in the kidney. The kidney lesions have been interpreted to be the result of a general vascular disturbance, resulting in focal areas of ischemia and fibrosis. In another study, using immunohistochemical techniques, glomerular changes were evaluated in guinea pigs collected from several sources. Spontaneous deposits of IgG and complement (C3) were demonstrated along the mesangial and peripheral glomerular basement membranes. It was suggested that the antigen-antibody complexes might

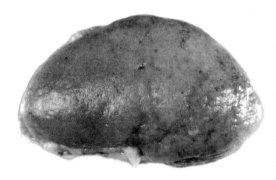

FIG. 5.37—Kidney from aged guinea pig with nephrosclerosis. A finely granular, pitted cortical surface is evident macroscopically.

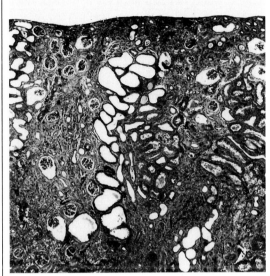

FIG. 5.38—Section of kidney illustrating a typical case of segmental nephrosclerosis. Note the interstitial fibrosis and the convoluted tubules lined by poorly differentiated epithelial cells.

be due to an infectious agent or endogenous tissue antigen. In a search for possible infectious agents, cultures for bacteria are usually unrewarding. In one study, a herpesvirus was isolated from affected kidneys. However, the virus was also recovered from normal kidneys, and the renal lesions in inoculated guinea pigs were not reproduced. An accelerated disease process in guinea pigs fed an unusually high protein diet has been observed. Elevated blood pressures consistent with a mild degree of hypertension have been recorded in animals with renal lesions.

PATHOLOGY. At necropsy, there are multiple, granular, pitted areas on the surface of the kidney, resulting in irregular contours in severely affected animals (Fig. 5.37). On the cut surface, pale linear streaks extend down into the cortex, with some involvement of the medulla in advanced lesions. On microscopic examination, there is segmental to diffuse interstitial fibrosis, with distortion and obliteration of the normal architecture (Figs. 5.38 and 5.39). Tubular lesions are concentrated primarily in the regions of the convoluted tubules and Henle's loop. Scattered tubules are dilated and lined by poorly differentiated, cuboidal to squamous epithelial cells. Some nephrons, interpreted to be nonfunctional, consist of tubular remnants lined by poorly differentiated cuboidal epithelium with lightly eosinophilic to amphophilic cytoplasm. Tubules are occasionally dilated and contain proteinaceous material and

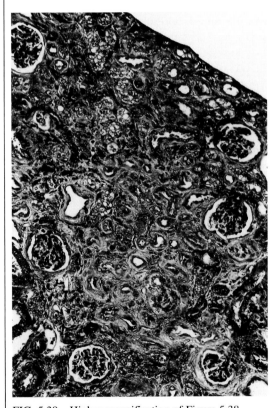

FIG. 5.39—Higher magnification of Figure 5.38, showing thickening of basement membranes and marked interstitial fibrosis.

cellular debris. In nephrons interpreted to be fully functional, convoluted tubules are lined by hypertrophied epithelial cells with abundant, eosinophilic cytoplasm. Most glomeruli are essentially normal histologically. Occasionally there is atrophy of individual glomeruli, with regional fibrosis. In advanced lesions, there is diffuse to segmental infiltration with fibroblasts and collagenous tissue formation. There are minimal focal aggregations of mononuclear cells consisting mainly of lymphocytes. Arterioles and arteries may have moderate medial hypertrophy, sometimes with prominent endothelial lining cells.

SIGNIFICANCE. Advanced cases of nephrosclerosis can cause disability in older guinea pigs. High BUN and serum creatinine values, nonregenerative anemia, and low urinary-specific gravity are clinical findings recorded in animals with advanced nephrosclerosis. The pathogenesis of the renal changes has not been resolved.

Cystitis and Urolithiasis. Urinary tract infections occur occasionally in this species, particularly in older sows. This may be due primarily to the proximity of the urethral orifice to the anus in females, with the likelihood of infection with fecal contaminants such as *Escherichia coli.*

PATHOLOGY. At necropsy, changes may vary from thickening of the bladder mucosa with congestion in chronic cases to intramural and/or intraluminal hemorrhage in animals with acute cystitis. Microscopic changes seen in chronic cases are characterized by leukocytic infiltration in the lamina propria, mononuclear cells predominating, and occasionally fibroblast proliferation. In acute cases, there may be ulceration, hemorrhage, and infiltration with heterophils. Urinary calculi, which occur most frequently in females, may vary in size from sandlike to large concentric bladder stones.

SIGNIFICANCE. Predisposing factors identified in urinary tract infections in guinea pigs include age, sex, and immunosuppression.

Ovarian Cysts (Cystic Rete Ovarii/Serous Cysts). Multiple cystic areas are frequently pres-

ent on the ovaries at necropsy, particularly in sows 1 or more years of age. Small ovarian cysts less than 1 mm in diameter may also be present on the ovaries of younger females, but they are frequently missed at necropsy. In older sows, on gross examination thin-walled, fluid-filled, fluctuant cysts up to 2 cm in diameter may be present on the ovaries. Smaller cysts are usually concentrated in the cephalic pole near the hilus of the ovary. Occasionally, there is one large cyst, with no recognizable ovarian tissue (Fig. 5.40). Cysts contain clear, serous fluid. On microscopic examination, cysts are of variable size and are lined by low cuboidal to columnar epithelial cells (Fig. 5.41). Solitary cilia or tufts of cilia are present on the luminal surface of some cells (Fig. 5.42). Depending on the size of the cysts, there may be marked compression of the ovarian tissue, and in advanced cases only remnants of the ovary remain. Serial sections have revealed continuity between rete ovarii, follicles, and ovarian mesothelium, and the large serous cysts appear to develop from the rete ovarii.

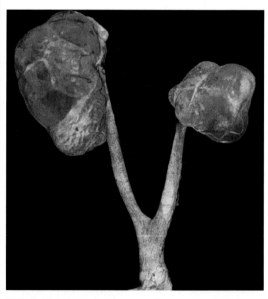

FIG. 5.40—Reproductive tract from an aged adult sow, illustrating changes consistent with cystic rete ovarii. There are large, fluid filled cysts on the surface of the ovaries.

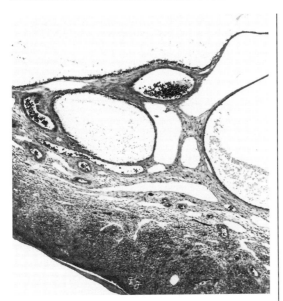

FIG. 5.41—Histological section, illustrating fluid-filled cysts lined by cuboidal epithelial cells, with compression of remnants of ovarian parenchyma.

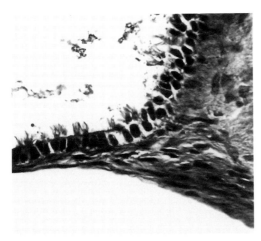

FIG. 5.42—Cystic rete ovarii, higher magnification. Cystic areas are lined by ciliated cuboidal epithelial cells.

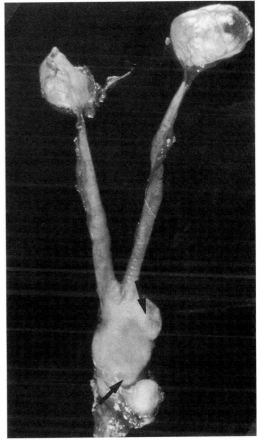

FIG. 5.43—Cystic rete ovarii and uterine leiomyoma in old sow. There is an irregular, multilobulated mass at the uterocervical junction (*arrows*), with extension into the vaginal area.

SIGNIFICANCE. Cystic rete ovarii have been associated with reduced reproductive performance in sows at 15 mo of age and older. Cystic endometrial hyperplasia, mucometra, endometritis, fibroleiomyomas (Figs. 5.43 and 5.44), and alopecia are the other changes associated with the disease.

Fatty Infiltration of the Pancreas. Fatty deposits occur in the pancreas in older guinea pigs as a normal part of the aging process. The proportion of the exocrine pancreas decreases with age, with no apparent impairment of function. Histologically, there are large areas of adipose tissue interposed between normal pancreatic tissue (Fig. 5.45). Fatty infiltration can also occur within the islets.

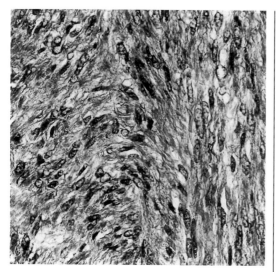

FIG. 5.44—Microscopic section of uterine leiomyoma, illustrating the pallisading bands of fusiform cells.

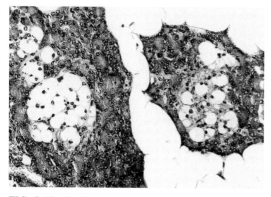

FIG. 5.45—Section of pancreas from mature guinea pig. There is fatty infiltration of the interstitium and fatty change in the islet cells. This is a relatively common finding in guinea pigs.

BIBLIOGRAPHY FOR DISEASES ASSOCIATED WITH AGING

Bauch, L., and Stefkovic, G. 1986. Searching the records for clues about kidney disease in guinea pigs. Vet. Med. 81:1127–30.

Bhatt, P.N., et al. 1971. Isolation and characterization of a herpes-like (Hsiung-Kaplow) virus from guinea pigs. J. Infect. Dis. 123:178–89.

Keller, L.S.F., and Lang, C.M. 1987. Reproductive failure associated with cystic rete ovarii in guinea pigs. Vet. Pathol. 24:335–39.

Peng, X., et al. 1990. Cystitis, urolithiasis and cystic calculi in aging guinea pigs. Lab. Anim. 24:159–63.

Quattropani, S.L. 1977. Serous cysts in aging guinea pig ovary: Light microscopy and origin. Anat. Rec. 188:351–60.

Steblay, R.W., and Rudofsky, U. 1971. Spontaneous renal lesions and glomerular deposits of IgG and complement in guinea pigs. J. Immunol. 107:1192–96.

Takeda, T., and Grollman, A. 1970. Spontaneously occurring renal disease in the guinea pig. Am. J. Pathol. 40:103–17.

NEOPLASMS

Spontaneous tumors are rare in guinea pigs under 3 yr of age and uncommon even in older animals. There appear to be variations in genetic susceptibility to spontaneous neoplasia. A serum factor (probably asparaginase) that has antitumor activity has been demonstrated in the sera of normal guinea pigs. In addition, splenic preparations containing large numbers of Foa-Kurloff cells have been shown to inhibit transformed human epithelial cells in vitro.

Cavian Leukemia. On rare occasions, leukemia occurs as a spontaneous disease in various inbred and noninbred strains of guinea pigs. Cases are most frequently seen in young adult animals. Leukocyte counts in the peripheral blood are relatively high, varying from 50,000 to over 200,000/mm^3. Leukemia has been produced experimentally with transplanted cells and cell-free filtrates. Leukocyte counts of up to 350,000 mm^3 have been observed. Although retrovirus appears to play an important role in this disease, C-type virus particles have also been observed in the germinal centers of lymph nodes from normal guinea pigs.

PATHOLOGY. Leukocytosis (up to 180,000 mm^3 or greater) with a preponderance of lymphoblastic cells is the typical picture seen in blood samples. At necropsy, lymph nodes, such as cervical, axillary, and inguinal, are enlarged and firm, homogeneous, and tan on the cut surface. There is marked splenomegaly and hepatomegaly. Microscopically, there is usually moderate to marked infiltration of lymphoblastic cells in the spleen,

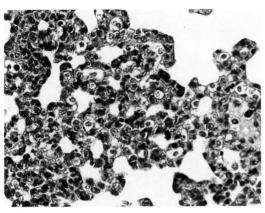

FIG. 5.46—Section of lung from young adult guinea pig with cavian leukemia. Note the marked hypercellularity of the alveolar septa.

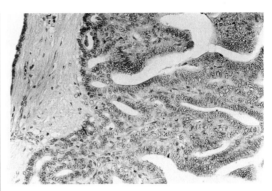

FIG. 5.48—Section from mammary adenocarcinoma in older sow. Mammary tumors of this type also occur occasionally in males.

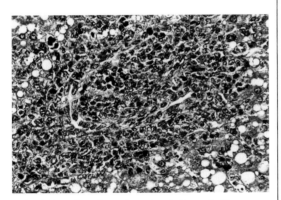

FIG. 5.47—Liver from the animal shown in Figure 5.46. There is a marked periportal infiltrate consisting of poorly differentiated lymphopoietic cells.

liver, bone marrow, interstitium of the lung, thymus, alimentary tract lymphoid tissue, heart, eyes, and adrenals. (Figs. 5.46 and 5.47).

SIGNIFICANCE. Guinea pig leukemia is associated with, but not necessarily caused by, an endogenous retrovirus of the lymphopoietic system.

Tumors of the Reproductive Tract. Tumors of the reproductive tract represent approximately 25% of spontaneous tumors in this species. Of the ovarian tumors, the majority are teratomas. A variety of tissue types may be evident in these tumors, including ciliated and mucous epithelial cells, striated muscle, and cells of ectodermal origin. These tumors should not be confused with cystic rete tubules seen commonly in older sows. Uterine tumors are primarily benign and of mesenchymal origin. Most are fibromas, or leiomyomas (see Figs. 5.43 and 5.44). Rarely, malignant uterine tumors such as myxosarcomas or leiomyosarcomas have been described. Primary malignant uterine tumors may consist of poorly differentiated mesenchymal cells, with extension into the peritoneal cavity. Mammary adenocarcinomas occur in both male and female guinea pigs. The majority are interpreted to be of ductal origin (Fig. 5.48). Metastases may occur to regional lymph nodes. Some are of low-grade malignancy and remain localized to the original site.

Pulmonary Tumors. Pulmonary tumors represented approximately 35% of reported tumors in one survey. The majority were benign papillary adenomas, and most were interpreted to be of bronchogenic origin. The changes were similar to those produced by certain infectious agents, and it was suggested that there may be hyperplastic and adenomatous changes in airways and alveoli in response to various stimuli, not bona fide primary pulmonary tumors. Small, white, circumscribed nodules, visible macroscopically, on microscopic examination consist of papillary

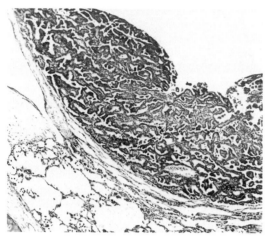

FIG. 5.49—Section of lung from aged sow with multiple bronchial adenomas. Affected airways are lined by poorly differentiated respiratory epithelial cells.

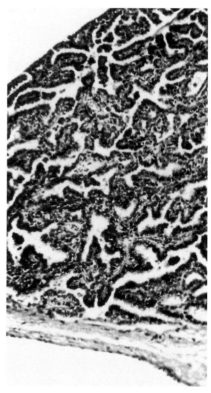

FIG. 5.50—Higher magnification of Figure 5.49, illustrating the papillary pattern and the cuboidal epithelial cells lining the underlying stroma.

structures lined by a single layer of hyperchromatic cuboidal epithelium (Figs. 5.49 and 5.50). Primary malignant tumors of the lung are rare in guinea pigs.

Tumors of the Skin. Skin tumors represent a small percentage of neoplasms reported in this species. The majority are benign. Trichoepitheliomas are the most common tumors of the skin (Figs. 5.51 and 5.52). Cutaneous papillomas, sebaceous gland adenomas, penile papillomas, lipomas, fibrosarcomas, fibromas, and carcinomas have also been described.

Tumors of the Endocrine and Cardiovascular Systems. Tumors of the endocrine system occur in guinea pigs; these include benign adrenocortical tumors. Benign mixed tumors (myxomas) are the most commonly reported tumors of the cardiovascular system. They may include well-differentiated mesenchymal components, such as cartilage, bone, and fat. Primary myocardial tumors should not be confused with rhabdomyomatosis, a congenital condition characterized by vacuolation of myofibers and glycogen deposition (see Heart: Rhabdomyomatosis [Nodular Glycogen Infiltration], discussed in Anatomic Features). For an excellent summary of primary cavian tumors, see Manning (1976).

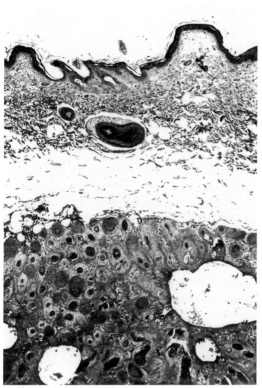

FIG. 5.51—Trichofolliculoma/trichoepithelioma from adult guinea pig. Note the aggregations of follicular structures in the subcutis and the intact epidermis overlying the tumor.

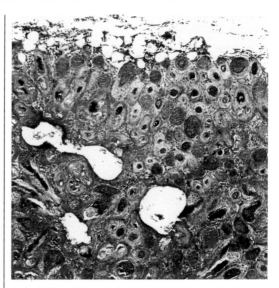

FIG. 5.52—Higher magnification of Figure 5.51, illustrating the numerous follicular structures within the mass.

BIBLIOGRAPHY FOR NEOPLASMS

Bimes, C., et al. 1981. Demonstration of a principle ensuring destruction of human cancer cells in culture. C.R. Hebd. Seances Acad. Sci. 292:293–98.

Brackie, G., et al. Cutaneous papilloma arising from trichepitheliomas in a guinea pig. Contemp. Top. 34(6):91–93.

Field, K.J., et al. 1989. Spontaneous reproductive tract leiomyomas in aged guinea pigs. J. Comp. Pathol. 101:287–94.

Hong, C.C., et al. 1980. Naturally occurring lymphoblastic leukemia in guinea pigs. Lab. Anim. Sci. 30:222–26.

Jungeblut, C.W., and Opler, S.R. 1967. On the pathogenesis of cavian leukemia. Am. J. Pathol. 51:1153–60.

Manning, P.J. 1976. Neoplastic diseases. In *The Biology of the Guinea Pig,* ed. J.E. Wagner and P.J. Manning, pp. 211–25. New York: Academic.

Opler, S.R. 1967. Pathology of cavian leukemia. Am. J. Pathol. 51:1135–47.

Prattis, S.M., et al. 1989. Cutaneous penile mass in a guinea pig. Lab. Anim. (USA) 18(April):15–17.

Wriston, J.C., and Yellin, T.O. 1973. L-asparaginase: A review. Adv. Enzymol. 39:185–248.

Zwart, P., et al. 1981. Cutaneous tumors in the guinea pig. Lab. Anim. 15:375–77.

6

RABBIT

Rabbits are classified as members of the order Lagomorpha. An additional pair of incisor teeth are present directly behind the large incisors on the upper jaw, thus placing them in a different category than the order Rodentia. Domestic rabbits used in the research laboratory and for meat production in the commercial rabbitry are descendants of the European wild rabbit, *Oryctolagus cuniculus.* Their size and readily accessible vessels of the ear make them ideal candidates for antibody production and blood collection. Under natural conditions, the blood flow to their large ears also represents the primary means of temperature control in the domestic rabbit. There are over 100 breeds of rabbits recognized worldwide. However, the majority of rabbits seen in the research facility are the New Zealand White breed. Does are induced ovulators and, following parturition ("kindling"), usually nurse the kits only once daily. The practice of cecotrophy, or reingestion of the mucus-coated "night feces," occurs daily and appears to be one method of recycling cecotrophs, which are relatively high in protein and B complex vitamins. Domestic rabbits in the laboratory animal facility or the commercial rabbitry are frequently nervous and easily frightened. Careful, firm handling, including support of the hindlegs, is essential in order to avoid unrestrained kicking, which may result in accidental fracture of the vertebral column. For additional information on necropsy technique, see Feldman and Seely (1988).

ANATOMIC FEATURES

Hematology. Erythrocytes are approximately 6.5–7.5 μm in diameter, and polychromasia may be evident in a few erythrocytes. The normal value for reticulocytes in adult rabbits is 2–5%, and the estimated mean life span for erythrocytes in circulation is approximately 50 d. By convention, the counterpart of neutrophils is called heterophils in this species. Some experts suggest that the neutrophil name should be retained in rabbits, since the characteristics of this cell resemble neutrophils more closely than the heterophils seen in some of the lower species. Heterophils are 9–15 μm in diameter and have distinct, acidophilic granules present in the cytoplasm. Eosinophils are 12–16 μm in diameter, with large cytoplasmic granules that stain a dull pink-orange with conventional hematology stains. Basophils may be relatively numerous and occasionally represent up to 30% of circulating leukocytes. Lymphocytes are usually the predominant leukocyte in the peripheral blood of domestic rabbits. Small lymphocytes are approximately 7–10 μm in diameter; large lymphocytes may vary from 10 to 15 μm in diameter and sometimes have a few azurophilic cytoplasmic granules. Hematological values have been compared in healthy rabbits and in animals with various disease states (Hinton et al. 1982; Toth and Krueger 1989).

Alimentary Tract. As with other herbivores, rabbits have a large and relatively complex digestive system. The stomach is thin-walled, and typically contains approximately 15% of the ingesta present in the alimentary tract. The small intestine is short compared with that in many species, representing roughly 12% of the total volume of the gastrointestinal tract. Rabbits are hind gut fermenters, and the cecum typically holds around 40% of the ingesta present in the digestive system. Fine particulate materials are selectively channeled into the cecum during passage through the large intestine, while larger particulate material is usually directed into the colon and passed as fecal pellets. The sacculus rotundus is a spherical, thick-walled

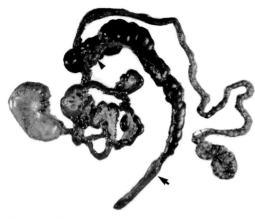

FIG. 6.1—Alimentary tract from mature rabbit, illustrating the prominent cecum and colon. Note the sacculus rotundus at the ileocecal junction (*arrowhead*) and the appendix at the tip of the cecum (*arrow*).

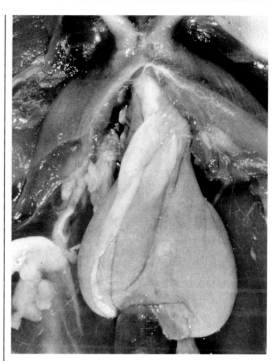

FIG. 6.2—Open urinary bladder from domestic rabbit, illustrating the typical crystalline material seen in the urine of this species (primarily calcium carbonate and triple phosphate crystals).

enlargement at the ileocecal junction (Fig. 6.1). The adjacent cecum has a round patch of lymphoid tissue called the cecal tonsil. The increased thickness of the wall in these lymphoid structures is due to aggregates of organized lymphoid tissue and macrophages in the lamina propria and submucosa. The appendix constitutes the tip of the cecum. It is thick-walled and has abundant lymphoid tissue, which accounts for the marked thickness evident on gross examination. The gut-associated lymphoid tissue (GALT) represents over 50% of the total mass of lymphoid tissue in the body, which accounts for the relatively small spleen seen macroscopically in this species. A common incidental finding in rabbits is the presence of large histiocytes filled with particulate debris in the follicular centers of GALT. Brunner's glands are distributed throughout the length of the duodenum. In the liver, cytoplasmic vacuolation of hepatocytes associated with glycogen accumulation is a variable finding seen microscopically in rabbits fed commercial diets.

Urinary Tract. Once rabbits begin eating solid rations, the alkaline urine normally contains quantities of dull yellow to brown calcium carbonate and triple phosphate crystals (ammonium magnesium phosphate and calcium carbonate monohydrate) (Fig. 6.2). Whereas in most mammals calcium absorption is regulated according to metabolic needs, in the domestic rabbit, calcium is reported to be absorbed in proportion to the amount in the diet. In addition, calcium and magnesium are excreted primarily in the urine in this species, while in most mammals calcium is excreted mainly in the bile. Occasionally the urine is pigmented, the color varying from dark red to orange. This may occur as an incidental finding in normal rabbits, and the color change may be due to dietary porphyrins. Hyperpigmented urine has also been associated with elevated levels of urobilin, the oxidative product of urobilinogen. Urinalysis and microscopic examination of urine will enable the pathologist to differentiate this condition from hematuria. Causes of hematuria in this species include uterine adenocarcinoma, uterine polyps, episodic bleeding from endometrial venous aneurysms, cystitis, polyps in the urinary bladder, pyelonephritis, and renal infarction with hemorrhage.

Skeletal System. In the domestic rabbit, bones are relatively fragile in comparison with the muscle mass. The skeleton of New Zealand White rabbit represents approximately 6–7% of the total body weight. On the other hand, skeletal muscle constitutes over 50% of the body weight in this species. Fractures, particularly those of the vertebral column, may readily occur, particularly when the hindlegs are not restrained properly during handling.

Cardiovascular System. The right chambers of the heart are relatively thin-walled, and a frequent postmortem finding is a quantity of clotted blood in the right ventricle, with no evidence of postmortem contraction.

BIBLIOGRAPHY
FOR ANATOMIC FEATURES

Bray, M.V., et al. 1992. Endometrial venous aneurysms in three New Zealand rabbits. Lab. Anim. Sci. 42:360–62.

Cheeke, P.R. 1994. Nutrition and nutritional diseases of the rabbit. In *The Biology of the Laboratory Rabbit,* ed. P.J. Manning et al., pp. 321–33. New York: Academic.

———. 1987. *Rabbit Feeding and Nutrition.* New York: Academic.

Cheeke, P.R., and Amberg, J.W. 1973. Comparative calcium excretion by rats and rabbits. J. Anim. Sci. 37:450–54.

Cruise, L.J., and Brewer, N.R. 1994. Anatomy. In *Biology of the Laboratory Rabbit,* ed. P.J. Manning et al., pp. 47–62. New York: Academic Press.

Feldman, D.B., and Seely, J.C. 1988. *Necropsy Guide: Rodents and the Rabbit.* Boca Raton, Fla.: CRC.

Garibaldi, B.A., et al. 1987. Hematuria in rabbits. Lab. Anim. Sci. 37:769–72.

Hinton, M., et al. 1982. Haematological findings in healthy and diseased rabbits: A multivariate analysis. Lab. Anim. 16:123–29.

Jelenko, C., et al. 1971. Organ weights and water composition of the New Zealand albino rabbit (*Oryctolagus cuniculus*). Am. J. Vet. Res. 32:1637–39.

Manning, P.J., et al. 1994. *The Biology of the Laboratory Rabbit.* New York. Academic.

Sanderson, J.H., and Phillips, C.E. 1981. *An Atlas of Laboratory Animal Hematology.* Oxford, Engl.: Clarendon.

Toth, L.A., and Krueger, J.M. 1989. Hematologic effects of exposure to three infective agents in rabbits. J. Am. Vet. Med. Assoc. 195:981–86.

Wells, M.Y., et al. 1988. Variable hepatocellular vacuolization associated with glycogen in rabbits. 16:360–65.

Yu, B, and Chiou, W.S. 1996. The morphological changes of intestinal mucosa in growing rabbits. Lab. Anim. 31: 254–63.

VIRAL INFECTIONS

DNA VIRAL INFECTIONS

Adenovirus Infection. Adenoviral enteritis has been identified in commercial rabbits in Hungary. Peak losses occurred at 6–8 wk of age. Profuse diarrhea was observed in severely affected animals, with low mortality. There was a dramatic increase in the numbers of *Escherichia coli* in the small intestine and cecum in rabbits that succumbed to the disease.

PATHOLOGY. Severely affected animals are dehydrated, with fluid contents in the cecum.

DIAGNOSIS. The adenovirus was isolated from the intestinal wall and gut contents, spleen, kidney, and lung when inoculated onto rabbit kidney cell cultures. A significant rise in adenoviral antibody levels was detected in convalescent sera.

SIGNIFICANCE. To date, confirmed cases of adenoviral enteritis in rabbits appear to be confined to Europe. In the outbreak described, a marked increase in coliforms was observed, indicating that *Escherichia coli* may have played a significant role in the disease process.

Papillomaviral Infections

RABBIT (SHOPE) PAPILLOMATOSIS. The Shope cottontail rabbit papilloma virus is the type species of the papilloma virus subgroup of Papoviridae. The virus has been, and continues to be, extensively used as a model for papillomatosis and virus-induced malignancy. Infectious clones of viral DNA are now used extensively.

EPIZOOTIOLOGY. Primarily a benign disease of cottontail rabbits, this disease has occurred in spontaneous outbreaks in domestic rabbits. Insect vectors are probably the usual means of mechanical spread of the causative agent from cottontail rabbits to domestic rabbits. When the cottontail papilloma virus is inoculated into domestic (*Oryctolagus*) rabbits, it produces papillomas with a high incidence of progression to squamous cell carcinomas. Papillomas induced by this virus in *Oryctolagus* rabbits produce minimal or no infectious virus, in contrast to papillomas induced in the natural host (*Sylvilagus*). Papillomas typically undergo immune-mediated resolution if they do not progress to carcinomas. Host immunity has been shown to have two distinct targets: virus structural antigens, invoking protection against virus reinfection, and tumor antigens, invoking papilloma regression. If rabbits are immunized against virus, viral immunity does not affect papilloma status, and rabbits remain susceptible to induction of papillomas with infectious DNA. Once rabbits are immune to the tumor, they resist virus and DNA challenge.

PATHOLOGY. Naturally occurring papillomas occur most frequently on the eyelids and ears and consist of a pedunculated, cornified surface overlying a fleshy central area. The histologic findings are consistent with a squamous papilloma. *Differential diagnosis* must discriminate from spontaneous nonviral papillomas.

Oral Papillomatosis

EPIZOOTIOLOGY. The causative agent, rabbit oral papillomavirus, is the only member of this group with the domestic rabbit as the natural host.

PATHOLOGY. The virus is probably spread by direct contact, and oral abrasions may permit the initial entry. Lesions most frequently occur in rabbits between 2 and 18 mo of age. Pedunculated lesions most commonly occur along the ventral aspect of the tongue (Fig. 6.3). These papillomas usually regress spontaneously within a few weeks. They are typical squamous papillomas on microscopic examination. Basophilic intranuclear inclusions and viral antigen may be present in the stratum spinosum. Fibromas have been produced in hamsters inoculated with homogenates of oral papilloma material collected from rabbits.

Papovaviral Infection. Cottontail rabbits are frequently subclinically infected with rabbit kidney vacuolating virus, which has been isolated from primary rabbit kidney cultures. This virus has no known pathogenic effect in cottontail or domestic rabbits but can be a contaminant of papilloma virus stocks. It belongs to the polyoma virus subgroup of Papoviridae.

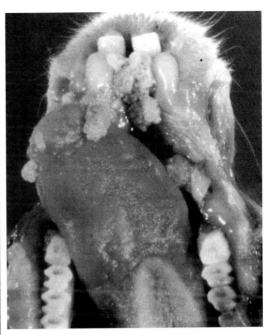

FIG. 6.3—Multiple oral papillomas in a juvenile New Zealand White domestic rabbit. There are multiple papillomas involving both the tongue and buccal cavity.

Parvoviral Infection. A parvovirus has been isolated from clinically normal rabbits in Japan. In a serological survey of commercial rabbits, approximately 60% of animals evaluated had antibody to lapine parvovirus. Oral or intravenous inoculation of young rabbits with lapine parvovirus may result in transient depression and anorexia, with no mortality. The virus may be isolated from a variety of organs for up to 2 wk postinoculation and from the small intestine on day 30 postinoculation. On microscopic examination, a mild to moderate enteritis was present in the small intestine, with exfoliation of enterocytes. In a survey of laboratory rabbits from commercial and private sources in the United States, the majority had relatively high antibody titers to lapine parvovirus. In addition, rabbit parvovirus has been isolated from the kidneys of neonatal rabbits. Thus the inadvertent use of parvovirus-contaminated rabbits or primary cell cultures represents a potential complicating factor when used in research.

SIGNIFICANCE. The role, and importance (if any), of lapine parvovirus in the enteritis complex currently is unknown.

Poxviral Infections

MYXOMATOSIS

EPIZOOTIOLOGY AND PATHOGENESIS. Myxomatosis was first recognized in European rabbits of the genus *Oryctolagus* acquired for experiments in a South American laboratory in the late nineteenth century. The name "infectious myxomatosis" was used to denote the myxoid appearance of the subcutaneous masses associated with the disease. In the original cases described, the virus was believed to have been transmitted by insect vectors from the relatively resistant tropical forest rabbit (*Sylvilagus braziliensis*). Myxomatosis was first recognized in North America in 1930, where outbreaks of the disease occurred in rabbitries in southern California. Myxomatosis remains enzootic in the western United States, and sporadic cases occasionally occur in domestic rabbits. The brush rabbit (*Sylvilagus bachmani*) has been implicated as a reservoir host in that area. Myxomatosis virus is an example of an infectious agent used as a means of biological control of a specific population. Around 1950, the virus was introduced into the wildlife population in Australia in an effort to reduce (or eliminate) the massive numbers of European rabbits (*Oryctolagus cuniculus*), which had become a major economic problem in that country. Mortality rates of up to 99% subsequently dropped to around 25% within a few years. The dramatic reduction in mortality appears to be related both to the emergence of less-virulent strains of the virus and to the natural selection for genetically resistant rabbits in the wild. In 1953, myxomatosis virus was released into the rabbit population in France by a citizen who was disenchanted with the wild rabbit problem. The virus subsequently spread to other countries in Western Europe, including England. Transmission of the virus is usually mechanical and by arthropod vectors, primarily mosquitoes in North and South America and Australia and fleas in Europe.

ETIOLOGY. Myxomatosis virus is a poxvirus morphologically indistinguishable from vaccinia virus. This large DNA virus is closely related antigenically to strains of rabbit fibroma virus.

PATHOGENESIS AND NECROPSY FINDINGS. Following inoculation by an arthropod vector, viral replication results in the development of a primary subcutaneous myxoid mass, usually within 3–4 d. Within 6–8 d, mucopurulent conjunctivitis, subcutaneous edema, and multiple subcutaneous skin tumors are usually observed. In rabbits that die with a peracute form of the disease, the animal may be found dead, and other than redness of the conjunctiva, there may be no other evidence of disease.

PATHOLOGY. Microscopically, in the subcutaneous masses there is proliferation of large, stellate mesenchymal cells ("myxoma cells") interspersed within a homogeneous matrix of mucinous material, with a sprinkling of inflammatory cells (Fig. 6.4). Hypertrophy and proliferation of endothelial cells occur, and changes in

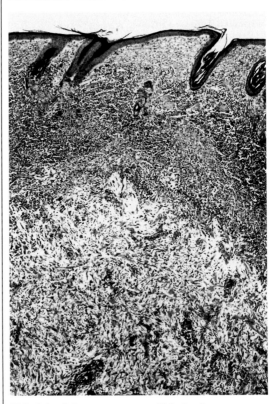

FIG. 6.4—Subcutaneous myxoid lesion in spontaneous case of myxomatosis in New Zealand White rabbit. (Courtesy N.I. Patton)

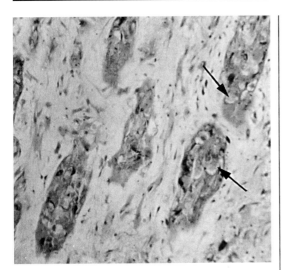

FIG. 6.5—Higher magnification of skin from myxomatosis lesion. Intracytoplasmic inclusions (*arrows*) are present in many cells of follicular epithelium. (Courtesy J.A. Yager)

the epithelium overlying the lesions may vary from hyperplasia to degeneration. Intracytoplasmic inclusions may be present in the affected epidermis (Fig. 6.5) and in epithelial cells of the conjunctiva. Proliferation of alveolar epithelium, hypertrophy and hyperplasia of reticulum cells in lymph nodes and spleen, focal necrosis, hemorrhage, and proliferative vasculitis have also been described. Lymphoid depletion of the spleen is a common finding.

DIAGNOSIS. The presence of characteristic gross and microscopic lesions in rabbits of the genus *Oryctolagus,* particularly in areas where the disease is known to occur, are useful diagnostic criteria. Demonstration of the virus by intracutaneous inoculation of young susceptible rabbits with suspect material, or recovery and identification of the virus from lesions, following inoculation onto chorioallantoic membrane or cell culture, has been used to confirm the diagnosis.

SIGNIFICANCE. In confirmed cases of myxomatosis, identification of the source of the virus, including possible wildlife reservoirs, and the elimination and exclusion of insect vectors are primary considerations.

RABBIT (SHOPE) FIBROMATOSIS. The tumor-producing, transmissible agent was first isolated from a cottontail rabbit (*Sylvilagus floridanus*) in the United States in 1932. The virus is transmissible to European rabbits (*Oryctolagus cuniculus*) and cottontails, producing localized fibromas. Shope fibroma virus infections are relatively widespread in wild cottontail rabbits in the United States and Canada. It is regarded as a benign, self-limiting disease in the wildlife population. The virus may persist for several months within lesions, and mechanical transmission by arthropod vectors appears to be the primary means of spread. In rare occasions, Shope fibromatosis has been diagnosed in commercial rabbitries. Wild cottontail rabbits in the area are the likely reservoir host, with spread by insect vectors.

ETIOLOGY. Rabbit fibroma virus is a poxvirus closely related antigenically to myxomatosis virus and to the hare and squirrel fibroma viruses.

PATHOLOGY. In naturally infected cottontail and European rabbits, firm, flattened tumors occur on the legs and feet, sometimes with involvement of the muzzle, periorbital, and perineal regions (Fig. 6.6). These subcutaneous tumors may be up to 7 cm in diameter, are usually freely movable, and may persist for several months. In young rabbits, metastases to abdominal viscera and bone marrow may also occur.

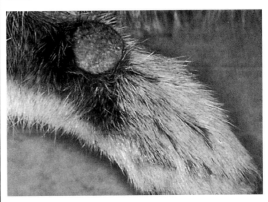

FIG. 6.6—Discrete nodular fibromatous growth on the forepaw of a *Sylvilagus* (cottontail) rabbit naturally infected with Shope's rabbit fibroma virus.

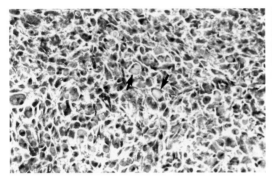

FIG. 6.7—Skin biopsy from domestic rabbit with Shope fibromatosis. There is a dense network of fusiform to polyhedral fibroblasts in the dermis, with prominent intracytoplasmic inclusion bodies (*arrows*).

MICROSCOPIC FEATURES. There is localized fibroblast proliferation, with mononuclear and polymorphonuclear cell infiltration. Fibroblasts characteristically are fusiform to polygonal. In European domestic rabbits (*O. cuniculus*), subcutaneous masses may vary from myxoid in type to typical fibromas. Intracytoplasmic, eosinophilic inclusion bodies may be present in reactive mesenchymal cells (Fig. 6.7) and in epidermal cells overlying the tumors. *Differential diagnoses:* The typical gross and histological appearance of the circumscribed fibrous masses should facilitate the differentiation of Shope fibroma from myxomatosis and from the raised, horny, epidermal growths seen in papillomatosis. However, the myxoid forms sometimes seen histologically can be confused with myxomatosis. Considerable variation in microscopic appearance may occur.

RABBIT POX. The disease is relatively rare and is characterized by the presence of localized to confluent papules on the skin, sometimes accompanied by necrosis and hemorrhage. Papular lesions may also occur in the oropharynx, respiratory tract, spleen, and liver. In the "pockless" form, a few pocks were present in the oral cavity, and focal hepatic necrosis, pleuritis, and splenomegaly were also observed. Histologic changes described have included focal necrosis with leukocytic infiltration in the skin and affected viscera, as well as necrosis of lymphoid tissue. The diagnosis has been confirmed by virus isolation and fluorescent antibody procedures. In a comparison of the pathogenesis of the Utrecht and the Rockefeller strains of rabbit pox, it was concluded that the primary site for viral replication in the naturally occurring disease is the respiratory tract. There is a subsequent viremia, with replication in lymphoid tissues and skin.

Herpesviral Infections

LEPORID HERPESVIRUS 1 (HERPESVIRUS SYLVILAGUS) INFECTION. H. sylvilagus was first isolated from primary kidney cell cultures harvested from weanling cottontail rabbits. Inoculation of young cottontail rabbits with the virus by the parenteral route produces a chronic infection with persistent viremia. Within 6–8 wk following inoculation, changes consistent with a lymphoproliferative disease are observed grossly and microscopically. Histological examination reveals alterations, which may vary from lymphoid hyperplasia to lymphosarcoma. In the malignant form of the disease, diffuse infiltration of various tissues with immature lymphocytes commonly occurs. *H. sylvilagus* infection has been proposed as a model to compare the changes that occur in Epstein-Barr virus infections in humans. Although *H. sylvilagus* replicates in kidney cells prepared from the domestic rabbit, attempts to infect New Zealand White rabbits with the virus have been unsuccessful.

HERPES SIMPLEX VIRUS INFECTION. For decades, domestic rabbits have served as a useful animal model for experimental herpes simplex encephalitis. A naturally occurring case of fatal encephalitis due to herpes simplex virus infection was observed in a 1-year-old pet rabbit. There was a nonsuppurative meningoencephalitis with necrosis of neurons and prominent intranuclear inclusion bodies in neurons and astroglial cells (Fig. 6.8). Typical herpesvirus particles were observed in affected cells by electron microscopy, and herpes simplex was identified as the causative agent using the appropriate diagnostic techniques. Contact with human shedder of herpes simplex virus was the most likely source of the infection. Additional sporadic cases of herpes encephalitis in pet rabbits associated with human contact have been observed by the authors.

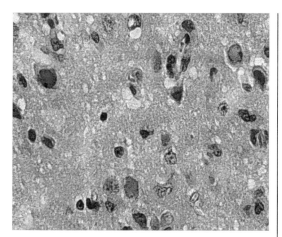

FIG. 6.8—Section of cerebrum from spontaneous case of fatal herpes simplex encephalitis. Note the prominent intranuclear inclusions in the neuropil.

HERPESVIRUS-LIKE VIRAL INFECTIONS. Systemic infections with a herpesvirus-like agent have been observed in several commercial rabbitries in Canada. The disease, which affects animals of various ages, is characterized by sudden onset. Frequently animals are found dead, with no previous evidence of disease. At necropsy, multiple hemorrhages are present in the skin, abdominal viscera, and heart with hydropericardium. Microscopically, there are multiple foci of necrosis in the spleen, dermis, lungs, and adrenal glands. Intranuclear eosinophilic to amphophilic inclusions are present in affected areas in the lung, spleen, and skin. Typical herpesviral particles have been observed in affected tissues and in inoculated rabbit kidney cell culture.

RNA VIRAL INFECTIONS

Caliciviral Infection: Rabbit Hemorrhagic Disease (RHD); Viral Hemorrhagic Disease; Rabbit Calicivirus Disease

EPIZOOTIOLOGY AND CHARACTERISTICS OF THE VIRUS. The disease was first recognized in the People's Republic of China in 1984 and subsequently has been diagnosed in many other countries, including Germany, Italy, Switzerland, Russia, Spain, Republic of North Korea, Poland, Hungary, several countries in Africa, Mexico, and the United Kingdom. The first confirmed report of calicivirus infection in domestic rabbits in the United States occurred in a small rabbitry in Iowa in March 2000, with high mortality. There had been no introductions of rabbits to the premises in 2 yr, and it had been over 6 mo since any rabbits had left the facility and returned. As of this writing, the origin of the virus had not been determined. The problem of systematic characterization has been hampered by the inability to grow the virus in cell culture. The causative agent is now recognized to be a calicivirus. The virus is closely related to the calicivirus causing the European Brown Hare Syndrome (EBHS). However, attempts to infect rabbits and hares with the heterologous virus have failed to result in clinical disease. Scientists in Australia recognized the potential of RHD virus as a means of biological control for the wild rabbit population in that country. The initial inoculation trials began on Wardang Island off the southern coast of Australia. The virus escaped to the mainland in 1995, and subsequently, millions of wild rabbits have succumbed to the disease. RHD virus appears to be species-specific, and the small mammals and domestic animals tested to date have been resistant to the infection. The virus can be spread in a variety of ways including direct contact, aerosols, insect and animal vectors, fomites, and contaminated carcasses. Following outbreaks of the disease in commercial rabbitries, slaughter, disinfection, and using inactivated virus to immunize replacement stock are the steps recommended to eliminate the infection.

CLINICAL SIGNS. There frequently is an explosive outbreak of the disease. The morbidity may vary from 30% to 80% or higher. After an incubation period of 1–2 d, clinical signs are characterized by incoordination, shaking, and a variety of other nervous signs, and death in 2–3 d. Mortality in affected rabbits may be up to 90% or more. The highest mortality rates occur in adult rabbits.

PATHOGENESIS AND PATHOLOGY. Following oral inoculation, the virus replicates in tissues such as liver, small intestine, and spleen, with subsequent viremia. Disseminated intravascular coagulation is considered to play an important role in the pathogenesis of this disease. At necropsy, frequently there is blood-stained nasal discharge, hepatomegaly, splenomegaly, perirenal hemorrhage, and serosal hemorrhage on areas such as pericardium and intestine. Histological findings usually include necrosis of hepatocytes with striking dissociation of hepatic cords (Fig.6.9). Cryptal necrosis occurs in areas of the small intestine. Pulmonary edema, hemorrhage, and necrosis of lymphocytes in splenic follicles and lymph nodes frequently occur. Fibrin thrombi are present in small vessels of multiple organs, including kidney, brain, adrenals, heart, testes, and lung (Fig.6.10). Erythrophagocytosis may be evident in the spleen. Viral antigen can be demonstrated in liver, spleen, small intestine, and mesenteric lymph nodes by immunohistochemistry. The liver is the organ of choice for the detection of viral antigen or the visualization of viral particles by electron microscopy.

SIGNIFICANCE. RHD is a disease of major economic importance to the rabbit industry in many parts of the world. Additional characterization of the virus, the epizootiology of the disease, and the potential of RHD virus as a means of long-term biological control remain under study. Based on 1999 data, there is no evidence that the virus is becoming attenuated in the wild in Australia.

Coronaviral Infections

CORONAVIRAL ENTERITIS

EPIZOOTIOLOGY. Enteritis with mortality has been associated with a coronaviral infection in a barrier-maintained breeding colony in Germany. The epizootic occurred in young rabbits 3–8 wk of age, with peak mortality at 6 wk of age. Typical coronaviral particles were demonstrated by electron microscopy. Coronavirus-associated enteritis in young rabbits has been reported elsewhere, usually with low mortality. In one reported serological survey of selected commercial rabbitries in North America, the prevalence of detectable antibody varied from 3 to 40%.

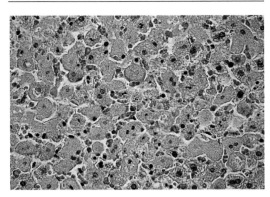

FIG. 6.9—Section of liver from a fatal case of rabbit hemorrhagic disease in a feral *Oryctolagus* rabbit from Australia. Note the vacuolation of hepatocytes and the striking dissociation of hepatic cords. (Courtesy M. Kabay, Animal Health Laboratories, Agriculture Western Australia)

PATHOLOGY. Affected animals may be thin and dehydrated, with fecal staining in the perineal region. The cecum may be distended, containing watery, off-white to tan feces. Microscopic changes are confined to the small and large intestine. Villous blunting; vacuolation and necrosis of enterocytes; mucosal edema; and polymorphonuclear and mononuclear cell infiltration are characteristic findings.

DIAGNOSIS. Characteristic clinical and pathologic findings are important considerations. Confirmation of the diagnosis requires the demonstration of coronaviral particles by electron microscopic examination of gut contents, preferably by immunoelectron microscopy. To date, the virus has not been replicated in cell culture. *Differential diagnoses* include *Escherichia coli*

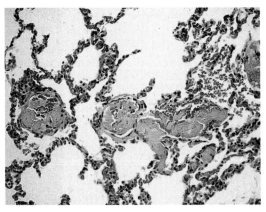

FIG. 6.10—Section of lung from the same animal as in FIGure 6.9. Note the multiple thrombosed vessels. (Courtesy M. Kabay, Animal Health Laboratories, Agriculture Western Australia)

infections, coccidiosis, rotaviral infections, and clostridial enteropathies.

SIGNIFICANCE. The presence of typical coronaviral particles in the feces of young diarrheic rabbits indicates that the virus is likely to play a role in the disease. However, coronaviral particles have also been observed in the gut contents of asymptomatic animals, indicating that inapparent infections occur. Frequently only mild symptoms occur in rabbits inoculated with infectious virus. Although coronaviral enteritis may occur in the absence of identifiable copathogens, simultaneous infection with an enteropathogenic strain of *E. coli* or other enteric pathogens may occur. Thus careful screening for concurrent infections is essential.

CORONAVIRAL PLEURAL EFFUSION DISEASE AND CARDIOMYOPATHY

EPIZOOTIOLOGY. Pleural effusion disease and cardiomyopathy have been associated with coronaviral infections in laboratory rabbits in the United States and Europe. In the Scandinavian reports, pleural effusion was recognized in rabbits following inoculation with a coronavirus-contaminated stock of the Nichols strain of *Treponema pallidum*. The virus is related antigenically to human coronavirus strain 229E.

PATHOLOGY. Fatal infections were characterized by lymphoid depletion of the splenic follicles, focal degenerative changes in the thymus and lymph nodes, proliferative changes in glomerular tufts, and uveitis. In rabbits inoculated with material containing the same strain of *T. pallidum* in the United States, multifocal myocardial degeneration and necrosis were typical changes observed. Viral particles were demonstrated in the sera of infected rabbits postinoculation. Antibodies to two human strains of coronavirus were demonstrated in convalescent rabbit sera, and antigen was detected in myocardial lesions using antisera to human 229E coronavirus.

SIGNIFICANCE. Currently there is no evidence that the causative agent occurs as a natural pathogen of rabbits. Rabbit coronavirus–associated myocarditis has been recognized as one animal model for cardiomyopathy and congestive heart failure.

Rotaviral Infection

ETIOLOGY. Rotaviruses (from the Latin *rota*, "wheel") are double-stranded, nonenveloped RNA viruses of the family Reoviridae. Cultivatable rabbit strains of rotavirus isolated to date have been identified as serotype 3.

EPIZOOTIOLOGY AND PATHOGENESIS. Rotaviral infections are recognized to be a major cause of enteritis in human and veterinary medicine. In the domestic rabbit, outbreaks of rotaviral enteritis are usually confined to suckling and weanling animals. Serological surveys have indicated that rotaviral infections are enzootic in many commercial rabbitries. A high percentage of animals, including preweaning animals, may be seropositive. Epidemiology studies have indicated that protection may be afforded by transplacentally derived maternal antibodies, which subsequently decline to low levels by 1 mo of age. However, on exposure to the virus at 30–45 d of age, there may be sufficient residual antibody to protect them from overt disease. Viral shedding in conventional diarrheic rabbits is frequently seen at 35–42 d of age. Based on serological surveys, clinically healthy rabbits may have a subclinical infection at around 4 wk, with subsequent rise in antibodies to rotavirus. In one epizootic of rotaviral enteritis in a specific-pathogen-free rabbitry, sucklings 1–3 wk of age were affected. The disease was characterized by rapid spread, with high morbidity and mortality. This was interpreted to be consistent with the introduction of a new infectious agent into a colony not previously exposed, thus with no maternal immunity to afford protection during the neonatal period. Following ingestion, rotaviruses replicate in the relatively mature enterocytes lining villi, particularly in the jejunum and ileum. Due to damage to cells that synthesize disaccharidases, lactose and other disaccharides remain in the gut lumen, causing an osmotic drain and attracting fluid into the lumen. Only the monosaccharides may be absorbed. Viral infections of enterocytes may also facilitate bacterial adhesion to damaged cells. In weanling rabbits inoculated with an enteropathogenic strain

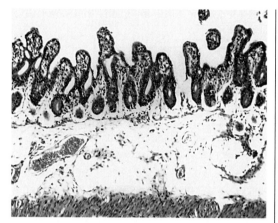

FIG. 6.11—Section of small intestine from young rabbit with a confirmed epizootic of rotaviral enteritis. There is blunting and fusion of villi. Enterocytes lining villi are cuboidal and poorly differentiated. (Courtesy T.R. Schoeb)

of *Escherichia coli,* superimposed rotaviral infections have been shown to have an additive effect, resulting in increased morbidity and mortality.

PATHOLOGY. On gross examination, typically animals are dehydrated, and fluid contents are present in the cecum. Other organs are usually grossly normal. In the small intestine, there may be moderate to severe villous blunting, fusion of adjacent villi, and vacuolation to flattening of apical enterocytes in the jejunum and ileum, sometimes with denuding (Fig. 6.11). There may be focal areas of desquamation in the cecum, frequently with basophilic debris in the cytoplasm of affected enterocytes. Lesions may be similar in coronaviral enteritides. Depending on the availability of diagnostic laboratory facilities, demonstration of the virus (usually by examination of intestinal contents for viral particles by electron microscopy or by the demonstration of viral antigen by enzyme-linked immunosorbent assay [ELISA] techniques), virus isolation, and serology are procedures that should enable one to identify the causative viral agent. In cases of *bacterial enteritis,* villous blunting may occur with attaching strains of *E. coli* in this species. Microscopic examination of the small intestine for evidence of bacterial attachment to enterocytes may be of assistance, but isolation and serotyping are essential steps if a primary or concomitant infec-

tion with *E. coli* is suspected. Fecal flotation and/or microscopic examination of the small and large intestines are essential steps to determine whether coccidia are playing a role in the disease.

DIAGNOSIS. Diagnosis is based on the history, age, and characteristic gross and microscopic features and on the demonstration of rotavirus by direct electron microscopy of fecal samples, by the ELISA technique or virus isolation, or by a rise in antibody titer to the virus. *Differential diagnoses* include coronaviral enteritis, coliform enteritis, coccidiosis, and clostridial enteropathies. ELISA kits, marketed for human rotavirus antigen, are available from commercial suppliers and work well for testing fecal samples for rabbit rotaviral antigen.

SIGNIFICANCE. Demonstration of rotaviral particles in the feces does not constitute a definitive diagnosis but should be confirmed by microscopic examination of the gastrointestinal tract for characteristic lesions. In one study, rotavirus was detected in 25% of diarrheic feces and 10% of normal feces. Frequently there are other factors, including infectious agents, contributing to the disease. Infections with copathogens such as enteropathogenic *E. coli* and/or coccidia frequently play a significant role in this disease. The disease in rabbits has been studied as an animal model for rotaviral infections in other species.

Sendai Viral Infection. Laboratory rabbits have been shown to be susceptible to experimental Sendai virus infection, although viral replication appeared to be confined to the upper respiratory tract. Following intranasal inoculation with the MN strain of Sendai virus, there was transient viral shedding postinoculation, and animals seroconverted. Viral antigen was detected in the nasal epithelium for up to 10 d postexposure. Infected rabbits remained asymptomatic throughout the study.

BIBLIOGRAPHY FOR VIRAL INFECTIONS

DNA Viral Infections

Adenoviral Enteritis
Bondon, L., and Prohaska, P. 1980. Isolation of adenovirus from rabbits with diarrhea. Acta Vet. Acad. Sci. Hung. 28:247–55.

Papillomaviral Infections

DiGiacomo, R.F., and Mare, C.J. 1994. Viral diseases. In *The Biology of the Laboratory Rabbit,* ed. S.H. Weisbroth et al., pp. 171–204. New York: Academic.

Sundberg, J.P., et al. 1985. Oral papillomatosis in New Zealand White rabbits. Am. J. Vet. Res. 46:664–68.

Weisbroth, S.H., and Scher, S. 1970. Spontaneous oral papillomatosis in rabbits. J. Am. Vet. Med. Assoc. 157:1940–44.

Shope, R.E. 1937. Immunization of rabbits to infectious papillomatosis. J. Exp. Med. 65:607–24.

Papovaviral Infection

Hartley, J.W., and Rowe, W.P. 1966. New papovavirus contaminating Shope papillomata. Science 143:258–61.

Parvoviral Infection

Matsunaga, Y., and Chino, I. 1981. Experimental infection of young rabbits with rabbit parvovirus. Arch. Virol. 68:257–64.

Matsunaga, Y., et al. 1977. Isolation and characterization of a parvovirus of rabbits. Infect. Immun. 18:495–500.

Metcalf, J.B., et al. 1989. Natural parvovirus infection in laboratory rabbits. Am. J. Vet. Res. 50:1048–51.

Poxviral Infections

Bedson, H.S., and Duckworth, M.J. 1963. Rabbit pox: An experimental study of the pathways of infection in rabbits. J. Pathol. Bacteriol. 85:1–20.

Christensen, L.R., et al. 1967. Pockless rabbit pox. Lab. Anim. Care 17:281–96.

DiGiacomo, R.F., and Mare, J.C. 1994. Viral diseases. In *The Biology of the Laboratory Rabbit,* ed. P.J. Manning et al., pp. 171–204. New York: Academic.

Fenner, F. 1990. Poxviruses of laboratory animals. Lab. Anim. Sci. 40:469–80.

Fenner, F., and Radcliffe, F.N. 1965. *Myxomatosis.* London and New York: Cambridge University Press.

Hurst, E.W. 1937. Myxoma and Shope fibroma. 1. The histology of myxoma. Br. J. Exp. Pathol. 18:1–15.

Joiner, G.N., et al. 1971. An epizootic of fibromatosis in a commercial rabbitry. J. Am. Vet. Assoc. 159:1583–87.

Patton, N.M., and Holmes, H.T. 1977. Myxomatosis in domestic rabbits in Oregon. J. Am. Vet. Med. Assoc. 171:560–62.

Herpesviral Infections

Hesselton, R.M., et al. 1988. Pathogenesis of *Herpesvirus sylvilagus* infection in cottontail rabbits. Am. J. Pathol. 133:639–47.

Hinze, H.C. 1971a. Induction of lymphoid hyperplasia and lymphoma-like disease in rabbits by *Herpesvirus sylvilagus.* Int. J. Cancer 8:514–22.

————. 1971b. A new member of the herpesvirus group isolated from wild cottontail rabbits. Infect. Immun. 3:350–54.

Swan, C., et al. 1991. *Herpesvirus*-like viral infection in a rabbit. Can. Vet. J. 32:627–28.

Weissenbock, J.A., et al. 1997. Naturally-occurring herpes simplex encephalitis in a domestic rabbit. Vet. Pathol. 34:44–47.

RNA Viral Infections

Caliciviral Infection

Chasey, D. 1996. Rabbit hemorrhagic disease: The new scourge of *Oryctolagus cuniculus.* Lab. Anim. 31:33–44.

Finkel, E. 1999. Australian biocontrol beats rabbits, but not rules. Science 285:1842.

Marcato, P.S., et al. 1991. Clinical and pathological features of viral hemorrhagic disease of rabbits and the European brown hare syndrome. Rev. Sci. Tech. Off. Int. Epizoot. 10:371–92.

Ohlinger, V.F., et al. 1990. Identification and characterization of the virus causing rabbit hemorrhagic disease. J. Virol. 64:3331–36.

Smid, L., et al. 1991. Rabbit hemorrhagic disease: An investigation of properties of the virus and evaluation of an inactivated vaccine. Vet. Microbiol. 26:77–85.

Coronaviral and Rotaviral Infections

Christensen, N., et al. 1978. Pleural effusion disease in rabbits: Histopathological observations. Acta Pathol. Microbiol. Scand.(A) 86:251–56.

Conner, M.E., et al. 1988. Rabbit model of rotavirus infection. J. Virol. 62:1625–33.

Deeb, B.J., et al. 1993. Prevalence of coronavirus antibodies in rabbits. Lab. Anim. Sci. 43:431–33.

Descoteaux, J.-P., and Lussier, G. 1990. Experimental infection of young rabbits with a rabbit enteric coronavirus. Can. J. Vet. Res. 54:473–76.

DiGiacomo, R.F., and Thouless, M.E. 1986. Epidemiology of naturally occurring rotavirus infection in rabbits. Lab. Anim. Sci. 36:153–56.

Eaton, P. 1984. Preliminary observations on enteritis associated with a coronavirus-like agent in rabbits. Lab. Anim. 18:71–74.

Edwards, S., et al. 1992. An experimental model for myocarditis and congestive heart failure after rabbit coronavirus infection. J. Infect. Dis. 165:134–40.

LaPierre, J., et al. 1980. Preliminary report of a coronavirus in the intestine of the laboratory rabbit. Can. J. Microbiol. 26:1204–8.

Osterhaus, A.D.M.E., et al. 1982. Coronavirus-like particles in laboratory rabbits with different syndromes in the Netherlands. Lab. Anim. Sci. 32:663–65.

Peeters, J.E., et al. 1984. Infectious agents associated with diarrhea in commercial rabbits: A field study. Ann. Rech. Vet. 15:335–40.

Schoeb, T.R., et al. 1986. Rotavirus-associated diarrhea in a commercial rabbitry. Lab. Anim. Sci. 36:149–52.

Small, J.D., et al. 1979. Rabbit cardiomyopathy associated with a virus antigenically related to human coronavirus strain 229E. Am. J. Pathol. 95:709–29.

Thouless, M.E., et al. 1996. The effect of combined rotavirus and *Escherichia coli* infections in rabbits. Lab. Anim. Sci. 46:381–85.

Sendai Viral Infection
Machii, K., et al. 1989. Infection in rabbits with Sendai virus. Lab. Anim. Sci. 39:334–37.

General Bibliography
DiGiacomo, R.F., and Mare, C.J. 1994. Viral diseases. In *The Biology of the Laboratory Rabbit,* ed. S.H. Weisbroth et al., pp. 171–204. New York: Academic.

BACTERIAL INFECTIONS

RESPIRATORY BACTERIAL INFECTIONS

Pasteurella multocida **Infection: Pasteurellosis.** Infections with *P. multocida* remain a major cause of disease and mortality in commercial rabbitries. Webster's articles on the epidemiology and characteristics of pasteurellosis, published in the 1920s, remain classic descriptions of the various manifestations of the disease. Patterns of disease associated with infections with *P. multocida* in the rabbit include "snuffles," atrophic rhinitis, otitis media, conjunctivitis, bronchopneumonia, abscessation, genital tract infections, abortions and neonatal mortality, and acute septicemia. In conventional, non–barrier-maintained rabbitries with a history of pasteurellosis, the majority of animals may be harboring the organism in the upper respiratory tract and tympanic bullae.

ETIOLOGY. The causative agent is a small, gram-negative rod with bipolar-staining properties. On initial isolation, colonies may be mucoid in appearance due to the abundant capsular material. Serotyping entails the identification of the capsular antigen (type A), and serotypes 12:A, 3:A, and 3:D are the usual types identified.

EPIZOOTIOLOGY AND PATHOGENESIS. Snuffles is most frequently associated with infection with serotype 12:A. Serotypes 3:A, and occasionally 3:D, have been more frequently associated with disease of the lower respiratory tract. Inapparent carriers of *P. multocida* frequently occur, and even deep nasal swabs may fail to detect all animals carrying the organism in the nasal passages and nasopharynx on culture. Rabbits negative on nasal culture may be harboring *P. multocida* in the tympanic bullae, and the organism may be as readily recoverable from the middle ear as from the nasopharynx. Subclinical infections involving the tympanic bullae are relatively common, and rabbits that are asymptomatic may have typical lesions of otitis media when examined macroscopically. The organism may be acquired through various sources. Direct nasal contact with a shedder animal is the most likely route of exposure. Contact with infected vaginal secretions is another possible source of infection, and the organism may be recovered from this site in a relatively high percentage of carrier animals. The vagina may serve as an important reservoir for the organism and a means of venereal spread to breeding males. Similarly, bucks may harbor *Pasteurella* in the genital tract, and the organism may be transmitted to the doe at mating. In young rabbits born to infected does, colonization with *P. multocida* may occur as early as 3 wk of age, although 3 mo is considered the usual time for the establishment of the infection in young rabbits. A significant percentage of *Pasteurella*-free rabbits are likely to become infected when introduced into an infected colony. Aerosols do not appear to play a major role in the spread of the disease in facilities with adequate air exchange. In one study of contact and airborne transmission of *Pasteurella,* some animals became infected when caged with shedders, but rabbits in adjacent cages separated by a distance of 75 cm remained free from the infection. Whether similar slow rates of spread occur under less than ideal field conditions is unknown. Certainly housing and husbandry practices may have a significant influence on the incidence of pasteurellosis in commercial and laboratory facilities. The reduction of air changes during colder months, poor sanitation, and overcrowding are all conditions that promote the elevation of the ammonia levels above a critical level of 25 ppm, increasing the likelihood of respiratory disease. The role of fomites in the transmission of the organism under field conditions is not known. *Pasteurella* may be readily recoverable from the watering nipples used by rabbits with snuffles. In view of the demonstrated adherence of type A *P. multocida* to rabbit pharyngeal cells, this may be one means of spread. The possibility of interspecies transmission is an important consideration. In one report, two strains of *P. multocida* from other species (bovine and turkey isolates) were passed in mice and rabbits. Following conjunctival inoculation in susceptible New Zealand White rabbits with either of the strains, acute pasteurellosis occurred. Identical phage types have been isolated from European hares and from wild rats on the same premises.

In the laboratory setting, experimental manipulations may enhance susceptibility to the disease. For example, in one study, inoculation of clinically normal rabbits with a variant of Shope fibroma virus resulted in an exacerbation of acute pasteurellosis. Changes were attributed to the immunosuppressant effects of the experimental procedure. Host factors play a key role in susceptibility to the disease, and it is difficult to consistently produce significant lesions in nonmanipulated "healthy" rabbits inoculated intranasally with virulent strains of *P. multocida*.

The upper respiratory tract is usually the primary nidus of infection in affected rabbits. The organism can be spread by various routes from this site: for example, to the lower respiratory tract by the aerogenous route; to the middle ear by the eustachian tube, hematogenously, or by local extension; to the external genital tract by venereal spread or nasal inoculation; and to other areas of the body by the hematogenous route or by local spread. In addition, infections of the upper and lower respiratory tract have been produced experimentally by subcutaneous or intravenous inoculations.

PATHOLOGY. *Chronic rhinitis,* with catarrhal to mucopurulent exudate, is associated with the typical upper respiratory tract form of the disease. When performing a necropsy, it is essential that the nasal bones overlying the turbinates be removed to provide adequate exposure for a thorough examination of this area. Turbinate atrophy has been observed in rabbits naturally or experimentally infected with a 12:A strain of *P. multocida* (Fig. 6.12). The prevalence of this manifestation of the disease has not been determined. *Suppurative otitis media* is a common manifesta-

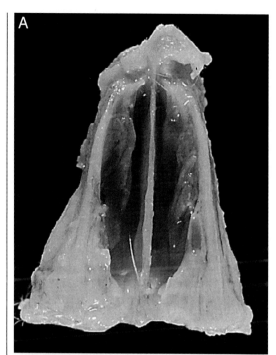
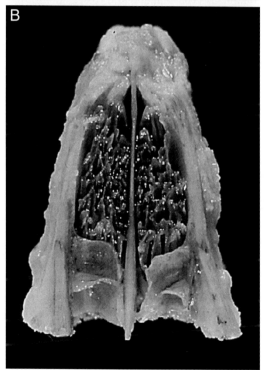

FIG. 6.12—Turbinate atrophy associated with chronic rhinitis due to *Pasteurella multocida* infection. Note the striking loss of turbinates in the affected (**A**) compared with the normal control rabbit (**B**). (Courtesy R.F. DiGiacomo and *American Journal of Veterinary Research*)

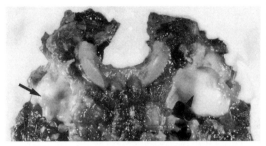

FIG. 6.13—Bilateral otitis media associated with chronic pasteurellosis in an adult rabbit. Thick suppurative exudate is present in both tympanic bullae (*arrows*), with thickening of the tympanic membrane.

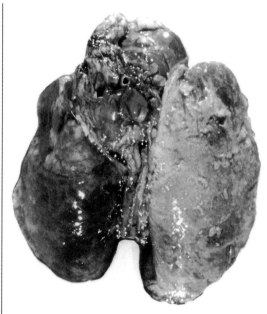

FIG. 6.14—Fibrinohemorrhagic bronchopneumonia in peracute pulmonary pasteurellosis. Fibrinous exudate is present on the pleural surface.

tion of pasteurellosis in this species. In many cases, there may be no clinical evidence of middle ear infection; thus it is essential that the tympanic bullae be opened and examined routinely at necropsy. Grossly, the affected middle ears contain a dull yellow to gray, thick, viscid exudate (Fig. 6.13). The lining of the tympanic bullae is light tan and opaque. On microscopic examination, there is frequently squamous metaplasia of the epithelium lining the tympanic bulla, with leukocytic infiltration into the submucosa and tympanic cavity, heterophils predominating. Rupture of the tympanic membrane may also occur. The inflammatory process may also extend into the inner ear.

Suppurative conjunctivitis is another common manifestation of the disease. With *bronchopneumonia,* the degree of consolidation may vary from localized cranioventral bronchopneumonia to acute necrotizing fibrinopurulent bronchopneumonia (Fig. 6.14). Affected lung tissue in the acute necrotizing form is swollen and moderately firm, frequently with concurrent fibrinous pleuritis and pericarditis. In some cases, pulmonary lesions may be confined to one lung. Similarly, *empyema* associated with pasteurellosis may be unilateral or bilateral in distribution. Microscopically, in animals with localized lower respiratory tract disease, the lesions may vary from chronic bronchitis with peribronchial lymphocytic infiltration to alveolitis with infiltrating leukocytes, heterophils predominating. In the acute, necrotizing form of the disease, destruction of alveoli and small airways, alveolar flooding with fibrinous exudate and erythrocytes, and infiltration with heterophils are typical findings (Fig. 6.15). Multinucleated giant cells may be present in affected alveoli. Pleuritis and pericarditis are frequently observed (Fig. 6.16).

When there is involvement of the *reproductive tract,* macroscopic changes may include pyometra, with chronic suppurative salpingitis and perioophoritis or localized suppurative lesions in the genital system. Acute, transmural, necrotizing metritis has been associated with peracute pasteurellosis. This form occurs during the perinatal period, presumably due to invasion via the dilated cervices. Abortions and stillbirths may precede the death of the doe. Affected does usually die within a few hours after showing signs of disease. At necropsy, fibrinous exudate may be adherent to the uterine serosa, with ecchymoses. The uterine wall is thickened and contains necrotic material (Fig. 6.17). There may be concurrent serositis. Microscopically, there is acute, necrotizing transmural metritis and serositis, with changes in other organs consistent with a bacterial septicemia. In bucks with genital tract lesions associated with *Pasteurella* infections, there may be suppurative orchitis with abscessation.

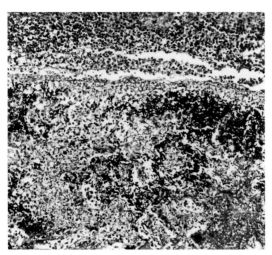

FIG. 6.15—Acute necrotizing bronchopneumonia associated with the respiratory form of acute pasteurellosis. There is destruction of alveoli, fibrinous exudation, and leukocytic infiltration, heterophils predominating.

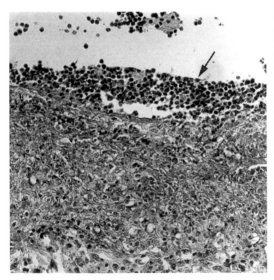

FIG. 6.16—Section of heart from a case of acute pleuritis and pericarditis associated with *Pasteurella multocida* infection. Note the marked infiltrate, consisting of heterophils.

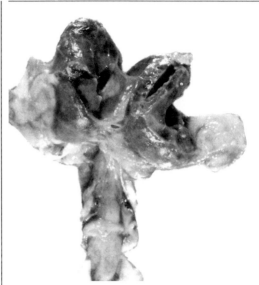

FIG. 6.17—Acute necrotizing transmural metritis in doe that died within a few hours of kindling (peracute pasteurellosis). Fibrinous exudate is adherent to the serosal surface of the uterine horns.

since they tend to excavate bone and are difficult to drain because of the viscid nature of pus in this species. Localized infections may spread to other sites, resulting in manifestations such as vegetative endocarditis.

Acute septicemia is a frequent finding in some rabbitries where chronic *Pasteurella* infections occur. Affected animals may be found dead, with no previous evidence of disease. There may be a concurrent rhinitis and/or otitis media evident at necropsy, but frequently there is no gross evidence of lesions at necropsy. Microscopically, there should be changes consistent with an acute bacterial septicemia, including hemorrhage, variable thromboses of small vessels, and focal cellular degeneration in organs such as liver and adrenal glands. Acute *suppurative meningoencephalomyelitis* is another possible manifestation of pasteurellosis, occasionally with concomitant optic neuritis and iritis.

Circumscribed *abscesses* containing thick, yellow-gray exudate may involve various sites, including subcutaneous tissue, mammary glands, brain, lung, visceral organs, and bone. Abscesses involving the jaw are particularly difficult to treat,

DIAGNOSIS. The diagnosis should be confirmed by bacterial culture. In cases of suspected septicemic pasteurellosis, the organism should be recoverable from a variety of parenchymatous organs and heart blood. Nasal cultures, although useful in identifying carriers/shedders of the organism, will not necessarily detect all infected animals. The ELISA technique has been used to identify animals that were consistently negative for *Pasteurella* on deep nasal culture. *Differential Diagnoses:* With suppurative lesions, bacterial culture should facilitate differentiation of *Pasteurella* infections from other pyogenic infections, such as staphylococcosis. Other bacterial infections associated with respiratory disease in this species are due to *Bordetella bronchiseptica, Staphylococcus,* and rarely, organisms such as *Klebsiella pneumoniae.*

SIGNIFICANCE. *Pasteurella* infections remain a major cause of disease and mortality in commercial rabbitries. With the increased usage of specific pathogen-free rabbits, pasteurellosis should become uncommon in the well-managed research laboratory. The diagnosis of pasteurellosis has serious implications for the researcher. Unexpected deaths during routine procedures such as antibody production may represent immeasurable losses of valuable antigens and personnel time. Experimental manipulations may exacerbate a subclinical infection with *P. multocida,* resulting in clinical disease and possibly mortality. Aside from mortality associated with *Pasteurella* infections, the effects of the disease on various physiological functions, including the immune response, have not been studied adequately.

Bordetella bronchiseptica Infection

EPIZOOTIOLOGY AND PATHOGENESIS. The role played by *B. bronchiseptica* in respiratory infections in the rabbit has not been resolved. The organism may be recovered from the upper and lower respiratory tracts in both clinically normal and diseased animals, suggesting that it is relatively nonpathogenic in this species. However, localized suppurative bronchopneumonia has been produced experimentally in cortisone-treated rabbits inoculated intranasally with *B. bronchiseptica,* and *Bordetella* has been isolated in pure culture from localized pneumonic lesions. A relatively high percentage of conventional commercial and laboratory-reared rabbits may have detectable antibodies to *B. bronchiseptica.* Cultures of *B. bronchiseptica* tend to localize along the cilia of the respiratory epithelial cells in rab-

bits, and *Bordetella* infections have been demonstrated to cause ciliostasis in the canine trachea. It is likely that initial or co-infections with *Bordetella* in airways will impair clearance mechanisms and thus facilitate the establishment of *Pasteurella* in the lower respiratory tract. In chronic infections, there may be prominent peribronchial lymphoid hyperplasia, although this change is not specific for *B. bronchiseptica* infections.

PATHOLOGY AND DIAGNOSIS. Lesions associated with *Bordetella* infections are suppurative bronchopneumonia and interstitial pneumonitis (Fig. 6.18). In chronic infections, there may be prominent peribronchial and perivascular cuffing with lymphocytes. The organism can be recovered in large numbers from lesions in the respiratory tract.

SIGNIFICANCE. *B. bronchiseptica* on occasion may be considered to be a significant opportunistic infection or to act as a copathogen in this species.

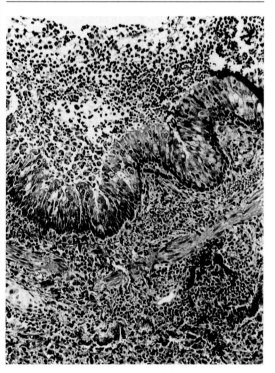

FIG. 6.18—Chronic suppurative bronchitis in weanling rabbit associated with *Bordetella bronchiseptica* infection. There is prominent peribronchial cuffing with lymphocytes. Lesions are similar to those seen in chronic *Pasteurella* infections of the respiratory tract.

Chronic lesions in the lower respiratory tract are a relatively common finding in clinically healthy conventional rabbits. These changes have been associated with chronic infections with *B. bronchiseptica,* but lesions of this type have also been observed with chronic *Pasteurella* infections and in the absence of bacterial isolates from the lung. Occasionally in young rabbits outbreaks of respiratory disease occur that are attributed to *Bordetella* infections. Until proven otherwise, *B. bronchiseptica* should be regarded as a potential pathogen, particularly in rabbits 4–12 wk of age. Perhaps the most significant issue with *B. bronchiseptica* is that rabbits can serve as a source of infection of guinea pigs, which are highly susceptible to this xbacterium.

Cilia-Associated Respiratory (CAR) Bacillus Infection.

Colonization of the apices of the respiratory cells lining the larynx, trachea, and bronchi has been observed in laboratory rabbits. The bacilli were demonstrated both in silver-stained preparations and by electron microscopy. The animals were asymptomatic, suggesting that rabbits may not necessarily develop clinical disease postexposure as readily as do rats and mice. However, in one study, inoculated rabbits developed rhinitis postinoculation with a rabbit isolate, but not with a rat isolate. Mild to moderate peribronchial lymphoid hyperplasia and hyperplasia of epithelial cells lining airways were described.

SIGNIFICANCE. Based on serological studies, the organism is relatively common in commercial rabbitries, but the significance of the CAR bacillus as a respiratory tract pathogen is currently not known. 16S rRNA analysis indicates that the rabbit isolate belongs to a different genus than the rat CAR bacillus and is closely related to *Helicobacter* spp.

BACTERIAL INFECTIONS OF THE ENTERITIS COMPLEX IN RABBITS.

"Enteritis complex" is a term used to encompass a multifactorial complex that commonly occurs in rabbits, particularly in rabbits 5–12 wk of age. Many factors are recognized to play a role in the enteritis complex in domestic rabbits. Frequently, an epizootic (or enzootic) of the disease coincides with recent weaning or changes in feed, environment, or management practices. Important infectious agents now recognized to play a role in this disease complex include rotaviruses and coronaviruses (see RNA viruses), *Clostridia, Escherichia coli, Lawsonia, Salmonella, Vibrio,* and coccidia (see protozoal infections). In addition, mucoid enteropathy, which has an incompletely understood pathogenesis, is a major component of the enteritis complex of rabbits. Thus, the following section encompasses the bacteria of the enteritis complex and includes mucoid enteropathy because of its suspected association with bacterial toxins.

Clostridial Infections

CLOSTRIDIAL ENTEROPATHIES/ENTEROTOXEMIA. Species of *Clostridium* implicated in the enteritis complex in domestic rabbits include *C. perfringens, C. difficile,* and *C. spiroforme* (in addition to *C. piliforme,* which is covered in a separate section). They are gram-positive bacilli that reside in the gut and grow under anaerobic conditions. Pathogenic strains are capable of producing powerful enterotoxins (or cytotoxins) that can alter normal gut function and produce severe, often fatal, enteric disease.

EPIZOOTIOLOGY AND PATHOGENESIS. For years, *C. perfringens* has been regarded as a likely participant in the enterotoxemia/enteritis complex in domestic rabbits. Type E iota toxin has been demonstrated in fatal cases of enterotoxemia, and the disease was attributed to *C. perfringens.* The term "carbohydrate overload" has been associated with the syndrome. The proposed sequence of events was as follows: Rabbits ingesting high-energy feed may fail to degrade and digest the majority of carbohydrates in the small intestine. Significant amounts of carbohydrate may then reach the level of the large intestine, promoting the overgrowth of organisms such as clostridia. This may cause disturbances in the osmolality of intestinal contents, production of enterotoxins, diarrhea, and death. Some previously reported outbreaks of enteropathies associated with *C. perfringens* may have been due to *C. spiroforme,* since antitoxin prepared against *C. perfringens* type E iota toxin will also neutralize similar toxins produced by pathogenic strains of *C. spiroforme.* Fatal colitis and enterotoxemia associated with overgrowth of *C. difficile* has occurred following prolonged treatment with penicillin and ampicillin. Subsequent experimental reproduction of the disease following treatment with lincomycin was attributed to *C. difficile* or *C. perfringens*. Spontaneous enterotoxemia with mortality due to *C. difficile* infection has been reported in specific pathogen-free rabbits in the absence of prior antibiotic treatment. The organism was recovered from the small intestine and cecum, and toxins A and B were demonstrated in vitro.

C. spiroforme is now recognized to be the most common clostridial pathogen associated with the enteritis complex in juvenile rabbits. In one survey of diarrheic rabbits, *C. spiroforme* was isolated from over 50% at necropsy, and 90% of the strains isolated were toxigenic. Although this organism is not considered to be a normal inhabitant of the alimentary tract in rabbits, it frequently is difficult to produce disease experimentally in healthy rabbits inoculated orally with *C. spiroforme*. The normal gut flora appears to act as a microbial barrier, and disruption of the normal gut microflora is considered to be an important predisposing factor. Changes in feed, weaning, previous antibiotic treatment, and concurrent infections are examples of events that may permit colonization with *C. spiroforme* and thus trigger an epizootic of enteric disease. In outbreaks of the disease, the organism may be the sole identified pathogen. However, there may be concurrent infections with other pathogens, such as *Escherichia coli, Eimeria* spp., rotavirus, and cryptosporidia. In one survey, *C. spiroforme* was considered to be the sole pathogen in 13% of the samples examined, and a copathogen in 33% of samples studied (Peeters et al. 1986). Following the multiplication of pathogenic strains of clostridia in the large intestine, enterotoxins may be produced, resulting in damage to enterocytes, impaired function, profuse diarrhea, subsequent depression, dehydration, and death. In peracute cases, rabbits may be found dead in their cages, with little or no prior evidence of disease. A chronic form may also occur. Anorexia, wasting, and intermittent diarrhea may occur over a period of several days.

PATHOLOGY. In peracute cases, the carcass is usually in good condition, and perineal soiling with diarrheic feces is a variable finding. In suba-cute to chronic cases, carcasses are frequently thin and dehydrated. Staining of the perineum, belly, and rear legs with watery green to tarry brown feces commonly occurs. Internally, straw-colored fluid may be present in the peritoneal cavity. Extensive ecchymoses are usually present in the cecal serosa, sometimes with involvement of the distal ileum and proximal colon. Epicardial and thymic ecchymoses may also occur. The cecum and adjacent areas are frequently dilated, with watery to mucoid, green to dark brown contents and with gas formation. There may be marked thickening of affected areas due to submucosal edema, and mucosal changes vary from hemorrhage to ulceration and fibrinous exudation (Fig. 6.19).

Typical microscopic changes present in the cecum of affected animals are those of a necrotiz-

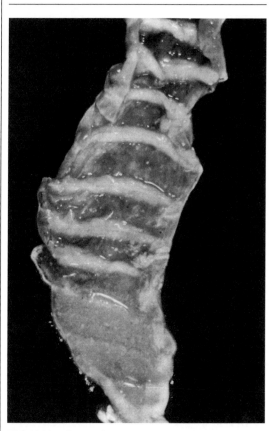

FIG. 6.19—Cecum from a case of spontaneous typhlitis, illustrating changes compatible with clostridial enteropathy. Note the mucosal hemorrhage and the fibrinous exudate on the surface of the mucosa.

ing typhlitis, with irregular denuding of the mucosa, ulceration, fibrinous exudation, and leukocytic infiltration, heterophils predominating (Fig. 6.20). Changes observed in enterocytes vary, including swelling, vacuolation, flattening, denuding, and proliferation. The mucosa and submucosa are congested, frequently with focal hemorrhage, and thrombi may be present in adjacent vessels. Gram-positive bacilli may be present in large numbers on the surface of affected areas of gut mucosa (Fig. 6.21).

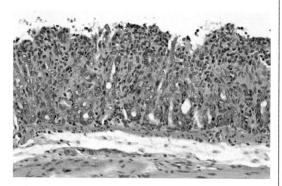

FIG. 6.20—Necrotizing typhlitis from a fatal case of clostridial enteropathy due to *Clostridium spiroforme*. There is degeneration of mucosal cells, sloughing, and disruption of the normal architecture.

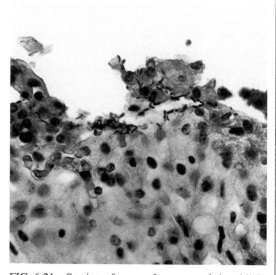

FIG. 6.21—Section of cecum from case of clostridial enteropathy (Brown and Brenn stain). Large numbers of bacilli are adherent to the intestinal mucosa. *Clostridium spiroforme* was isolated in large numbers from the affected areas of gut.

The optimal lesion (for diagnosis) is selective necrosis of mucosal epithelium, with relative sparing of the crypt bases and lamina propria, with submucosal edema, and mucosal/submucosal/serosal hemorrhage. All of these features relate to the effects of luminal toxin penetrating to various depths of the intestinal wall. In subacute to chronic lesions, necrotizing changes are replaced by hyperplasia as the mucosa undergoes repair. In this stage, clinical signs of malabsorption and diarrhea continue. Clinical support of the rabbit has often been stopped at this stage, under the erroneous assumption that the rabbit was not improving. When rabbits are presented for necropsy following death, autolysis and postmortem bacterial overgrowth can obscure mucosal lesions, but a presumptive diagnosis of clostridial enteropathy can still be made on the basis of submucosal edema and hemorrhage.

DIAGNOSIS. The typical age (usually juvenile) and history of a change in feed, management, or environment may be helpful, particularly if coinciding with an explosive outbreak of diarrhea. Clinical signs may include watery diarrhea, depression, and hypothermia, sometimes with terminal convulsions. Gram-stained smears from the ileum and cecum are helpful. Typical curved and coiled gram-positive organisms are associated with *C. spiroforme* infections (Fig. 6.22). Anaerobic cultures are recommended for positive identification of the organism. Several procedures are available for the identification of the clostridial toxin recovered from gut contents or bacterial culture using specific antitoxins. They include skin testing, mouse protection tests, cytotoxicity assay using Vero cells, ELISA testing using antibodies to purified toxin antigens, and rocket immunoelectrophoresis. High-speed centrifugation has been used to separate the organism in intestinal contents. Aerobic bacterial cultures, fecal flotation, and virology screening are procedures recommended in order to search for possible concurrent infections. *Differential diagnoses* include coccidiosis, *E. coli* infections, and Tyzzer's disease.

SIGNIFICANCE. Clostridial infections are recognized as important pathogens in the enteritis complex in this species. A thorough investigation is

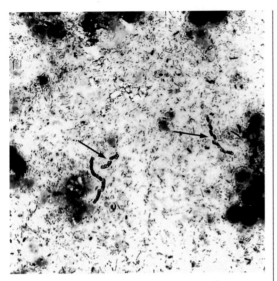

FIG. 6.22—Smear from intestinal contents demonstrating the typical curved and coiled appearance (*arrows*) of *Clostridium spiroforme* (Gram stain).

required in order to identify possible predisposing factors that could upset the normal microbial population of the gut and precipitate an outbreak of the disease. Examples are changes in feed, recent weaning, poor sanitation, adverse environmental conditions, and concurrent infections with other pathogens. Increasing the dietary fiber is recommended as one important means of controlling clostridial enteropathies. Natural diets for this species are high in fiber content, unlike the contrived high-energy diets commonly fed to domestic rabbits today.

CLOSTRIDIUM PILIFORME INFECTION: TYZZER'S DISEASE. The disease was first recognized by Ernest Tyzzer, who described a fatal epizootic in the Japanese waltzing mouse. He noted miliary focal necrosis of the liver and demonstrated bundles of pleomorphic, gram-negative bacilli within the cytoplasm of hepatocytes and in intestinal epithelial cells. He failed to culture the organism but reproduced the disease in mice inoculated with material from fatal cases of the disease. The original article remains a classic description of the disease. The disease has now been recognized in a variety of laboratory animals, wildlife, and domestic species, including the domestic rabbit and cottontail, rat, mouse, hamster, gerbil, guinea pig, rhesus monkey, foal, dog, kitten, and calf.

EPIZOOTIOLOGY AND PATHOGENESIS. Formerly classified as *Bacillus piliformis,* based on 16S rRNA analysis, the organism is now classified as *Clostridium piliforme.* It is relatively labile in the vegetative phase and replicates only in embryonated chick eggs and selected cell lines. The organism may survive for long periods in the spore state and has been shown to remain infectious in contaminated bedding for at least 1 yr. Antigenic differences have been demonstrated in strains of *C. piliforme* isolated from different species. The antigenic differences observed may be due to host-associated antigens, not because of the distinctly different host organisms. It is likely that interspecies infections can occur. Typical lesions have been produced in laboratory animals inoculated orally with isolates from other species. The organism is passed in the feces, and the infection usually occurs by ingestion. There has been speculation, but no proof, that intrauterine transmission may occur in rabbits. Inapparent infections occur, and cortisone treatment has been used to detect subclinically infected animals. There appears to be considerable natural resistance to the organism; frequently, corticosteroid treatment is required in order to reproduce the disease consistently. Following oral inoculation in rodents, intestinal and hepatic lesions have been observed by 3 and 4 d, respectively. On the other hand, there may be local multiplication in the gut mucosa only, with minimal tissue damage. Following oral exposure, the usual sequence of events is multiplication of *C. piliforme* in the intestinal mucosa, with tissue damage, dissemination to the liver by the portal circulation with bacteremia, subsequent hepatitis, and on occasion, myocarditis.

Predisposing factors are an important consideration. In rabbits, "stress factors" include shipping, changes in diet, high environmental temperatures, and poor sanitation. Alterations in the gut flora may enhance susceptibility to the disease. All ages may be affected during epizootics in domestic rabbits, but young weanlings are most frequently affected. The morbidity may vary from 10% to over 50%. The mortality rate in affected animals is high, and rabbits that sur-

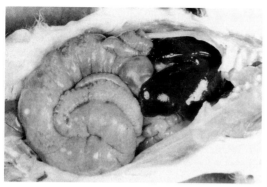

FIG. 6.23—Acute Tyzzer's disease in 12-week-old domestic rabbit. There is marked dilation of the cecum, and fibrinous exudate is adherent to the serosal surface. (Courtesy R.J. Julian)

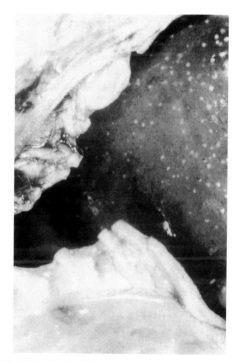

FIG. 6.24—Typical circumscribed focal hepatic lesions in a fatal case of Tyzzer's disease in adult domestic rabbit.

vive may be permanently stunted because of residual lesions, particularly stenosis of the gut. The disease is characterized by a sudden outbreak of profuse, watery diarrhea, a short course, and high mortality in affected animals. Rabbits may be found dead with no prior evidence of clinical disease.

PATHOLOGY. On external examination, dehydration and fecal staining in the perineal region are typical findings. There are usually extensive ecchymoses and occasionally fibrinous exudate on the serosal surface of the cecum and colon (Fig. 6.23). The walls of affected areas, particularly the cecum, are markedly thickened and edematous. The cecum and colon contain dirty brown, watery contents, and the mucosal surface is discolored and dull, frequently with an irregular, granular appearance. Fibrinous strands and debris often adhere to the mucosa. Disseminated pale miliary foci up to 2 mm in diameter are frequently present in the liver (Fig. 6.24). Myocardial lesions, when present, occur as pale, linear streaks, particularly near the apex of the left ventricle. In affected rabbits that survive, carcasses are thin, usually with identifiable circumferential regions of fibrosis and stenosis in the terminal ileum or large intestine.

Microscopic changes are found consistently in the intestinal tract, usually in the liver, and infrequently in the myocardium. In the intestinal tract, there is focal to segmental necrosis of the mucosa of the cecum, with variable involvement of distal ileum and proximal colon. There is sloughing of enterocytes, and large numbers of bacteria are often present on the surface of the damaged mucosa. Lesions are frequently transmural. There is extensive submucosal edema, necrosis of muscular layers, and concurrent leukocytic infiltration, heterophils predominating (Fig. 6.25). In the liver, focal lesions occur most often adjacent to the periportal areas. Circumscribed areas of coagulation to caseation necrosis contain variable numbers of identifiable heterophils, macrophages, and cell debris. In the myocardium, focal to linear areas of coagulation necrosis may be present, usually accompanied by minimal inflammatory response. In rabbits examined during the acute stages of the disease, variable numbers of bacilli are usually demonstrable in the cytoplasm of hepatocytes at the periphery of the focal lesions, more frequently in enterocytes, and sometimes in the adjacent smooth muscle of the gut. Occasionally bacilli are also visible in myofibers associated with myocardial lesions. Intracytoplasmic, eosinophilic bacilli should be

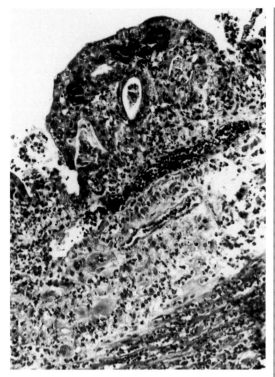

FIG. 6.25—Cecum from a spontaneous epizootic of Tyzzer's disease in a commercial rabbitry. There is a necrotizing transmural typhlitis, with effacement of the mucosal surface and leukocytic infiltration.

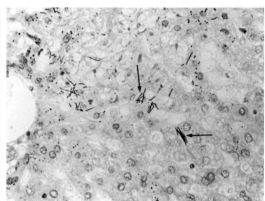

FIG. 6.26—Section of liver in lapine Tyzzer's disease. Bacilli (*arrows*) are present in cytoplasm of hepatocytes (Warthin-Starry stain).

evident in H & E–stained sections. However, paraffin-embedded sections stained with the Warthin-Starry silver method or Giemsa are much better procedures to demonstrate the characteristic bundles of filamentous bacilli associated with the disease (Fig. 6.26). In the rabbit, a careful search may be required in order to locate the organisms.

Microscopic changes seen in the livers of rabbits that survive the acute stages of the disease include focal fibrosis, with infiltrating macrophages and the presence of multinucleated giant cells and mineralized debris. Focal to segmental fibrosis, with disruption of the architecture, occurs in the large intestine, and occasionally in the myocardium, in surviving animals. Tyzzer's bacilli are not present in lesions examined during the convalescent stages of the disease.

DIAGNOSIS. Giemsa-stained impression smears of the hepatic lesions may reveal the typical intra-cytoplasmic fascicles of beaded filamentous bacilli. The presence of the extensive transmural cecal damage, together with the focal hepatic and myocardial lesions, should enable the pathologist to differentiate Tyzzer's disease from other infectious diseases. The demonstration of the typical bacilli in tissue sections are required to confirm the diagnosis. Serological assays are now used to detect seropositive animals. *Differential diagnoses* include listeriosis, staphylococcosis, other bacterial infections of the large intestine, and coccidiosis.

SIGNIFICANCE. It is essential that routine bacteriology and fecal flotations be performed to eliminate the possibility of concurrent infections. Elevated intestinal *Escherichia coli* counts and coccidia oocysts have been observed in some outbreaks of Tyzzer's in rabbits. The significance of these findings has not been determined. The organism may be harbored as an inapparent infection, which may be activated by manipulations or adverse environmental conditions. In view of speculation regarding interspecies transmission, possible sources of the organism should be investigated; wild rodents have been proposed as one source. The organism is relatively refractory to antibiotic treatment.

***Escherichia coli* Infection.** Enteropathogenic strains of *E. coli* are a major cause of enteritis in rabbits from commercial rabbitries and occasionally in research facilities.

EPIZOOTIOLOGY AND PATHOGENESIS. *E. coli* is normally absent or present in small numbers in the alimentary tract of suckling and weanling rabbits. It has been attributed to the low pH of the stomach so that the stomach and small intestine are relatively free from bacteria in this species. Under certain conditions, there may be a marked proliferation of the organisms, and up to 30 million colony-forming units of *E. coli* per gram of feces have been recovered from diarrheic rabbits. Several factors may promote this phenomenal growth of *E. coli*. For example, in intestinal coccidiosis, frequently there is a striking concurrent rise in fecal output of *E. coli*. The mucosal damage associated with intestinal coccidiosis may enhance proliferation of *E. coli* and the resorption of endotoxins. A rise in cecal pH occurs in intestinal coccidiosis, and when diets are fed with a high digestive hydrochloride requirement, this may promote the dissociation of volatile cecal fatty acids, which normally exert an antibacterial effect in the gut.

Isolates of *E. coli* recovered from diarrheic rabbits have been categorized as enteropathogenic strains. They cause intestinal disease, do not produce enterotoxins (currently designated as heat-stable or heat-labile), and are not considered to be enteroinvasive. There appear to be significant variations in the pathogenicity of lapine isolates. Strains of low virulence cause problems primarily in rabbitries with poor sanitation and are usually responsive to antibiotic treatment and improved hygiene. On the other hand, highly virulent strains are often refractory to antibiotic therapy. A large number of strains have been isolated from suckling and weanling rabbits with diarrhea, serotyped, and characterized. In general, strains of *E. coli* isolated from naturally occurring diarrheas in suckling or weanling animals produce disease experimentally only in the same age group. For example, strain RDEC-1, isolated from weanling rabbits, attaches only to the enterocytes of weanling rabbits and produces disease in this age group but not in sucklings. This may be due to the absence of the sucrose-isomaltose enzyme complex on the enterocyte brush border

of suckling rabbits. The complex develops after weaning and has been shown to permit binding of this strain to enterocytes. In studies of the virulence of strains of *E. coli* isolated from sucklings, the organism attached to the enterocytes in both the large and small intestine. In weaned rabbits with experimental coliform enteritis, bacterial attachment occurred in the ileum, cecum, and colon. In rabbits, the adhesins responsible for the attachment of the enteropathogenic strains of *E. coli* to enterocytes are an antigenically diverse group.

In experimental coliform enteritis in suckling rabbits, mortality occurred within 3 d, while in weaned animals, diarrhea and mortality usually occurred after 1 wk. Isolates of *E. coli* from clinically normal rabbits usually failed to produce detectable disease. In experimental coliform enteritis in susceptible weanlings, the organism initially attaches to the Peyer's patch dome epithelium, and later to the enterocytes of the ileum and large intestine. Intestinal lesions were most extensive at 7–14 d postinoculation, with a corresponding significant rise in fecal *E. coli*.

PATHOLOGY. At necropsy, the carcass may be dehydrated, and the perineal region is frequently stained with watery yellow to brown fecal material. The small intestine is usually grossly normal. The cecum and colon frequently are distended with watery yellow to gray-brown contents. There may be serosal ecchymoses, edema of the walls of the cecum and colon, edematous mesenteric lymph nodes, and prominent lymphoid tissue in the Peyer's patches and sacculus rotundus. Microscopically, in sucklings with coliform enteritis, large numbers of coccobacilli are usually attached to enterocytes in both the small and large intestine, with polymorphonuclear cell infiltration in the lamina propria. Microscopic changes are normally more extensive in weanlings with the disease. In the small intestine, ileal villi are often blunted, and the lamina propria is edematous, with leukocytic infiltration, heterophils predominating. Enterocytes at the tips of villi are swollen, and bacterial colonies may be attached to these cells, with effacement of the microvillous brush border. In the cecum and colon, there is bacterial attachment and swelling of affected enterocytes, frequently with

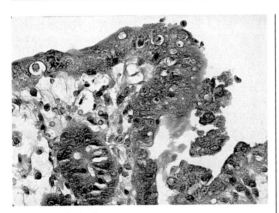

FIG. 6.27—Section of cecum from case of acute col-iform enterotyphlitis in weanling rabbit. The surface of exfoliated epithelial cells and intact enterocytes is covered with numerous attaching *Escherichia coli*.

detachment and ulceration involving primarily the tips of the cecal folds (Fig. 6.27).

DIAGNOSIS. The age, history, clinical signs, and gross and microscopic findings are useful criteria in making the diagnosis. The characterization of the isolate of *E. coli* is recommended in order to determine whether the strain is likely to be a primary pathogen. Isolates of *E. coli* have been divided into biotypes according to their carbohydrate fermentation patterns. There is a good correlation between biotype and serotype in identified pathogenic strains. *Differential diagnoses* include acute coccidiosis, clostridial enteropathies, viral enteritides, and Tyzzer's disease. Concurrent infection of *E. coli* and *Lawsonia intracellularis* has been associated with proliferative enterocolitis (see *Lawsonia intracellularis* Infection).

SIGNIFICANCE. Coliform enteritis is an important cause of disease and mortality in commercial rabbitries and occasionally in research facilities. Diagnostic procedures should include screening for other infectious agents, since more than one pathogen may be contributing to the disease. For example, oral inoculation of weanling rabbits with either lapine rotavirus or an enteropathogenic strain of *E. coli* resulted in mild diarrhea or no disease. In contrast, rabbits inoculated with both agents developed clinical disease with mortality. In outbreaks of intestinal coccidiosis, fre-

quently there is a marked elevation of fecal *E. coli* counts, and it is likely that they are having an additive effect on the disease. The investigation should include a careful review of possible predisposing factors. These would include management and environmental changes, poor sanitation, recent additions to the rabbitry, and acclimatization associated with the postweaning period.

***Lawsonia intracellularis* Infection: Proliferative Enteritis/Histiocytic Enteritis.** The rabbit is among a growing number of species, including rats, hamsters, and guinea pigs, that develop small intestinal proliferative and histiocytic lesions associated with *L. intracellularis* infection. For a number of years, the causative agent was called an intracellular *Campylobacter*-like organism (CLO). *Campylobacter* continues to be incriminated in this disease in some species (but not the rabbit) because it is often a copathogen, or at the very least, a co-infection. *L. intracellularis* is an obligate intracellular bacterium that does not grow in cell-free medium, although some success has been achieved with growth in cell cultures.

EPIZOOTIOLOGY AND PATHOGENESIS. Based upon 16S rRNA sequencing of amplicons from lesions from various species, there appears to be little genetic variation among organisms from one host species to another, and interspecies susceptibility (swine to hamster, horse to hamster) suggests that there is a close relationship among the organisms that infect various host species. Transmission is likely to be by ingestion of fecal material, and experimental transmission has been achieved in this manner. There is no evidence that the organism infects tissue other than enteric mucosa. Location of lesions (gut segment) varies with species. In the rabbit, the jejunum and proximal ileum are typically affected. The fact that the location of lesions is typical for each host species suggests that intestinal microenvironment or host receptors may be critical to pathogenesis. The means of cellular invasion is not known, but in vitro studies indicate that it involves receptor-ligand mechanisms. Regardless of host species, *L. intracellularis* organisms grow to large numbers within the apical cytoplasm of enterocytes, which is a diagnostic feature.

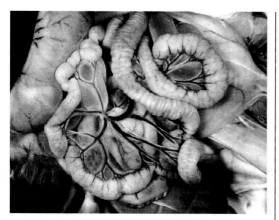

FIG. 6.28—Histiocytic enteritis in domestic rabbit associated with *Lawsonia intracellularis* infection. Note the marked thickening and rugose appearance of serosal surface of the small intestine.

PATHOLOGY. The quality of intestinal lesions varies with the stage of infection. In acute infection, diarrhea with mortality occurs in suckling, weanling, and young adult domestic rabbits. At necropsy of rabbits with acute disease, there may be semifluid mucinous contents present, particularly in the colon and rectum. Animals with more chronic lesions have thickened opaque loops of small intestine (Fig. 6.28). The mucosal surfaces are rugose in character. Microscopically, mucosal lesions vary from suppurative and erosive to primarily proliferative in nature. Lesions of the erosive type ranged from focal denuding to segmental loss of enterocytes, with polymorphonuclear cell infiltration in the underlying areas. Proliferative lesions are characterized by multifocal to diffuse hyperplasia of enterocytes lining crypts and villi, with mononuclear cell infiltration. Histiocytes with abundant granular cytoplasm, and occasionally multinucleated giant cells, are often prominent in the lamina propria (Fig. 6.29). Silver- and PAS-stained sections of affected mucosa reveal typical intracytoplasmic clusters of small bacteria in the apical cytoplasm of the crypt-villus column (Fig. 6.30). Histiocytes within the lamina propria have PAS-positive granular material in their cytoplasm. Electron microscopy reveals typical organisms in enterocytes, and histiocytes contain degenerating bacterial debris.

SIGNIFICANCE. The prevalence of the organism and the incidence of clinical disease due to this

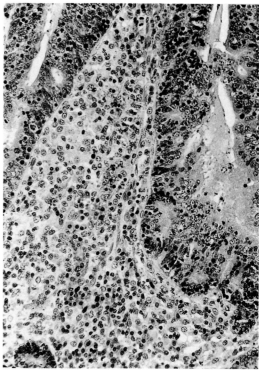

FIG. 6.29—Section of ileum from juvenile rabbit with histiocytic enteritis. There is distortion of the normal mucosal architecture, with marked mononuclear cell infiltration in the lamina propria.

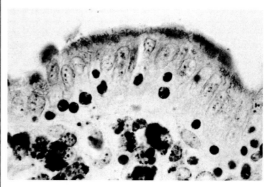

FIG. 6.30—Warthin-Starry stain of intestinal mucosa from rabbit infected with *Lawsonia intracellularis.* Note staining of organisms in the apical cytoplasm of enterocytes and in the histiocytes in the lamina propria.

bacterium in lagomorphs are currently unknown. *Lawsonia* infection can be common in some rabbit colonies. Lesions can often be mild and found as an incidental finding in some rabbits. As with other host species, there may be other viral, bacterial, or protozoal precipitating factors involved. Co-infection with enteropathogenic *Escherichia coli* has been documented in rabbits.

Salmonella Infection. Salmonellosis is relatively rare in domestic rabbits housed in well-managed facilities. Septicemia, diarrhea, abortions, and rapid death have been associated with organisms such as *Salmonella typhimurium* and *S. enteritidis.* Salmonellosis has been identified in specific-pathogen-free rabbits following experimental surgery and irradiation. Pathologic changes associated with lapine salmonellosis include polyserositis, focal hepatic necrosis, splenomegaly, acute enteritis with fibrinous exudation, and suppurative metritis. Laboratory rabbits have been implicated as reservoirs of *S. mbandaka* infection. In view of the public health aspects, and the dangers of interspecies spread, the diagnosis of salmonellosis warrants a thorough investigation and eradication procedures.

Vibrio Infection. *Vibrio* organisms have been associated with at least one reported outbreak of enteritis in weanling rabbits. In the cecum, submucosal edema with polymorphonuclear cell infiltration was observed. Enterocytes were flattened and irregular, with focal ulceration. Cecal crypts were hyperplastic, and some crypts were distended with bacteria and cell debris. In Levaditi-stained tissue sections, *Vibrio*-like organisms were demonstrated on the surface and within the cytoplasm of damaged mucosal cells. The organisms in the cecum were confirmed to be *Vibrio* by electron microscopy. Vibrios were rarely observed in the ceca of controls, and when present, there was no evidence of invasion. Thus vibrios appeared to play a role as a primary pathogen (or copathogen) in these reported cases of acute typhlitis. The prevalence of *Vibrio* infections and the significance of this organism in the enteritis complex have not been determined.

Mucoid Enteropathy. Mucoid enteropathy (ME) is recognized to be a major cause of disease

and mortality in young domestic rabbits. Other names for the syndrome have included "mucoid enteritis," "bloat," and "hypoamylasemia." Clinical signs associated with the disease are as follows: anorexia, lethargy, crouched stance, diarrhea, succussion splash, teeth grinding, cecal impaction, and accumulation of large quantities of clear gelatinous mucus in the colon. Cecal impaction and mucous production occur most often in rabbits that live for 7–14 d after the onset of disease. The morbidity is variable but may be high, particularly in rabbits affected during the postweaning period. There is usually a high mortality rate in affected animals regardless of the treatment used. Rabbits 7–10 wk of age are most often affected, but ages ranging from 5 to 20 wk may be involved in outbreaks of ME.

EPIZOOTIOLOGY AND PATHOGENESIS. Many theories have been proposed to explain the etiopathogenesis of the disease. Dietary factors have frequently been implicated in ME. This condition was relatively uncommon prior to the feeding of high-energy commercial rations, and rabbits fed a low-fiber diet have been shown to have a higher incidence of the disease than those fed diets high in fiber. It was suggested that dietary components such as lectins or "allergens" may create an unfavorable environment in the cecum, permitting opportunistic bacteria to proliferate. Rabbits on low-fiber diets have lower cecal acetate levels. This short-chain fatty acid is reported to inhibit the growth of potentially harmful opportunistic bacteria in the cecum. With lower acetate levels, "secretagogues" produced by these bacteria may then stimulate the colonic cells to secrete large quantities of mucus. Ligation of the cecum or colon will also induce excessive mucous production similar to the naturally occurring disease. In this study, local antibiotic treatment prevented the disease. It was concluded that ME is a toxin-induced secretory disease occurring secondary to constipation and impaction. Bacteria such as *Escherichia coli* and clostridia have been isolated from the small and large intestine in large numbers in some cases of acute onset ME. Such cases may be accompanied by an acute enterotyphlitis. However, inoculation of susceptible rabbits with these isolates seldom produces disease.

Studies of the cecal microbial flora have revealed that striking changes occur in rabbits with ME. In normal animals, large numbers of ciliated protozoa and large, metachromatically staining bacilli are present in the cecal contents. Rabbits with ME have a dramatic cecal dysbiosis. Large metachromatic bacilli and ciliated protozoa may be present in small numbers or completely absent, and there is a marked rise in coliform bacteria in the cecal contents in ME. Using cannulated animals, cecal inoculation with cecal contents from affected animals resulted in the disease only after acidification of the cecum. Cecal acidification in cannulated animals resulted in a dysbiosis similar to that present in the naturally occurring disease. The cecum normally provides a relatively constant internal environment; disruption of this internal milieu may precipitate severe disease. Certain rations promote cecal hyperacidosis and subsequent dysbiosis. The resultant changes may lead to the hypersecretion of intestinal fluid; the loss of water, potassium, and bicarbonates; and frequently death. Microbial instability may occur more often in young animals, where homeostatic mechanisms are poorly developed, thus increasing susceptibility to dietary changes associated with weaning.

PATHOLOGY. At necropsy, the stomach may be distended with fluid and gas. The jejunum is frequently distended with translucent, watery fluid, and the cecum is impacted with dried contents and gas. The colon is usually distended with characteristic clear, gelatinous mucus (Fig. 6.31). Microscopically, there is massive discharge of mucin from goblet cells in the mucosa of affected small and large intestine, with minimal or no inflammatory response. Based on lectin-binding studies, the goblet cell mucus glycoprotein is altered during the course of the disease. Lesions are usually minimal to absent in the cecum. In the colon, crypts and the lumen of the gut are distended with mucus and mucous plugs (Fig. 6.32). *Differential diagnoses* include any infectious or management problem that may lead to disruption of the intestinal microflora or function, such as coccidiosis, clostridial infections, hairballs, and constipation of questionable or unknown etiology.

SIGNIFICANCE. The history, clinical signs, and characteristic gross and microscopic findings should provide the basis for a definitive diagnosis. Feeding practices should be investigated. Bacterial culture, fecal flotation, and other procedures deemed appropriate should be used to screen for concurrent infections by pathogenic agents.

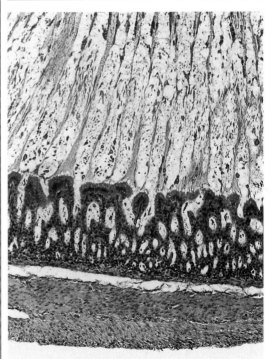

FIG. 6.32—Section from colon of rabbit with mucoid enteropathy. Note the abundant mucus within the lumen and adherent to enterocytes, with minimal inflammatory reaction.

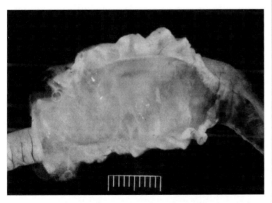

FIG. 6.31—Sacculated colon from juvenile domestic rabbit with mucoid enteropathy. The opened sacculated colon is filled with clear gelatinous material.

Note: For additional information on viral and protozoal agents associated with the enteritis complex, see the appropriate sections.

OTHER BACTERIAL INFECTIONS

***Listeria* Infection: Listeriosis.** Listeriosis is characterized by abortions and sudden deaths, particularly in does in advanced pregnancy. *Listeria monocytogenes* is a small gram-positive, non–spore-forming rod. In 1926, Murray et al. described an acute, fatal disease in young rabbits. Focal hepatitis, ascites, and enlarged mesenteric lymph nodes were typical findings. They observed a marked rise in circulating blood monocytes in both the spontaneous and experimental disease and proposed the name *Bacterium monocytogenes* for the newly recognized organism. The reactive monocytes were observed to phagocytize the organism in vitro with the same avidity as did heterophils.

EPIZOOTIOLOGY AND PATHOGENESIS. In sporadic outbreaks of the disease, the source of the organism is frequently attributed to contaminated feed or water. Inapparent carriers and shedders also occur. *Listeria monocytogenes* has a specific predilection for the gravid uterus in advanced pregnancy. Adult, nonpregnant does and bucks are usually resistant to the infection. Following oral or conjunctival inoculation of females in advanced pregnancy, abortions, stillbirths, and mortality in the dam usually occur. Pregnancy may be interrupted as early as 24 hr postinoculation. However, inoculation of females by the intravaginal, oral, or conjunctival route either prior to mating or early in pregnancy failed to produce disease. The organism can cross the placental barrier in advanced pregnancy. Uterine infections may persist postkindling and may serve as the source of infection for the next pregnancy. Newborn kits born to infected dams that survive may subsequently develop systemic listeriosis, and stunting and meningoencephalitis are other possible sequelae. On the other hand, young rabbits may shed *Listeria* as an inapparent infection for several weeks postkindling.

PATHOLOGY. Deaths typically occur in does in advanced pregnancy. Straw-colored fluid is frequently present in the peritoneal cavity, occasion-

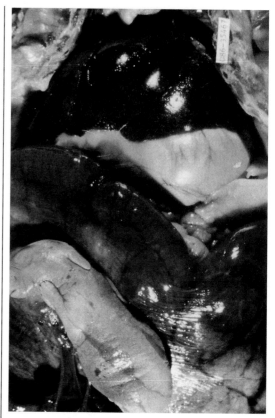

FIG. 6.33—New Zealand White doe that died near-term with acute listeriosis. There are pinpoint-size foci of hepatic necrosis. The kits are intact, with no evidence of maceration. (Courtesy R.J. Hampson)

ally with fibrinous exudate and ecchymoses on the serosal surface of the uterus. Disseminated pale, miliary foci of necrosis on the liver, edema of regional lymph nodes, splenomegaly, and visceral congestion are the usual macroscopic findings. The uterus may contain relatively intact, near-term kits (Fig. 6.33) or fetuses in various stages of decomposition or mummification. In acute cases, the placenta may be edematous and hemorrhagic, but in an infection of longer duration, the placenta is usually thickened, friable, and dull dirty gray, with an irregular surface. Focal miliary hepatic lesions may be evident in stillborn kits. Characteristic microscopic changes seen in adult cases of listeriosis include focal suppurative hepatitis and marked infiltration with heterophils (Fig. 6.34). There may be focal inflammatory lesions in the adrenal cortices, congestion and thromboses in the

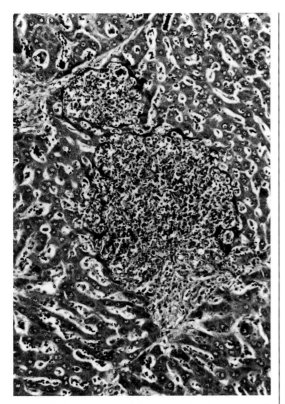

FIG. 6.34—Focal suppurative hepatitis from a case of listeriosis in pregnant doe. There is a clearly delineated lesion, with marked infiltration with heterophils.

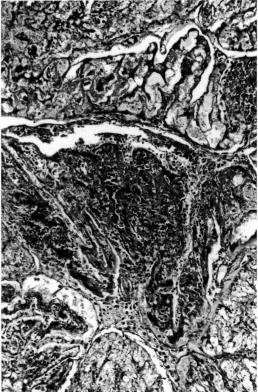

FIG. 6.35—Section of placenta from animal in Figure 6.34. There is marked placental edema and degeneration of trophoblastic cells, with leukocytic infiltration.

splenic sinusoids and blood vessels, and acute necrotizing to chronic suppurative metritis and placentitis (Fig. 6.35). In rabbits that die with the acute form of the disease, large numbers of gram-positive bacilli are usually visible, particularly in the placenta. Focal hepatitis and occasionally meningitis have been observed in newborn animals and in kits that succumb within a few days of birth with listeriosis.

DIAGNOSIS. In acute cases of listeriosis, the organism can usually be readily recovered from the uterine wall, placenta, and fetuses. Blood, liver, and spleen are other likely sources of the organism at necropsy. Recovery of the organism is considered to be a much more satisfactory method to confirm the diagnosis than are serological techniques. *Differential diagnoses:* Diseases causing disseminated foci of hepatic necrosis in the rabbit include Tyzzer's disease, tularemia, and salmonellosis. In perinatal deaths seen in does

with acute pasteurellosis and metritis, there may be acute necrotizing uterine lesions, but liver lesions are normally absent.

SIGNIFICANCE. In addition to the mortality associated with lapine listeriosis, the dangers of inadvertent exposure by human contacts should be emphasized.

Staphylococcal Infections. Outbreaks of staphylococcosis occur sporadically in commercial rabbitries and in laboratory animal facilities. Manifestations of the disease vary from localized abscessation to an acute septicemic, frequently fatal form of the disease.

EPIZOOTIOLOGY AND PATHOGENESIS. Hemolytic, coagulase-positive strains of *Staphylococcus aureus,* particularly type C strains, have been associated with the disease. On rare occasions, staphylococcal infections have been associated with "snuffles" and lower respiratory tract disease. Virulent strains of the organism may be harbored as an inapparent infection in the upper respiratory tract. Such infections may spread by direct contact, but the organism has also been recovered from the air in contaminated facilities. In cases of abscessation, genital tract infection, or mastitis associated with pathogenic strains of *S. aureus,* possible routes of invasion include local inoculation or hematogenous spread. In the acute, systemic form of staphylococcosis, possible sites of entry include umbilical vessels, skin abrasions, or possibly the aerogenous route. Neonatal staphylococcal infections are a recognized cause of neonatal mortality in domestic rabbits in Europe, the United States, and Canada. In France, it is considered to be an important cause of mortality in suckling rabbits in commercial rabbitries. Disseminated staphylococcal infections have also been observed in wild rabbits. In some outbreaks, the same phage type isolated from the rabbits has been isolated from the nares of human contacts.

PATHOLOGY. In mature animals, *chronic suppurative lesions* may occur in the skin, mammary glands, genital tract, conjunctiva, footpads, and upper and lower respiratory tract. In neonatal infections, lesions may be confined to the skin and manifest as multiple raised suppurative lesions a few millimeters in diameter. These may involve a variety of areas, including the extremities, head, back, and sides (Fig. 6.36). The *acute septicemic form* of the disease usually occurs only in suckling kits during the first week of life, frequently with high mortality in affected litters. At necropsy, multifocal suppurative lesions may be present in the subcutaneous tissue and in viscera, including lung, kidney, spleen, heart, and liver (Fig. 6.37). Occasionally systemic staphylococcosis with focal suppurative lesions occurs in adult rabbits (Fig. 6.38). Microscopically, focal suppurative necrotizing lesions are present in affected organs. Bacterial colonies are usually associated with the lesions.

Bacterial culture is essential in order to confirm the diagnosis. In staphylococcal mastitis, affected glands may vary in appearance from swollen, red areas with induration of the overlying skin to chronic abscessation. *Respiratory tract lesions,*

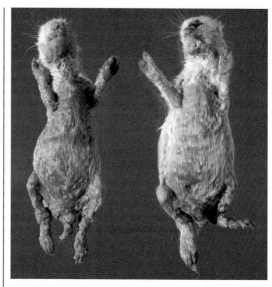

FIG. 6.36—Staphylococcal pyoderma in rabbit kits associated with acute staphylococcal infection.

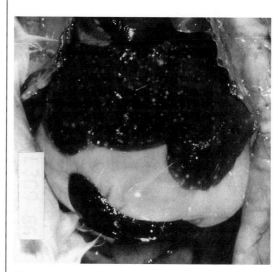

FIG. 6.37—Mortality associated with acute staphylococcal septicemia in 10-d-old kit. Note the multifocal suppurative lesions in the liver.

when present, may be characterized by mucopurulent rhinitis, occasionally with localized bronchopneumonia or abscessation of the lung.

DIAGNOSIS. Recovery of *S. aureus* from the lesions is essential to confirm the diagnosis. Gram-positive cocci are also readily demonstrated histologically in tissue sections. *Differen-*

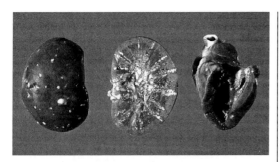

FIG. 6.38—Multifocal suppurative nephritis and myocarditis in an adult New Zealand White rabbit with systemic staphylococcal infection.

tial diagnoses include pasteurellosis, Tyzzer's disease, and listeriosis.

SIGNIFICANCE. Enzootics of neonatal staphylococcal infections may cause a high mortality rate in affected litters. With suppurative respiratory or genital tract lesions, or with abscessation suspected to be due to a virulent strain of *S. aureus,* bacterial culture is essential in order to differentiate the disease from other likely causative agents, such as *P. multocida.* In view of the widespread distribution of staphylococci in laboratory animals, characterization of the isolate is necessary in order to determine whether it is a potentially pathogenic strain. The possibility of human carriers warrants consideration.

PODODERMATITIS. Pododermatitis ("sore hocks") has been associated with staphylococcal infections. It may occur in association with staph abscesses or mastitis. The cellulitis and dermatitis present in pododermatitis is usually concentrated along the ventral hock region. For additional information, see Ulcerative Dermatitis ("Sore Hocks").

***Treponema paraluiscuniculi* (*cuniculi*) Infection: Venereal Spirochetosis.** The disease has several synonyms, including "vent disease" and "rabbit syphilis." The causative agent, *T. paraluiscuniculi* (formerly *T. cuniculi),* is a spirochete that has not been successfully grown in artificial media or cell culture. Based on serological surveys, treponematosis occurs occasionally in conventional facilities. However, the disease is seldom detected on cursory examination.

EPIZOOTIOLOGY AND PATHOGENESIS. The venereal route is the most important means of spread, although extragenital contact transmission may also occur. Young animals may develop the disease following contact with an infected dam. However, there is a demonstrated age-related susceptibility. Young rabbits have been shown to be relatively resistant to the infection, either by natural exposure or experimental inoculation. There is no evidence of intrauterine transmission. There appears to be a strain-related resistance/susceptibility to clinical disease postexposure. Treponematosis has also been diagnosed in wild rabbits in Britain.

PATHOLOGY. Lesions associated with treponematosis may occur in the vulva, prepuce, anal region, muzzle, and periorbital region. Initially, changes are characterized by edema, erythema, and papules at the mucocutaneous junctions. Syphilitic lesions later progress to ulceration and crusting. On microscopic examination, hyperplasia of the epidermis, necrosis of epithelial cells, and erosions and ulcerations, with infiltration by plasma cells, macrophages, and heterophils, are typical changes (Fig. 6.39). The infection is confined primarily to the epithelium, and other than hyperplasia of the regional lymph nodes, visceral involvement does not normally occur.

DIAGNOSIS. Scrapings from lesions, with wet mount preparation and *dark-field examination,* is the recommended method for confirming the diagnosis. Treponema spirochetes are recognized by their characteristic spiral shape and corkscrew movement. Demonstration of the spirochetes by silver staining of lesions in histology sections may be used (Fig. 6.40), but this is not as reliable as dark-field examination. *Serology* is a reliable diagnostic procedure. Tests available include the demonstration of reagin antibody (Wasserman antibody) and the fluorescent treponemal antigen test. Rabbits may seroconvert while still infected with the organism. *Differential diagnoses* include *Pasteurella* infections of the external genitalia and traumatic lesions.

SIGNIFICANCE. Treponematosis is considered to be a self-limiting disease. However, there appears to be increased susceptibility to other infectious

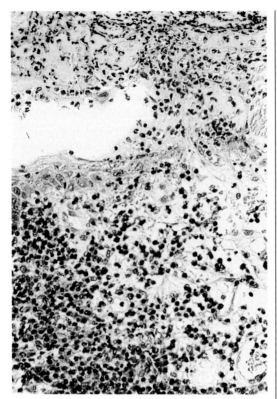

FIG. 6.39—Section of skin from the muzzle of laboratory rabbit with spontaneous treponematosis (rabbit syphilis). There is ulceration of the mucosa with leukocytic infiltration.

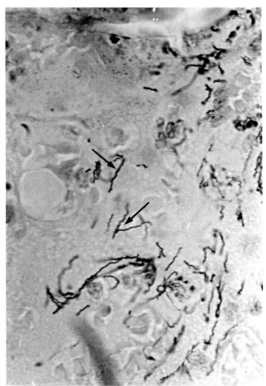

FIG. 6.40—Section from the lesion in Figure 6.39 (Warthin-Starry stain), illustrating the typical spirochetes (*arrows*) associated with the lesions.

agents in rabbits actively infected with *T. paraluiscuniculi.* The effect of treponematosis on fertility rates in rabbits has not been determined.

***Yersinia* Infection: Yersiniosis.** This disease is characterized by an acute to chronic infection in wild rodents and lagomorphs and in human patients. The bacterium, *Y. pseudotuberculosis,* is usually transmitted by the ingestion of contaminated food or water. Lesions are characterized by focal caseation necrosis of liver, spleen, cecum, and occasionally lymph nodes and reproductive tract. Although occasionally yersiniosis occurs in the wildlife population, it rarely occurs in domestic species.

MISCELLANEOUS BACTERIAL DISEASES. Mastitis occurs occasionally in recently kindled and heavily lactating does. The skin overlying the swollen, firm mammary gland(s) has a red to dark blue discoloration. On section, the gland may contain material varying from a fluid consistency to thick purulent exudate. Staphylococci, pasteurellae, or streptococci are the usual pathogens associated with mastitis in this species.

In **necrobacillosis ("Schmorl's disease"),** dermatitis can occur in does with large dewlaps subjected to excessive moisture due to salivation. Other predisposing factors include panting associated with high environmental temperatures, as well as malocclusion. The inflammatory process in the subcutaneous tissue may progress to suppuration with ulceration of the overlying skin. The most common bacterial agent associated with this syndrome is *Fusobacterium necrophorum.*

Streptococcal septicemia has been reported to occur in young rabbits. **Acute diplococcal infections** have been observed on rare occasions in domestic rabbits. In isolated cases, ***Klebsiella***

pneumonia has been associated with acute hemorrhagic bronchopneumonia in domestic rabbits. Suppurative and ulcerative skin lesions have been associated with various infections, including *Corynebacterium pyogenes*. For additional information on uncommon bacterial infections, see DeLong and Manning (1994).

BIBLIOGRAPHY
FOR BACTERIAL INFECTIONS

Respiratory Bacterial Infections

Pasteurella Infection

Al-Lebban, Z.S., et al. 1988. Rabbit pasteurellosis: Induced disease and vaccination. Am. J. Vet. Res. 49:312–16.

Chengappa, M.M., et al. 1980. A streptomycin-dependent live *Pasteurella multocida* vaccine for the prevention of rabbit pasteurellosis. Lab. Anim. Sci. 30:515–18.

Corbeil, L.B., et al. 1983. Immunity to pasteurellosis in compromised rabbits. Am. J. Vet. Res. 44:845–50.

Deeb, B.J., et al. 1990. *Pasteurella multocida* and *Bordetella bronchiseptica* infection in rabbits. J. Clin. Microbiol. 28:70–75.

DeLong, D., and Manning, P.J. 1994. Bacterial diseases. In *The Biology of the Laboratory Rabbit,* ed. P.J. Manning et al., pp. 131–70. New York: Academic.

Dhillon, A.S., and Andrews, D.K. 1982. Abortions, stillbirths, and infant mortality in a commercial rabbitry. J. Appl. Rabbit Res. 5:97–98.

DiGiacomo, R.F., et al. 1989. Atrophic rhinitis in New Zealand rabbits. Lab. Anim. Sci. 37:533.

———. 1987. Transmission of *Pasteurella multocida* in rabbits. Lab. Anim. Sci. 37:621–23.

———. 1983. Natural history of infection with *Pasteurella multocida* in rabbits. J. Am. Vet. Med. Assoc. 183:1172–75.

Flatt, R.E., et al. 1977. Suppurative otitis media in the rabbit: Prevalence, pathology and microbiology. Lab. Anim. Sci. 27:343–46.

Glass, L.S., and Beasley, J.N. 1990. Infection with and antibody response to *Pasteurella multocida* and *Bordetella bronchiseptica* in immature rabbits. Lab. Anim. Sci. 39:406–10.

Glorioso, J.C., et al. 1982. Adhesion of type A *Pasteurella multocida* to rabbit pharyngeal cells and its possible role in rabbit respiratory tract infections. Infect. Immun. 35:1103–9.

Holmes, H.T., et al. 1983a. The incidence of vaginal and nasal *Pasteurella multocida* in a commercial rabbitry. J. Appl. Rabbit Res. 6:95–96.

———. 1983b. Pasteurella contaminated water valves: Its incidence and implications. J. Appl. Rabbit Res. 6:123–24.

Lu, Y-S., and Pakes, S.P. 1981. Protection of rabbits against experimental pasteurellosis by a streptomycin-dependent *Pasteurella multocida* serotype 3A live mutant vaccine. Infect. Immun. 34:1018–24.

Mahler, M., et al. 1994. Inefficiency of enrofloxacin in the elimination of *Pasteurella multocida* in rabbits. Lab. Anim. 29:192–99.

Manning, P.J., et al. 1987. A dot-immunobinding assay for the serodiagnosis of *Pasteurella multocida* infection in laboratory rabbits. Lab. Anim. Sci. 37:615–20.

Nielsen, J.P. 1989. Personal communication. National Veterinary Laboratory, Copenhagen, Denmark.

Percy, D.H., et al. 1988. Incidence of *Pasteurella* and *Bordetella* infections in fryer rabbits: An abattoir survey. J. Appl. Rabbit Res. 11:245–46.

———. 1984. Characterization of *Pasteurella* isolated from rabbits in Canada. Can. J. Comp. Med. 48:36–41.

Scharf, R.A., et al. 1981. A modified barrier system for the maintenance of *Pasteurella*-free rabbits. Lab. Anim. Sci. 31:513–15.

Watson, W.T., et al. 1975. Experimental respiratory infections with *Pasteurella multocida* and *Bordetella bronchiseptica* in rabbits. Lab. Anim. Sci. 25:459–64.

Webster, L.T. 1925. Epidemiological studies on respiratory infections of the rabbit. Pneumonia associated with *Bacterium leptisepticum*. J. Exp. Med. 43:555–72.

Zaoutis, T.E., et al. 1991. Screening rabbit colonies for antibodies to *Pasteurella multocida* by an ELISA. Lab. Anim. Sci. 41:419–22.

Bordetella bronchiseptica Infection

Bemis, D.A., and Wilson, S.A. 1985. Influence of potential virulence determinants on *Bordetella bronchiseptica*–induced ciliostasis. Infect. Immun. 50:35–42.

Feinstein, R.E., and Rehbinder, C. 1988. Health monitoring of purpose bred laboratory rabbits in Sweden: Major findings. Scand. J. Lab. Anim. Sci. 15:49–67.

Matsuyama, T., and Taking, T. 1980. Scanning electron microscopic studies of *Bordetella bronchiseptica* on the rabbit tracheal mucosa. J. Med. Microbiol. 13:159–61.

Percy, D.H., et al. 1988. Incidence of *Pasteurella* and *Bordetella* infections in fryer rabbits: An abattoir survey. J. Appl. Rabbit Res. 11:245–46.

Watson, W.T., et al. 1975. Experimental respiratory infections with *Pasteurella multocida* and *Bordetella bronchiseptica* in rabbits. Lab. Anim. Sci. 25:459–64.

CAR Bacillus Infection

Cundiff, D.D., et al. 1995. Characterization of cilia-associated respiratory bacillus in rabbits and analysis of the 16s rRNA gene sequence. Lab. Anim. Sci. 45:22–26.

Kurisu, K., et al. 1990. Cilia-associated respiratory bacillus infection in rabbits. Lab. Anim. Sci. 40:413–15.

Bacterial Infections of the Enteritis Complex in Rabbits

Clostridial Enteropathies/Enterotoxemia

Butt, M.T., et al. 1994. A cytotoxicity assay for *Clostridium spiroforme* enterotoxin in cecal fluid of rabbits. Lab. Anim. Sci. 44:52–54.

Carman, R.J., and Borriello, S.P. 1984. Infectious nature of *Clostridium spiroforme*–mediated rabbit enterotoxaemia. Vet. Microbiol. 9:497–502.

Carman, R.J., and Evans, R.H. 1984. Experimental and spontaneous clostridial enteropathies of laboratory and free living lagomorphs. Lab. Anim. Sci. 34:443–52.

Cheeke, P.R., and Patton, N.M. 1978. Effect of alfalfa and dietary fiber on the growth performance of weanling rabbits. Lab. Anim. Sci. 28:167–72.

Holmes, H.T., et al. 1988. Isolation of *Clostridium spiroforme* from rabbits. Lab. Anim. Sci. 39:167–68.

Patton, N.M., et al. 1978. Enterotoxemia in rabbits. Lab. Anim. Sci. 28:536–40.

Peeters, J.E., et al. 1986. Significance of *Clostridium spiroforme* in the enteritis-complex of commercial rabbits. Vet. Microbiol. 12:25–31.

Perkins, S.E., et al. 1995. Detection of *Clostridium difficile* toxins from small intestine and cecum of rabbits with naturally acquired enterotoxemia. Lab. Anim. Sci. 45:379–85.

Rehg, J.E., and Lu, Y-S. 1981. *Clostridium difficile* colitis in a rabbit following antibiotic therapy for pasteurellosis. J. Am. Vet. Med. Assoc. 179:1296–97.

Rehg, J.E., and Pakes, S.P. 1982. Implication of *Clostridium difficile* and *Clostridium perfringens* iota toxins in experimental lincomycin-associated colitis of rabbits. Lab. Anim. Sci. 32:253–57.

Clostridium piliforme Infection: Tyzzer's Disease

Allen, A.M., et al. 1965. Tyzzer's disease syndrome in laboratory rabbits. Am. J. Pathol. 46:859–82.

Cutlip, R.C., et al. 1971. An epizootic of Tyzzer's disease in rabbits. Lab. Anim. Sci. 21:356–61.

Duncan, A.J. 1993. Assignment of the agent of Tyzzer's disease to *Clostridium piliforme* comb. nov. on the basis of 16S rRNA sequence analysis. J. Syst. Bacteriol. 43:314–18.

Fries, A.S. 1977. Studies on Tyzzer's disease: Application of immunofluorescence for detection of *Bacillus piliformis* and for demonstration and determination of antibodies to it in sera from mice and rabbits. Lab. Anim. 11:69–73.

Fujiwara, K. 1978. Tyzzer's disease. Jap. J. Exp. Med. 48:467–80.

Fujiwara, K., et al. 1985. Antigenic relatedness of Tyzzer's disease occurring in Japan and other regions. Jap. J. Vet. Sci. 47:9–16.

Ganaway, J.R., et al. 1976. Tyzzer's disease in free-living cottontail rabbits (*Sylvilagus floridanus*) in Maryland. J. Wildl. Dis. 12:545–49.

———. 1971. Tyzzer's disease. Am. J. Pathol. 64:717–32.

Kovatch, R.M., and Zebarth, G. 1973. Naturally occurring Tyzzer's disease in a cat. J. Am. Vet. Med. Assoc. 162:136–38.

Peeters, J.E., et al. 1985. Naturally-occurring Tyzzer's disease (*Bacillus piliformis* infection) in commercial rabbits: A clinical and pathological study. Ann. Rech. Vet. 16:69–79.

Pulley, L.T., and Shively, J.N. 1974. Tyzzer's disease in a foal. Light and electron-microscopic observation. Vet. Pathol. 11:203–11.

Quereshi, S.R., et al. 1976. Tyzzer's disease in a dog. J. Am. Vet. Med. Assoc. 168:602–4.

Spencer, T.H., et al. 1990. Cultivation of *Bacillus piliformis* (Tyzzer) in mouse fibroblasts (3T3) cells. Vet. Microbiol. 29:291–97.

Tyzzer, E.E. 1917. A fatal disease of the Japanese waltzing mouse caused by a spore-bearing bacillus (*B. piliformis* n.sp.). J. Med. Res. 37:307–38.

Waggie, K.S., et al. 1987. Lesions of experimentally induced Tyzzer's disease in Syrian hamsters, guinea pigs, mice, and rats. Lab. Anim. 21:155–60.

Webb, D.M., et al. 1987. *Bacillus piliformis* infection (Tyzzer's disease) in a calf. J. Am. Vet. Med. Assoc. 191:431–34.

Coliform Enteritis

Blanco, J.E., et al. 1994. Serotypes, toxins and antibiotic resistance of *Escherichia coli* strains isolated from diarrheic and healthy rabbits in Spain. Vet. Microbiol. 38:193–201.

Moon, H.W., et al. 1983. Attaching and effacing of rabbit and human enteropathogenic *Escherichia coli* in pig and rabbit intestines. Infect. Immun. 41:1340–51.

Peeters, J.E., et al. 1988a. A selective citrate-sorbose medium for screening certain enteropathogenic attaching and effacing *Escherichia coli* in weaned rabbits. Tijdschrift Diergeneesk. 57:264–70.

———. 1988b. Biotype, serotype, and pathogenicity of attaching and effacing enteropathogenic *Escherichia coli* strains isolated from diarrheic commercial rabbits. Infect. Immun. 56:1442–48.

———. 1985. Scanning and transmission electron microscopy of attaching effacing *Escherichia coli* in weanling rabbits. Vet. Pathol. 22:54–59.

———. 1984a. Experimental *Escherichia coli* enteropathy in weanling rabbits: Clinical manifestations and pathological findings. J. Comp. Pathol. 94:521–28.

———. 1984b. Pathogenic properties of *Escherichia coli* strains isolated from diarrheic commercial rabbits. J. Clin. Microbiol. 20:34–39.

Prescott, J.F. 1978. *Escherichia coli* and diarrhea in the rabbit. Vet. Pathol. 15:237–48.

Prohaszka, L., and Baron, F. 1981. Studies on *E. coli*-enteropathy in weanling rabbits. Zbl. Vet. Med. B. 102–10.

Robins-Browne, R.M., et al. 1994. Adherence characteristics of attaching and effacing strains of *Escherichia coli* from rabbits. Infect. Immun. 62: 1584–92.

Schauer, D.B., et al. 1998. Proliferative enterocolitis associated with dual infection with enteropathogenic *Escherichia coli* and *Lawsonia intracellularis* in rabbits. J. Clin. Microbiol. 36:1700-1703

Smith, H.W. 1965. Observations on the flora of the alimentary tract of animals and factors affecting its composition. J. Pathol. Bacteriol. 89:95–122.

Thouless, M.E., et al. 1996. The effect of combined rotavirus and *Escherichia coli* infections in rabbits. Lab. Anim. Sci. 46:381–85.

Lawsonia Infection

Cooper, D.M., and Gebhart, C.J. 1998. Comparative aspects of proliferative enteritis. J. Am. Vet. Med. Assoc. 212:1446–51.

Duhamel, G.E., et al. 1998. Subclinical proliferative enteropathy in sentinel rabbits associated with *Lawsonia intracellularis*. Vet. Pathol. 35:300–303.

Hotchkiss, C.E., et al. 1996. Proliferative enteropathy of rabbits: The intracellular *Campylobacter*–like organism is closely related to *Lawsonia intracellularis*. Lab. Anim. Sci. 46:623–27.

McCathey, S., et al. 1996. Proliferative enterocolitis associated with a dual infection of *Lawsonia intracellularis* and an attaching and effacing *Escherichia coli* in a colony of New Zealand White rabbits. Lab. Anim. Sci. 46:461.

Schauer, D.B., et al. 1998. Proliferative enterocolitis associated with dual infection with enteropathogenic *Escherichia coli* and *Lawsonia intracellularis* in rabbits. J. Clin. Microbiol. 36:1700–1703

Schoeb, T.R., and Fox, J.G. 1990. Enterocolitis associated with intraepithelial *Campylobacter*-like bacteria in rabbits (*Oryctolagus cuniculus*). Vet. Pathol. 27:73–80.

Umemura, T., et al. 1982. Histiocytic enteritis of rabbits. Vet. Pathol. 19:326–29.

Salmonella Infection

Newcomer, C.E., et al. 1983. The laboratory rabbit as reservoirs of *Salmonella mbandaka*. J. Infect. Dis. 147:365.

Vibrio Infection

Moon, H.W., et al. 1974. Intraepithelial vibrio associated with acute typhlitis of young rabbits. Vet. Pathol. 11:313–26.

Mucoid Enteropathy

Hotchkiss, C. E., and Merritt, A.M. 1996a. Evaluation of cecal ligation as a model of mucoid enteropathy in specific-pathogen-free rabbits. Lab. Anim. Sci. 46:174–78.

———. 1996b. Mucus secretagogue activity in cecal contents of rabbits with mucoid enteropathy. Lab. Anim. Sci. 46:179–86.

Itagaki, S., et al. 1999. Lectin histochemical changes of the colon goblet cell mucin in rabbit mucoid enteropathy. Lab. Anim. Sci. 44:82–84.

Lelkes, L., and Chang, C-L. 1987. Microbial dysbiosis in rabbit mucoid enteropathy. Lab. Anim. Sci. 37:757–64.

McLeod, C.G., and Katz, W. 1986. Toxic components in commercial rabbit feeds and their role in mucoid enteritis. S. Afr. J. Sci. 82:375–79.

Toofanian, F., and Hamar, D.W. 1986. Cecal short-chain fatty acids in experimental rabbit mucoid enteropathy. Am. J. Vet. Res. 47:2423–25.

Toofanian, F., and Targowski, S. 1983. Experimental production of rabbit mucoid enteritis. Am. J. Vet. Res. 44:705–8.

van Kruiningen, H.J., and Williams, C.B. 1972. Mucoid enteritis in rabbits: Comparison to cholera and cystic fibrosis. Vet. Pathol. 9:53–77.

Other Bacterial Diseases

Listeria Infection

Gray, M.L., and Killinger, A.H. 1966. *Listeria monocytogenes* and listeriosis. Bacteriol. Rev. 30:309–82.

Murray, E.G.D., et al. 1926. A disease of rabbits characterized by a large mononuclear leucocytosis caused by a hitherto undescribed bacillus *Bacterium monocytogenes* (n. sp.). J. Pathol. Bacteriol. 40:407–39.

Vetesi, F., and Kemenes, F. 1967. Studies on listeriosis in pregnant rabbits. Acta Vet. Acad. Sci. Hung. 17:27–38.

Watson, G.L., and Evans, M.G. 1985. Listeriosis in a rabbit. Vet. Pathol. 22:191–93.

Staphylococcal Infections

Devries, L.A., et al. 1996. A new pathogenic *Staphylococcus aureus* type in commercial rabbits. Zentralbl. Vet. Med. B 43:313–15.

Hagen, K.W. 1963. Disseminated staphylococcal infection in young domestic rabbits. J. Am. Med. Assoc. 142:1421–22.

Okerman, L., et al. 1984. Cutaneous staphylococcosis in rabbits. Vet. Rec. 114:313–15.

Osebald, J.W., and Gray, D.M. 1960. Disseminated staphylococcal infection in wild jack rabbits. J. Infect. Dis. 106:91–94.

Renquist, D., and Soave, O. 1969. Staphylococcal pneumonia in a laboratory rabbit: An epidemiological follow-up study. J. Am. Med. Assoc. 155:1221–23.

Snyder, S.B., et al. 1976. Disseminated staphylococcal disease in the laboratory rabbit (*Oryctolagus cuniculus*). Lab. Anim. Sci. 26:86–88.

Treponema paraluiscuniculi (*cuniculi*) Infection: Venereal Spirochetosis

Cunliffe-Beamer, T.L., and Fox, R.R. 1981a. Venereal spirochaetosis of rabbits: Description and diagnosis. Lab. Anim. Sci. 31:366B71.

———. 1981b. Venereal spirochaetosis of rabbits: Epizootiology. Lab. Anim. Sci. 31:372–78.

DeLong, D., and Manning, P.J. 1994. Bacterial diseases. In *The Biology of the Laboratory Rabbit*, ed. P.J. Manning et al., pp. 131–70. New York: Academic.

Umemoto, T., et al. 1996. Immunological studies on venereal spirochetosis of rabbits (rabbit syphilis). J. Vet. Med. B. 43:267–76.

Yersiniosis, Bacterial Mastitis, and Other Bacterial Diseases

DeLong, D., and Manning, P.J. 1994. Bacterial diseases. In *The Biology of the Laboratory Rabbit,* ed. P.J. Manning et al., pp. 131–70. New York: Academic.

General Bibliography

DeLong, D., and Manning, P.J. 1994. Bacterial diseases. In *The Biology of the Laboratory Rabbit,* ed. P.J. Manning et al., pp. 131–70. New York: Academic.

Harkness, J.E., and Wagner, J.E. 1995. *The Biology and Medicine of Rabbits and Rodents.* Philadelphia: Lea and Febiger.

MYCOTIC INFECTIONS

Dermatophytosis ("Ringworm"). Clinical cases of dermatophytosis are uncommon in domestic lagomorphs. When present, lesions are usually located around the head and ears, sometimes with secondary spread to the paws. Affected areas are typically raised, circumscribed, and erythematous, with crusted surface and hair loss (Fig. 6.41). *Trichophyton mentagrophytes* is most frequently involved, but *Microsporum canis* infections have also been recognized in rabbits. Microscopic examination of skin scrapings from the periphery of lesions cleared in 10% KOH should reveal the typical arthrospores. Examination of tissue sections for the characteristic fungi and culture on the appropriate media

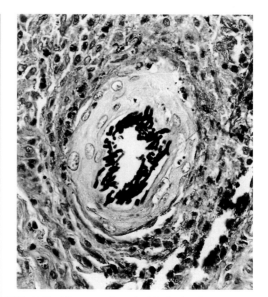

FIG. 6.42—Dermatophytosis. Typical arthrospores investing hair follicle in rabbit (PAS stain).

are both useful diagnostic procedures in confirming the diagnosis. On histopathology, characteristic changes include hyperkeratosis, epidermal hyperplasia, and folliculitis, with mononuclear and polymorphonuclear cell infiltration. Stains such as the methenamine silver and PAS-staining procedures are used to best demonstrate the typical arthrospores investing infected hair shafts (Fig. 6.42). *Differential diagnoses* include idiopathic "molt," hair loss in does during nest building, and "barbering" seen occasionally in group-housed juvenile rabbits.

SIGNIFICANCE. The diagnosis of dermatophytosis requires a thorough investigation to determine the possible sources of the infection. The disease is readily transmitted to susceptible human contacts; thus careful screening, culling, and slaughter are recommended. If animals are to be treated, oral griseofulvin has been used with some success, but it is potentially teratogenic in pregnant does. Rabbits may occasionally harbor pathogenic dermatophytes as an inapparent infection.

Aspergillus **Infection.** Pulmonary granulomas are occasionally encountered in rabbits at necropsy. They consist of circumscribed inflam-

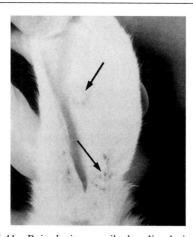

FIG. 6.41—Raised, circumscribed scaling lesions with reddened periphery (*arrows*) in a spontaneous case of dermatophytosis due to *Trichophyton mentagrophytes* infection.

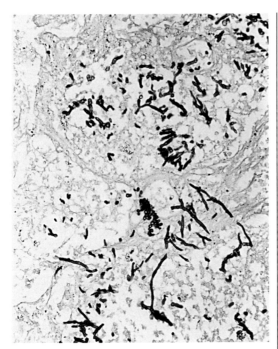

FIG. 6.43—Section of granuloma from lung of domestic rabbit (PAS stain), illustrating hyphae associated with focal pulmonary aspergillosis.

matory lesions with a central area of coagulation necrosis with mononuclear inflammatory cell response. Typical septate hyphae are evident, particularly with PAS or methenamine silver stains (Fig. 6.43). Pulmonary aspergillosis usually affects young rabbits, with elimination of the fungus as rabbits age, leaving pulmonary scars.

BIBLIOGRAPHY
FOR MYCOTIC INFECTIONS

Banks, K.L., and Clarkson, T.B. 1967. Naturally occurring dermatomycosis in the rabbit. J. Am. Med. Assoc. 151:926–29.
Hagen, K.W. 1969. Ringworm in domestic rabbits: Oral treatment with griseofulvin. Lab. Anim. Care 19:635–38.
Vogtsberger, L.M., et al. 1986. Spontaneous dermatomycosis due to *Microsporum canis* in rabbits. Lab. Anim. Sci. 36:294–97.

PARASITIC DISEASES

Protozoal Infections

INTESTINAL COCCIDIOSIS. Coccidiosis is a widespread, major disease problem in commer-cial rabbitries and in research facilities. Of the species of *Eimeria* associated with intestinal coccidiosis in the rabbit, *E. intestinalis* and *E. flavescens* are considered the most pathogenic; *E. magna, E. irresidua,* and *E. piriformis* moderately pathogenic; and *E. perforans, E. neoleporis,* and *E. media* the least pathogenic. In one survey in England, *E. magna, E. media,* and *E. perforans* were most frequently identified. Over 65% of the animals tested were carrying two to four species of *Eimeria.* In one study of experimental coccidiosis, 5-wk-old coccidia-free rabbits were inoculated with *E. intestinalis,* a relatively pathogenic species. Rabbits inoculated with 100 oocysts or less were asymptomatic. In animals receiving 10,000 or more sporulated oocysts, the mortality rate was around 50%. Hemodilution, hypokalemia, and a marked rise in *E. coli* bacterial counts occurred during the course of the disease. Enterocyte destruction and villous blunting were evident at 7–10 d postinoculation, with repair in survivors evident by 2 wk postinoculation.

LIFE CYCLE. Following passage in the feces, oocysts require 1 or more days to sporulate at room temperature before they are infective. When ingested, sporulated oocysts (sporocysts) release sporozoites, which invade enterocytes and multiply by schizogony. In rabbits inoculated with sporocysts directly into the duodenum, excystation and the invasion of enterocytes occurs as early as 10 min postinoculation. Sporozoites appear in the mucosa of the ileum within 6 hr, suggesting systemic rather than intraluminal migration. Depending on the species of *Eimeria,* one or more asexual cycles occur, followed by gametogony and oocyst passage in the feces. The prepatent period is from 5 to 12 d, depending on the species. There may be a phenomenal number of progeny from a single ingested oocyst. One oocyst of *E. magna* may produce over 25,000,000 oocysts in a susceptible host.

EPIZOOTIOLOGY AND PATHOGENESIS. Rabbits most frequently develop clinical disease during the postweaning period. The most damaging stage in the life cycle is the sexual cycle, where there may be extensive destruction of enterocytes and cells in the lamina propria in affected sections of the gut. Because oocysts require sporulation at room temperature before they are infective, reingestion of the "night feces" (cecotrophy) does not appear to play a role in the dissemination of the disease. In well-managed operations where coccidiostats are not used, control is dependent on rigorous sanitation practices. Exposure to relatively small numbers of oocysts should result in a subclinical infection, with appropriate immune response. However, immunity to one species of *Eimeria* is unlikely to provide good protection against other species. In many commercial operations, the feed is routinely medicated with anticoccidials to control the disease. However, this should not be considered an acceptable substitute for rigid sanitation practices.

PATHOLOGY. At necropsy, the perineal region and belly are frequently smeared with watery dark green to brown feces. The animal may be thin and dehydrated, depending on the duration of the disease. The cecum and colon contain dark green to brown watery, foul-smelling material. The mucosa of affected areas of the gut is congested and edematous, occasionally with hemorrhagic areas.

The location of microscopic changes varies with the species of *Eimeria* involved, but they are normally concentrated in the caudal half of the small intestine and in the cecum. In acute coccidiosis, there is destruction of enterocytes, villous atrophy in affected areas of small intestine, and marked leukocytic infiltration, heterophils predominating. Gametocytes and oocysts are usually evident in the intestinal mucosa in affected areas (Fig. 6.44).

DIAGNOSIS. Fecal flotations, mucosal scrapings, and microscopic examination for oocysts are standard diagnostic procedures. An approximate oocyst count and oocyst speciations are recommended, particularly in view of the recognized variation in pathogenicity among species of *Eimeria*. In acute cases of coccidiosis, oocysts may not be present in the feces but will be evident in sections of the appropriate areas of small and large intestine. Bacteriology cultures are essential, since there frequently is a significant rise in the bacterial count, especially coliforms. These bacteria may play an important role as opportunistic infections in clinical outbreaks of coc-

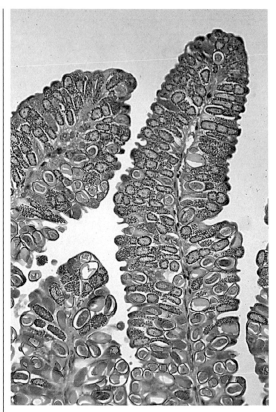

FIG. 6.44—Section of small intestine of juvenile rabbit with severe intestinal coccidiosis. Enterocytes are distorted due to massive numbers of micro- and macrogametocytes and oocysts.

cidiosis. *Differential diagnoses* include coliform enteritis, Tyzzer's disease, clostridial enteropathies, viral enteritides, and mucoid enteropathy.

SIGNIFICANCE. Coccidiosis is an important cause of clinical (or subclinical) disease in domestic rabbits, frequently causing weight loss and mortality. Events such as changes in management practices, feed changes, and experimental procedures may be sufficient to precipitate a clinical outbreak of the disease.

Hepatic Coccidiosis

EPIZOOTIOLOGY AND PATHOGENESIS. *Eimeria stiedae* infections occur in both domestic and wild rabbits and represent an important cause of poor weight gains, disease, and mortality in commercial rabbitries. Following the ingestion of sporulated oocysts (sporocysts), sporozoites invade the duodenal mucosa and migrate to the lamina propria prior to systemic migration. Sporozoites have been demonstrated in the regional mesenteric lymph nodes within 12 hr postexposure and in the liver by 48 hr. Organisms have been reported to migrate to the liver in mononuclear cells via lymphatics. However, viable sporozoites have also been demonstrated in the peripheral blood and bone marrow in *E. stiedae*–inoculated rabbits, and the hematogenous route has been proposed as means of migration to the liver. After migration, sporozoites invade the epithelial cells of the bile ducts and schizogony begins. Following the gametogeny, oocysts are formed, released into the bile ducts, and passed to the intestine. The prepatent period is approximately 15–18 d. Oocysts may be shed in the feces for up to 7 or more weeks postexposure. Oocysts are normally resistant to environmental change; thus contaminated premises and fomites may be a source of infective sporulated oocysts for several months. *E. stiedae* infestations may be manifest either as clinical or subclinical disease.

Weanling rabbits are most often affected. Frequently a significant number of livers collected from fryer rabbits in abattoirs are condemned because of hepatic coccidiosis. A dose-related effect has been observed in experimentally infected animals. In young rabbits inoculated orally with varying numbers of sporocysts (100 to 100,000 per animal), mortality rates in animals that received either 10,000 or 100,000 sporocysts were 40% or 80%, respectively. No fatalities occurred at lower dosages. Significant variations in liver enzymes and blood chemistry have been observed during the course of the disease. Four stages have been proposed: (1) the initial stage of metabolic dysfunction that coincides with hepatocyte damage during schizogony; (2) the cholestatic stage, with elevated transaminases and serum bilirubin; (3) the stage of metabolic dysfunction, characterized by hypoglycemia and hypoproteinemia; and (4) the period of immunodepression in heavily infected animals resulting in an inability to curtail the production of oocysts in the biliary system.

PATHOLOGY. At necropsy, affected animals are frequently thin and potbellied and lack body fat

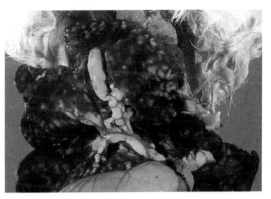

FIG. 6.45—Liver from juvenile rabbit with florid hepatic coccidiosis. In addition to the raised linear hepatic lesions, note the marked dilation and thickening of the gall bladder and common bile duct.

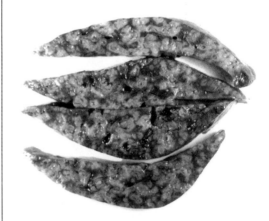

FIG. 6.46—Cut surface of liver from a case of hepatic coccidiosis (*Eimeria stiedae*). Bile ducts are dilated and filled with inspissated material.

reserves. There may be dark brown to green soiling in the perineal region. Ascites is a variable finding. Depending on the degree of liver involvement, there may be hepatomegaly and in severe cases icterus. In the liver, there are variable numbers of raised, linear bosselated, yellow to pearl gray circumscribed lesions 0.5–2 cm in diameter scattered throughout the parenchyma of the liver. The gallbladder is thickened and contains viscid green bile and debris (Fig. 6.45). On cut surface, lesions contain fluid green to inspissated, dark green to tan material (Fig. 6.46).

Microscopically, there is marked dilation of bile ducts, extensive periportal fibrosis, and mixed inflammatory cell infiltration in the periportal regions. In affected bile ducts, there is hyperplasia of epithelium, with papillary projections lined by reactive epithelial cells overlying collagenous tissue stroma. Infiltrating periductal inflammatory cells include lymphocytes, macrophages, and a sprinkling of polymorphs. Large numbers of gametocytes and oocysts are usually present in parasitized ducts (Fig. 6.47). In lesions of some duration, organisms may be sparse to absent in bile ducts, with prominent periportal fibrosis.

DIAGNOSIS. The diagnosis may be confirmed at necropsy by wet mount preparations. Oocysts are usually readily observed in aspirates from the gallbladder or in impression smears of sectioned

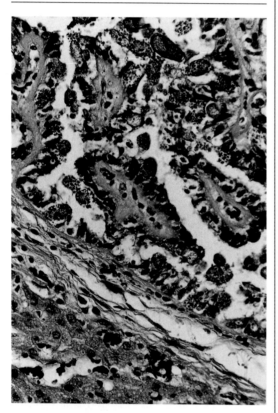

FIG. 6.47—Histological section, illustrating hepatic coccidiosis. There is a proliferative cholangitis with periportal fibrosis. Gametocytes and oocysts are present in bile duct epithelium and in the lumen of dilated ducts.

lesions. The characteristic proliferative biliary changes and organisms seen histologically are pathognomonic of the disease.

SIGNIFICANCE. Aside from clinical disease and mortality associated with hepatic coccidiosis, growth rates may be compromised significantly in affected rabbits. The changes in serum chemistry seen during the acute and convalescent stages of the disease indicate that significant metabolic aberrations do occur. There is some evidence that there may be an impaired immune response in rabbits heavily infected with *E. stiedae*. Improved sanitation is a major consideration in the effective control of the disease.

ENCEPHALITOZOON INFECTION: ENCEPHALITOZOONOSIS (NOSEMATOSIS). *E. cuniculi* is an obligate intracellular microsporidian parasite that affects a variety of mammalian hosts, most commonly the domestic rabbit. The organism is characterized by the presence of a coiled polar filament in the mature spore stage. Taxonomists have disagreed on the appropriate classification for the organism. When viewed by electron microscopy, the characteristic diplokarya seen during the developmental cycle in protozoa of the *Nosema* genus were absent, thus the designation to the genus *Encephalitozoon*. Following the extrusion of the sporoplasm from the spore coat, the sporoplasm may then invade a susceptible host cell. Penetration may be due to the mechanical forces exerted by the extruded polar filament or due to an active migratory process by the sporoplasm. Following entry into the cell, multiplication occurs in association with a cytoplasmic vacuole. Sporoblasts develop into mature spores, and finally the cell ruptures, releasing organisms that can then repeat the cycle.

EPIZOOTIOLOGY AND PATHOGENESIS. "Infectious motor paralysis" attributed to a protozoan parasite was first reported in laboratory rabbits by Wright and Craighead in 1922. The incidence of seropositive animals in some conventional rabbitries may be relatively high, and in the past, seroconversion has been detected in specific-pathogen-free rabbits. In one survey in Australia, approximately 25% of wild rabbits tested were seropositive for *E. cuniculi*. The organism has a wide host range. Susceptible species include the mouse, guinea pig, squirrel, monkey, cat, and dog. Encephalitozoonosis appears to be a more severe disease in species such as dogs and monkeys. In the large domestic rabbit, the disease is usually a subclinical infection, and renal lesions are frequently detected as an incidental finding. In surveys in the past, incidence of renal lesions attributed to *E. cuniculi* varied from approximately 5% to over 25%. Occasionally nervous signs, with mortality, occur in young New Zealand White rabbits with heavy infections. Dwarf rabbits appear to be especially susceptible to encephalitozoonosis, with clinical signs. Torticollis, other neurological manifestations, and renal lesions have been observed in infected pet dwarf rabbits.

PATHOGENESIS. The usual source of the infection is spores shed in the urine from rabbits actively infected with the disease. Transplacental infection has been reported to occur, although there is disagreement on this issue. Rabbits are readily infected experimentally by the oral or respiratory route, and invasion by inhalation has been identified as a possible portal of entry under field conditions. Following ingestion/oral inoculation, the spores appear to pass via infected mononuclear cells into the systemic circulation. Initially, target organs are those of high blood flow, such as lung, liver, and kidney. In rabbits inoculated orally with *E. cuniculi* and examined at 31 d postinoculation (pi), moderate to marked lesions were demonstrated primarily in the lung, liver, and kidney, and occasionally in the myocardium. No lesions were present in the central nervous system at 1 mo pi. At 3 mo pi, moderate to severe lesions were evident histologically in the kidney, and changes were minimal in the lung, liver, and heart. Lesions were evident in the brain at this stage postexposure. Serum titers may be detectable by 3–4 wk pi and reach high titers by 6–9 wk pi. Spores have been seen in the urine at 1 mo pi and may be excreted in large numbers up to 2 mo pi. Only small numbers are excreted thereafter. Shedding of spores is essentially terminated by 3 mo pi. Spores survive for less than 1 wk at 4° C but may remain viable for at least 6 wk at 22° C.

PATHOLOGY. At necropsy, affected animals are usually in good flesh, and frequently lesions seen macroscopically are regarded as an incidental finding. Lesions are usually confined to the kidney and appear as focal, irregular, depressed areas 1–100 mm in diameter. In severely affected kidneys, lesions frequently coalesce with adjacent foci (Figs. 6.48 and 6.49). On the cut surface, indistinct, linear, pale gray-white areas may extend into the underlying cortex.

On histopathology, granulomatous lesions are evident in the interstitium of the lung, kidney, and liver by 1 mo postexposure. In the lung, focal to

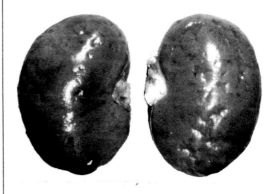

FIG. 6.48—Kidneys from rabbit with chronic encephalitozoonosis. There are multiple irregular, pitted areas on the surface of the cortices.

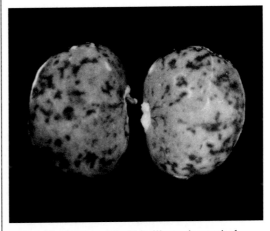

FIG. 6.49—Kidneys of rabbit, illustrating typical changes associated with recent infection with *Encephalitozoon cuniculi*. There are multiple dark red, depressed, irregular foci present in the cortex.

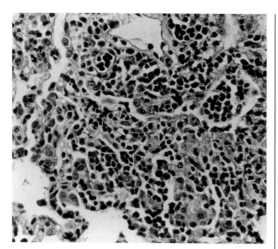

FIG. 6.50—Focal granulomatous interstitial pneumonitis, typical transient lesions associated with recent *Encephalitozoon* infection.

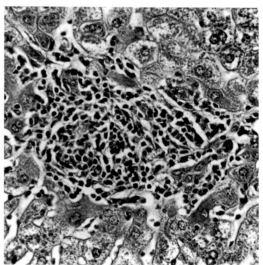

FIG. 6.51—Focal interstitial hepatitis associated with early *Encephalitozoon* infection. There is marked periportal infiltration with mononuclear cells.

diffuse interstitial pneumonitis, with mononuclear cell infiltration, may occur (Fig. 6.50). Hepatic lesions are characterized by a focal granulomatous inflammatory response (Fig. 6.51), with periportal lymphocytic infiltration. Focal lymphocytic infiltrates may also occur in the myocardium. In the kidney, early lesions consist of a focal to segmental granulomatous interstitial nephritis, with degeneration and sloughing of affected epithelial cells and mononuclear cell infiltration (Fig. 6.52). Lesions may be present at all levels of the renal tubule, usually with minimal involvement of the glomeruli. Using tissue Gram stains (e.g., Brown and Brenn), the spores are evident as ovoid, gram-positive organisms approximately 1.5 × 2.5–5 μm in size. Staining procedures using carbol fuchsin will stain the organisms a distinct purple color. Spores may be present within epithelial cells, in macrophages, in inflammatory foci, or free within collecting tubules. At 1–2 mo postexposure, organisms are usually readily demonstrated in the kidney. In renal lesions of longer duration, interstitial fibrosis, collapse of the parenchyma, and mononuclear cell infiltration are typical changes. The organism is usually eliminated from the kidney at this stage of the disease.

In the central nervous system, lesions normally do not occur until at least 30 d postexposure. Changes are those of a focal nonsuppurative granulomatous meningoencephalomyelitis, with

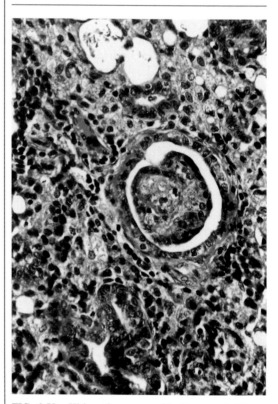

FIG. 6.52—Kidney from case of lapine encephalitozoonosis. There is a marked granulomatous interstitial nephritis, with mononuclear cell infiltration. There is degeneration of tubules, with mononuclear cell infiltration. Cellular debris is present in scattered tubules.

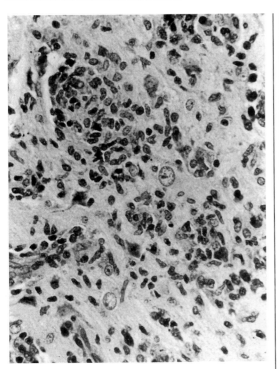

FIG. 6.53—Granulomatous encephalitis associated with chronic *Encephalitozoon* infection.

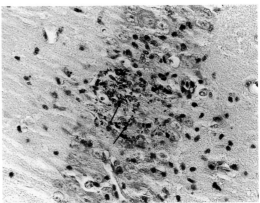

FIG. 6.54—Typical ovoid organisms are scattered in the neuropil (*arrows*) associated with encephalitozoonosis (Brown and Brenn stain).

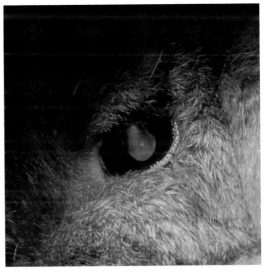

FIG. 6.55—Dwarf rabbit with cataract associated with chronic *Encephalitozoon cuniculi* infection (presumably a congenital infection). Some breeds of dwarf rabbits appear to be particularly susceptible to *Encephalitozoon* infection.

astrogliosis and perivascular lymphocytic infiltration (Fig. 6.53). Using appropriate stains, organisms may be evident as collections of spores within parasitized astroglial cells or as scattered organisms within granulomatous inflammatory foci (Fig. 6.54). Characteristic lesions may also be present in the central nervous system in the absence of identifiable organisms. Lesions observed in one dwarf rabbit with encephalitozoonosis included meningoencephalomyelitis with focal mineralization and fibrinoid necrosis of cerebral vessels, as well as focal radiculoneuritis. *E. cuniculi* infection has also been associated with cataractous change. In dwarf rabbits, there have been several cases of uveitis with cataract formation attributed to *E. cuniculi* infection (Fig.6.55). Typical organisms have been identified within the affected lens stroma. In rabbits with organisms present within the lens, such cases are likely due to intrauterine infections with *E. cuniculi*.

DIAGNOSIS. The identification of characteristic lesions and the demonstration of the organisms in tissue sections are the standard diagnostic procedures used to confirm the diagnosis. The organisms can be readily differentiated from other protozoal infections, such as toxoplasmosis, by the nature of the inflammatory response and staining properties of the organisms. *Toxoplasma* organisms are gram-negative and do not stain with carbol fuchsin stains. In addition, serology tests are available to identify animals that have been exposed to the organism. Serology tests currently used include the modified India ink immunoreaction test, indirect immunofluorescence microscopy, and a dot ELISA test. An intradermal skin test has also been used to detect infected rabbits. The serology tests have been the most widely used. Accurate tests have been made on single drops of blood and from tissues and fluids collected at necropsy.

CONTROL. The incidence of encephalitozoonosis is on the decline in many areas, particularly in well-managed facilities. Regular serological testing will readily identify infected animals. Since seroconversion precedes renal shedding, infected animals can be identified before they are excreting organisms.

SIGNIFICANCE. Although usually a subclinical infection, occasionally neurological disease and renal insufficiency may occur in heavily infected animals. In addition, it is likely that growth weights and feed conversion are compromised during the course of the disease. When present, the granulomatous lesions in the target tissues such as kidney and brain are a source of confusion and frustration for researchers doing histological evaluations of tissues during the course of an experiment. There is also evidence that alterations in the immune response may occur during the course of the disease. A variable response to implanted biomaterials has been observed in rabbits infected with *E. cuniculi*. Some strains of dwarf rabbits appear to be particularly likely to develop severe disease postexposure to *E. cuniculi*.

Antibodies to *Encephalitozoon* spp. have been detected in the sera of immunocompetent human subjects. Whether the seroconversion is due to exposure to *E. cuniculi* or another species has not been determined. Currently there is no convincing evidence that the organism causes disease in immunocompetent human contacts. However, there have been confirmed cases of *E. cuniculi* infection identified in AIDS patients. Manifestations vary from keratoconjunctivitis to pneumonia.

CRYPTOSPORIDIUM INFECTION: CRYPTOSPORIDIOSIS. Cryptosporidia have been identified in a variety of species, including calves, lambs, foals, mice, rats, and guinea pigs. An organism referred to as *C. cuniculus* has been identified in the small intestine of rabbits. Animals are usually asymptomatic, and the organism may be demonstrated as an incidental finding. When examined microscopically, occasionally the villi of the terminal small intestine are shortened and blunted. Round to ovoid bodies are present on the brush border of epithelial cells. Changes on enterocytes are minimal and consist of elongation or shortening of microvilli adjacent to attachment sites.

SIGNIFICANCE. Based on current information, cryptosporidia rarely occur as a primary pathogen in enteritis in rabbits. The role of *C. cuniculus* as a copathogen has not been fully studied. The organism can induce significant shortening of intestinal villi during the course of an infection and thus could produce a potential problem when intestinal changes are interpreted during experimental studies.

***Toxoplasma* Infection: Toxoplasmosis.** Antibodies to *T. gondii* have been detected in the sera of rabbits in the United States, but clinical disease rarely occurs. In one reported outbreak of the disease, anorexia, pyrexia, and neurological disorders were the usual presenting signs. At necropsy, there were multiple foci of necrosis with a granulomatous inflammatory response present in the lung, liver, and spleen. Both tachyzoites and tissue cysts were associated with the lesions.

Helminth Infestations

PINWORM INFESTATION: OXYURIOSIS

EPIZOOTIOLOGY AND PATHOGENESIS. Of the Oxyuridae, *Passalurus ambiguus* is a common parasite of domestic rabbits, and frequently the typical eggs, slightly flattened on one side, are observed on fecal flotation in asymptomatic rabbits. Adult worms are located in the cecum and other areas of the large intestine.

DIAGNOSIS. The identification of the typical pinworm eggs on fecal flotation and/or the adult worms in the large intestine will confirm the diagnosis.

SIGNIFICANCE. Infestations with moderate numbers of *Passalurus* are considered to be relatively harmless by most parasitologists, although clinicians frequently elect to treat affected animals. However, impaired weight gains, poor breeding performance, and occasionally death have been attributed to heavy infestations with pinworms.

BAYLISASCARIS INFECTION. Infections with *B. procyonis* commonly occur in the natural host, the raccoon. There appears to be a relatively amiable host-parasite relationship in the raccoon. However, when an unnatural host such as a rabbit (or a human being) accidentally ingests infective eggs, frequently a devastating cerebrospinal disorder results. Typical neurological signs include torticollis, ataxia, circling, opisthotonus, and recumbancy. If not euthanized, animals usually die as a result of the unremitting nervous signs.

EPIZOOTIOLOGY AND PATHOGENESIS. Hay or bedding contaminated with raccoon feces containing *B. procyonis* eggs is the usual source of the parasite. Following passage in raccoon feces, embryonation requires approximately 30 d before the eggs are infective. Eggs will remain infective for at least a year under appropriate environmental conditions. Following the accidental ingestion of embryonated eggs, the larvae are released in the intestine and undergo aggressive somatic and pulmonary migration. The severe damage, particularly in the central nervous system, is attributed to the rapid growth of the larvae and the ability to migrate into the brain, resulting in extensive trauma in target areas. In addition, metabolic wastes and enzymes elaborated by the parasite may evoke a vigorous inflammatory response.

PATHOLOGY. At necropsy, multiple, circumscribed, raised white nodules up to 1.5 mm in diameter are often present in the subepicardial and subendocardial regions of the heart and the serosal surface of the liver. Microscopic examination of the visceral lesions reveals focal granulomas, with mononuclear cells and polymorphs infiltrating the area. Remnants of the parasite are usually present within the lesions. In the central nervous system, lesions are most often present in the gray and white matter in the brain stem and cerebellar regions, but the cerebrum, including

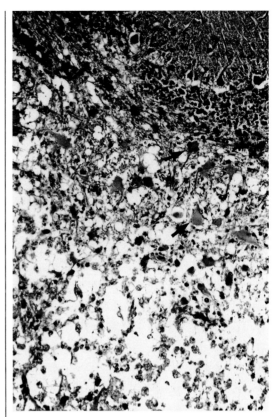

FIG. 6.56—Focus of leukomalacia in the cerebellum associated with cerebral *Baylisascaris procyonis* infection in domestic rabbit. There are prominent gemisocytic astrocytes (*arrows*) within the lesion. (Courtesy R.J. Hampson)

the hippocampus, may be involved. Sites of parasitic migration are characterized by extensive malacia and astrogliosis. Large numbers of Gitter cells and gemistocytic astrocytes may be present in lesions interpreted to be of several days duration (Fig. 6.56). Infiltrating inflammatory cells include lymphocytes, macrophages, eosinophils, and heterophils. Within the neuropil adjacent to the lesions, frequently there are nematode larvae with characteristic excretory columns and lateral alae (Fig. 6.57).

DIAGNOSIS. The lesions should be correlated with a possible source of *Baylisascaris* eggs. Larvae may be removed from the brain either by the Baermann method or by artificial digestion for positive identification.

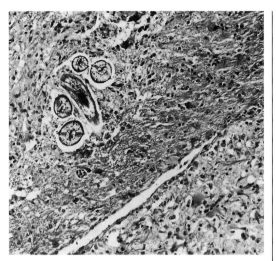

FIG. 6.57—Cerebral *Baylisascaris* infestation in New Zealand White rabbit. Note the focus of malacia with larvae present within lesion.

SIGNIFICANCE. *Baylisascaris* infection represents one possible cause of neurological disease in rabbits. Zoonotic aspects should be emphasized. However, rabbits are a "dead end" host and thus cannot serve as a source of infective eggs for human contacts.

OTHER HELMINTH INFECTIONS. In domestic rabbits, Trichostrongylidae include gastrointestinal helminths of the genera *Nematodirus* and *Trichostrongylus*. They are not considered to be a problem under normal circumstances. Of the cestodes, infestations with adult tapeworms are rare in the domestic rabbit. However, lagomorphs may serve as the intermediate host for *Taenia pisiformis*, a parasite whose definitive host is primarily the canine species. Raised, light tan, focal to linear, solitary or multiple lesions up to 3 mm in diameter are present on the surface of the liver. Microscopically, lesions often consist of a necrotic center containing cell debris, inflammatory cells, and remnants of the parasite. At the periphery, there is fibrosis, with multinucleated giant cell formation, epitheliod cells, polymorphs, and mononuclear cells. In older lesions, mineralization and fibrous tissue proliferation occur.

ECTOPARASITIC INFECTIONS

Mite Infestation: Acariasis

PSOROPTES CUNICULI INFECTION. *P. cuniculi* (ear mite) infestation is the most common and costliest disease due to an ectoparasite in domestic rabbits. The mites are obligate, nonburrowing parasites that chew and pierce the epidermal layers of the external ear, evoking a marked inflammatory response.

EPIZOOTIOLOGY AND PATHOGENESIS. The mite normally spends its entire life span in the external ear of the rabbit. The life cycle (egg to egg) is usually completed in around 3 wk. Up to 10,000 mites may be present in a severely infested ear.

PATHOLOGY. In heavily parasitized ears, foul-smelling branlike crusts may fill the external ear canal and extend up the ear (Fig. 6.58). The ear is often thickened and edematous. The mites can be easily demonstrated in wet mount preparations from the ear (Fig. 6.59).

CHEYLETIELLA INFESTATION. Cheyletid fur mites (*C. parasitovorax*) may be present without producing detectable disease. When lesions are present,

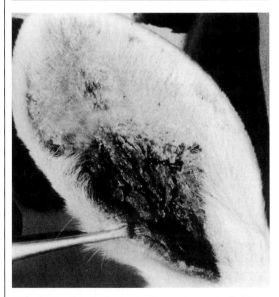

FIG. 6.58—Acariasis due to *Psoroptes cuniculi*. Note the crusting and oily debris present in the external ear canal.

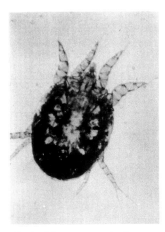

FIG. 6.59—Typical *Psoroptes* mite in a wet mount preparation collected from the affected ear.

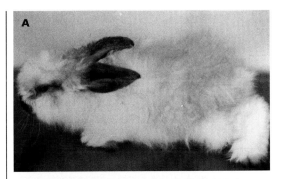

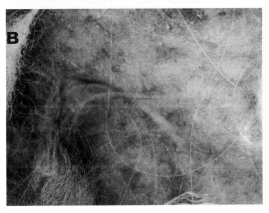

FIG. 6.60— (**A**) Dwarf rabbit with a history of doing poorly. Note the unkempt appearance of hair coat, *Cheyletiella* infestation. (**B**) Inguinal region, illustrating the scaling lesions with hair loss.

they are usually located on the dorsal trunk and scapular areas. They consist of areas of scaliness and hyperemia, with crusting and variable degrees of hair loss (Fig. 6.60). Pruritis is not intense, but careful observation reveals that rabbits are pruritic. There may be a relatively high prevalence of these mites in some commercial rabbitries.

OTHER MITE INFESTATIONS. *Notoedres cati* and *Sarcoptes scabiei* have been associated with alopecia and dermatitis involving the face, nose, lips, and external genitalia. Pruritis is common, and self-mutilation may occur. There have been isolated reports of infestation with another fur mite, *Listrophorus gibbus,* in domestic rabbits. The incidence of *L. gibbus* infections may be more common than currently realized. Infected rabbits are asymptomatic, there is usually no evidence of movement on the hair, and their preferred site of attachment is on the underside of the tail. For additional information on ectoparasites and helminths, see Hofing and Kraus (1994).

BIBLIOGRAPHY
FOR PARASITIC DISEASES

Coccidiosis

Abdel-Ghaffar, F.M., et al. 1990. Effects of *Eimeria labbeana* and *Eimeria stiedai* infection on the activity of some of the enzymes in the serum and liver of their hosts. Parasitol. Res. 76:440–43.

Barriga, O.O., and Arnoni, J.V. 1981. Pathophysiology of hepatic coccidiosis in rabbits. Vet. Parasitol. 8:201–10.

———. 1979. *Eimeria stiedae:* Oocyst output and hepatic function of rabbits with graded infections. Exp. Parasitol. 48:407–14.

Catchpole, J., and Norton, C.C. 1979. The species of *Eimeria* in rabbits for meat production in Britain. Parasitology 79:249–57.

Drouet-Viard, F., et al. 1994. The invasion of the rabbit intestinal tract by *Eimeria intestinalis* sporozoites. Parasitol. Res. 80:706–7.

Horton, R.J. 1967. The route of migration of *Eimeria stiedae* (Lindemann, 1865) sporozoites between the duodenum and bile ducts of the rabbit. Parasitology 57:9–17.

Owen, D. 1970. Life cycle of *Eimeria stiedae.* Nature 227:304.

Peeters, J.E., et al. 1984. Clinical and pathological changes after *Eimeria intestinalis* infection in rabbits. Zentralbl. Veterinaermed. (B) 31:9–24.

Rutherford, R.L. 1943. The life cycle of four intestinal coccidia of the domestic rabbit. J. Parasitol. 29:10–32.

Varga, I. 1982. Large-scale management systems and parasite populations: Coccidia in rabbits. Vet. Parasitol. 11:69–84.

Encephalitozoon Infection

Ansbacher, L., et al. 1988. The influence of *Encephalitozoon cuniculi* on neural tissue responses to implanted biomaterials in the rabbit. Lab. Anim. Sci. 38:689–95.

Anver, M.R., et al. 1972. Congenital encephalitozoonosis in a squirrel monkey. Vet. Pathol. 9:475–80.

Ashton, N., et al. 1976. Encephalitozoonosis (nosematosis) causing bilateral cataract in a rabbit. Br. J. Ophthalmol. 60:618–31.

Beckwith, C., et al. 1988. Dot enzyme-immunoabsorbent assay (dot ELISA) for antibodies to *Encepalitozoon cuniculi*. Lab. Anim. Sci. 38:573–76.

Bywater, J.E.C. 1979. Encephalitozoonosis a zoonosis? Lab. Anim. 13:149–51.

Bywater, J.E.C., and Kellett, B.S. 1978. The eradication of *Encephalitozoon cuniculi* from a specific pathogen-free rabbit colony. Lab. Anim. Sci. 28:402–4.

Cox, J.C. 1977. Altered immune responsiveness associated with *Encephalitozoon cuniculi* infection in rabbits. Infect. Immun. 15:392–95.

Cox, J.C., and Ross, J. 1980. A serological survey of *Encephalitozoon cuniculi* infection in the wild rabbit in England and Scotland. Res. Vet. Sci. 28:396.

Cox, J.C., et al. 1979. An investigation of the route and progression of *Encephalitozoon cuniculi* infection in adult rabbits. J. Protozool. 26L:260–65.

———. 1972. Presumptive diagnosis of *Nosema cuniculi* in rabbits by immunofluorescence. Res. Vet. Sci. 13:595–97.

De Groote, M.A., et al. 1995. Polymerase chain reaction and culture confirmation of disseminated *Encephalitozoon cuniculi* in a patient with AIDS: Successful therapy with albendazole. J. Infect. Dis. 171:1375–78.

Flatt, R.E., and Jackson, S.J. 1970. Renal nosematosis in young rabbits. Vet. Pathol. 7:492–97.

Hollister, W.S., et al. 1991. Evidence for widespread occurrence of antibodies to *Encephalitozoon cuniculi* (microspora) in man provided by ELISA and other serological tests. Parasitology 102:33–43.

Hunt, R.D., et al. 1972. Encephalitozoonosis: Evidence for vertical transmission. J. Infect. Dis. 126:212–14.

Kunstyr, I., and Naumann, S. 1985. Head tilt in rabbits caused by pasteurellosis and encephalitozoonosis. Lab. Anim. 19:208–13.

Kunstyr, I., et al. 1986. Humoral antibody response of rabbits to experimental infection with *Encephalitozoon cuniculi*. Vet. Parasitol. 21:223–32.

Lyngset, A. 1980. A survey of serum antibodies to *Encephalitozoon cuniculi* in breeding rabbits and their young. Lab. Anim. Sci. 30:558–61.

Moffat, R.E., and Schiefer, B. 1973. Microsporidiosis (encephalitozoonosis) in the guinea pig. Lab. Anim. Sci. 23:282–83.

Nast, R., et al. 1996. Generalized encephalitozoonosis in a Jersey wooly rabbit. Can. Vet. J. 37:303–5.

Owen, D.G. 1980. Investigation into the transplacental transmission of *Encephalitozoon cuniculi* in rabbits. Lab. Anim. 14:35–38.

Pakes, S.P., et al. 1972. A diagnostic skin test for encephalitozoonosis (nosematosis) in rabbits. Lab. Anim. Sci. 22:870–77.

Pakes, S.P., and Gerrity, L.W. 1994. Protozoal diseases. In *The Biology of the Laboratory Rabbit*, ed. P.J. Manning et al., pp. 205–30. New York: Academic Press.

Pattison, M., et al. 1971. An outbreak of encephalomyelitis in broiler rabbits caused by *Nosema cuniculi*. Vet. Rec. 88:404–5.

Plowright, W. 1952. An encephalitis-nephritis syndrome in the dog probably due to congenital *Encephalitozoon* infection. J. Comp. Pathol. 62:83–92.

Robinson, J.J. 1954. Common infectious disease of laboratory rabbits questionably attributed to *Encephalitozoon cuniculi*. Arch. Pathol. 58:71–84.

Rossi, P., et al. 1999. Resolution of microsporidial sinusitis and keratoconjunctivitis by itraconazol treatment. Am. J. Ophthalmol. 127:210–12.

Thomas, C., et al. 1997. Microsporidia (*Encephalitozoon cuniculi*) in wild rabbits in Australia. Aust. Vet. J. 75:808–10.

Van Gool, T., et al. 1997. High seroprevalence of *Encephalitozoon* species in immunocompetent subjects. J. Infect. Dis. 175:1020–24.

van Rensburg, I.B.J., and Du Plessis, J.L. 1971. Nosematosis in a cat: A case report. J. S. Afr. Med. Assoc. 42:327–31.

Waller, T., et al. 1980. Immunological diagnosis of encephalitozoonosis from postmortem specimens. Vet. Immunol. Immunopathol. 1:353–60.

Wolfer, J. 1992. Spontaneous lens capsule rupture in the rabbit. Vet. Pathol. 29:449.

Wolfer, J., et al. 1993. Phacoclastic uveitis in the rabbit. Prog. Comp. Vet. Ophthalmol. 3:92–97.

Wright, J.H., and Craighead, E.M. 1922. Infectious motor paralysis in young rabbits. J. Exp. Med. 36:135–40.

Cryptosporidium Infection

Inman, L.R., and Takeuchi, A. 1979. Spontaneous cryptosporidiosis in an adult female rabbit. Vet. Pathol. 16:89–95.

Rehg, J.E., et al. 1979. *Cryptosporidium cuniculus* in the rabbit (*Oryctolagus cuniculus*). Lab. Anim. Sci. 29:656–60.

Toxoplasma Infection

Dubey, J.P. 1988. *Toxoplasmosis of Animals and Man*. Boca Raton, Fla.: CRC.

Leland, M.M., et al. 1992. Clinical toxoplasmosis in domestic rabbits. Lab. Anim. Sci. 42:318–19.

Helminth Infestations

Dade, A.W., et al. 1975. An epizootic of cerebral nematodiasis in rabbits due to *Ascaris columnaris*. Lab. Anim. Sci. 25:65–69.

Duwel, D., and Brech, K. 1981. Control of oxyuriasis in rabbits by fenbendazole. Lab. Anim. 15:101–5.

Flatt, R.E., and Campbell, W.W. 1974. Cysticercosis in rabbits: Incidence and lesions of the naturally occurring disease in young domestic rabbits. Lab. Anim. Sci. 24:914–18.

Hofing, G.L., and Kraus, A.L. 1994. Arthropod and helminth parasites. In *The Biology of the Laboratory Rabbit,* ed. P.J. Manning et al., pp. 231–58. New York: Academic.

Kazacos, K.R., and Kazacos, E.A. 1988. Diagnostic exercise: Neuromuscular condition in rabbits. Lab. Anim. Sci. 38:187–89.

Kazacos, K.R., et al. 1983. Fatal cerebrospinal disease caused by *Baylisascaris procyonis* in domestic rabbits. J. Am. Vet. Med. Assoc. 183:967–71.

Ectoparasitic Infections

Flatt, R.E., and Weimers, J. 1976. A survey of fur mites in domestic rabbits. Lab. Anim. Sci. 26:758–61.

Hofing, G.L., and Kraus, A.L. 1994. Arthropod and helminth parasites. In *The Biology of the Laboratory Rabbit.* ed. P.J. Manning et al., pp. 231–58. New York: Academic.

Lin, S.L., et al. 1984. Diagnostic exercise (sarcoptic mange). Lab. Anim. Sci. 34:353–55.

Niekrasz, M.A. 1998. Rabbit fur mite (*Listophorus gibbus*) infestation in New Zealand White rabbits. Contemp. Top. 37(4):73–75.

Wright, F.C., and Riner, J.C. 1985. Comparative efficacy of injection routes and doses of ivermectin against *Psoroptes* in rabbits. Am. J. Vet. Res. 46:752–54.

MISCELLANEOUS DISORDERS

Hair Chewing (Barbering). Occasionally hair loss due to hair chewing (barbering) occurs. Patchy alopecia may be present on the face and back, with no evidence of a concurrent dermatitis. Hair chewing most commonly occurs in young, group-housed rabbits. Skin scrapings for microscopic examination and fungal culture are recommended in order to eliminate the possibility of dermatophyte infection. Boredom and low-roughage diets have been implicated as contributing factors to this condition.

Physical Injury. Fighting is common among group-housed rabbits that have reached sexual maturity. Abrasions and hair loss are common in the combatants, including lacerations around the external genitalia. Rarely, aggressive males may mutilate both bucks and does. Injuries observed include skin abrasions and amputation of the tips of the ears.

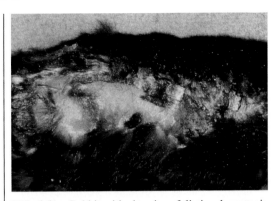

FIG. 6.61—Rabbit with chronic exfoliative dermatosis and sebaceous adenitis. Note the marked scaling lesions with hair loss over the dorsal aspects of the body. (Courtesy M. Taylor and K.E. Linder)

Exfoliative Dermatosis and Sebaceous Adenitis. This condition has been reported to occur in several different breeds of pet rabbits. In the cases reported to date, the disease occurs primarily in older adult animals. Typically, there is a nonpruritic scaling dermatosis with patchy to coalescing areas of alopecia (Fig. 6.61). Affected rabbits have proven to be refractory to a variety of treatments, including antimicrobial and anti-inflammatory drugs. Microscopic changes seen include hyperkeratosis, follicular interface dermatitis, interface folliculitis, reduction in the numbers of sebaceous glands with destruction and lymphocytic infiltration, and perifollicular to diffuse dermal fibrosis. *Differential diagnoses* would include screening for dermatophyte and ectoparasitic infections, as well as physical injury.

Ulcerative Dermatitis ("Sore Hocks"). The affected area of skin typically involves a circumscribed region of varying size on the plantar aspect of the metatarsal bones. Lesions consist of a circumscribed, ulcerated area covered by granulation tissue and necrotic debris (Fig. 6.62). Purulent exudate may be adherent to the lesions. The problem is most commonly seen in heavy, mature adults. Poor sanitation, trauma from poor-quality, wire-bottom cages, and hereditary predisposition are examples of factors that may influence the incidence of the disease. *Staphylococcus aureus* is the most frequent isolate from lesions.

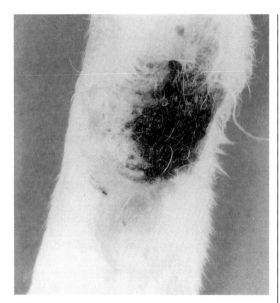

FIG. 6.62—Pododermatitis ("sore hock") in adult domestic rabbit.

Prolapse of the Deep Gland of the Third Eyelid. Swelling and protrusion of the third eyelid has been associated with prolapse of the deep bilobed gland of the third eyelid. Affected animals present with a unilateral or bilateral protrusion of the third eyelid from the medial canthus of the eye. Abnormal laxity of the connective tissue attaching the deep gland of the third eyelid to the bony orbital structures may be the underlying cause. Surgical removal of this gland is the recommended treatment.

Vertebral Fracture. Posterior paralysis due to vertebral fracture or dislocation occurs all too often in laboratory rabbits. The axial and appendicular skeletons of domestic rabbits are relatively fragile in proportion to their muscle mass. Thus an unsupported, sudden movement of the hindlimbs may exert sufficient leverage on the lumbosacral junction to cause a vertebral fracture. Depending on the duration of the problem prior to euthanasia and necropsy, the hindquarters may be soiled with urine and fecal material consistent with incontinence. The site of the fracture (or luxation) is usually the lumbosacral region (L7). There may be extensive hemorrhage in the underlying psoas muscles. Changes vary from luxation

to multiple fractures of the affected vertebra, with extensive damage to the lumbosacral spinal cord.

Gastric Trichobezoar (Hairball). Hairballs are frequently present as an incidental finding at necropsy in rabbits that have died from other causes. Depending on the size and location, however, anorexia, wasting, and occasionally death may occur in severely affected animals. In one study of clinically affected animals, hematology and blood chemistry values were within normal limits (Wagner et al. 1974). Animals are usually alert, with reduced feed and water consumption. The antemortem diagnosis is usually confirmed by palpation and sometimes by contrast radiography. Predisposing factors implicated include excessive grooming and hair chewing due to boredom. However, insufficient dietary roughage, poor gastric motility, and a sedentary lifestyle are considered to be more important contributing factors. Deaths do occur. At necropsy, animals may be in fair to poor condition. Large trichobezoars usually fill the stomach, extending into the pyloric region (Fig. 6.63). The intestinal tract usually contains scanty ingesta. Hepatic lipidosis is a characteristic finding. Gastric rupture and peritonitis may occur.

Intestinal Plasmacytosis. A syndrome characterized by marked plasma cell infiltration in the intestinal tract of domestic rabbits has been described. The intestinal lesions have been identi-

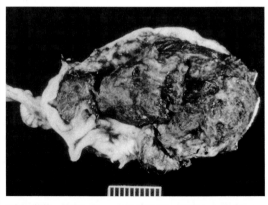

FIG. 6.63—Trichobezoar (hairball) and stomach from adult rabbit. The animal was alert but anorectic and was euthanized.

fied in New Zealand White, Dutch Belted, and Watanabe rabbits used in research projects. Older animals were particularly at risk, particularly rabbits used for antibody production or cholesterol studies. Affected animals are usually asymptomatic, and the changes are frequently detected only on histopathologic examination.

PATHOLOGY. At necropsy, there may be identifiable defects on the intestinal mucosa in severely affected animals. On microscopic examination, lesions are particularly prominent in the small intestine and cecum, with no apparent predilection to involve the sacculus rotundus or the cecal appendix. In the small intestine, mucosal erosions, dilation of lacteals, and blunting of the overlying villi are variable findings. In affected regions, there is marked infiltration of plasma cells in the lamina propria. The infiltrating cells are well differentiated and relatively uniform in size and shape. In severely affected rabbits, there is complete replacement of the normal architecture, the infiltrating cells forming dense aggregates in the lamina propria. In general, the infiltrates are confined to the intestinal tract, although in a few animals, increased numbers of plasma cells may be present in spleen and mesenteric lymph nodes.

ETIOPATHOGENESIS AND SIGNIFICANCE. The selective involvement of the intestinal tract and the nature of the cellular infiltrate are consistent with the response to antigenic stimuli at the local level. Microbial and/or food antigens would appear to be the logical candidates to evoke such a response, but the precise etiopathogenesis is currently unknown. The higher incidence of intestinal plasmacytosis in older rabbits suggests that length of antigenic exposure plays a role in this change. The prevalence of this condition in other research facilities warrants further study.

Myopathy Associated with Ketamine/Xylazine Administration. Multifocal myocardial degeneration with interstitial fibrosis has been observed in Dutch Belted rabbits following the administration of a ketamine/xylazine combination or the alpha$_2$ agonist, detomidine. This change is attributed to ischemia secondary to vasoconstriction with reduction in coronary blood flow, with sub-

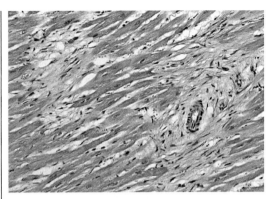

FIG. 6.64—Section of myocardium of Dutch Belted rabbit with multifocal myocardial degeneration with fibrosis postadministration of a regimen of ketamine/xylazine. (Courtesy R.P. Marini)

sequent myocardial degeneration and fibrosis. Collateral circulation in the myocardium is limited in this species. In lesions of recent onset, there is degeneration of myofibers with mononuclear and polymorphonuclear cell infiltration. In lesions of some duration, there is loss of myofibers and marked interstitial fibrosis (Fig. 6.64). Borderline vitamin E deficiency could also contribute to the development of the myocardial lesions.

BIBLIOGRAPHY
FOR MISCELLANEOUS DISORDERS
Bergdall, V.E., and Dysko, R.C. 1994. Metabolic, traumatic, mycotic, and miscellaneous diseases. In *The Biology of the Laboratory Rabbit,* ed. P.J. Manning et al., pp 336–53. New York: Academic.

Hillyer, E.V., and Quesenberry, K.E. 1997. Ferrets, Rabbits and Rodents: Clinical Medicine and Surgery. Philadelphia: W.B. Saunders.

Hurley, R.J., et al. 1994. Evaluation of detomidine anesthetic combinations in the rabbit. Lab. Anim. Sci. 44:472–77.

Janssens, G., et al. 1999. Bilateral prolapse of the deep gland of the third eyelid in the rabbit: Diagnosis and treatment. Lab. Anim. Sci. 49:105–9.

Jones, T., et al. 1982. Diagnostic exercise (vertebral fracture). Lab. Anim. Sci. 32:489–90.

Lee, K.P., et al. 1978. Acute peritonitis in the rabbit (*Oryctolagus cuniculi*) resulting from gastric trichobezoar. Lab. Anim. Sci. 28:202–4.

Li, X. 1996. Intestinal plasmacytosis in rabbits: A histologic and ultrastructural study. Vet. Path. 33:721–24.

Linder, K.E., et al. 1998. Generalized exfoliative dermatosis with sebaceous adenitis in three domestic rabbits. Fourteenth Proceedings of the AAVD/ACVD Meeting, pp. 89–90.

Marini, R.P., et al. 1999. Cardiovascular pathology possibly associated with ketamine/xylazine anesthesia in Dutch belted rabbits. Lab. Anim. Sci. 49:153–60.

Wagner, J.E., et al. 1974. Spontaneous deaths in rabbits resulting from gastric trichobezoars. Lab. Anim. Sci. 24:826–30.

White, S.D., et al. 2000. Sebaceous adenitis in four domestic rabbits (Oryctolagus cuniculi). Vet. Derm. 11:53–60.

NUTRITIONAL, TOXIC, AND METABOLIC DISEASES

Vitamin E Deficiency. With the current rigid quality-control standards for commercial feed production, confirmed nutritional problems are relatively rare. However, synthetic diets are prepared routinely by some researchers for specialized projects; thus there is also the possibility of human error in these formulations. There are several reports of nutritional muscular dystrophy due to vitamin E deficiency. In addition to stiffness and muscle weakness, neonatal mortality and infertility are manifestations of vitamin E deficiency in domestic rabbits. At necropsy pale, mineralized streaks may be present in musculature, such as the diaphragm, paravertebral regions, and hind limbs. Typical changes seen microscopically are hyaline degeneration of affected myofibers and clumping and mineralization of the sarcoplasm (Fig. 6.65). Macrophages may be present in reactive areas. Collapse of sarcolemmal sheaths and interstitial fibrosis frequently occur in lesions of some duration.

Calcium and Vitamin D Deficiency and Dental Disorders. The feeding of pelleted rations formulated for this species should provide the required levels for a healthy skeletal system. However, some pet owners may feed treats or poorly formulated rations, resulting eventually in borderline osteomalacia. Clinical signs include drooling of saliva, overgrowth and ridging of the incisor teeth, distorted growth of the premolar and molar teeth, anorexia, and weight loss. In cases of malocclusion, particularly if accompanied by other compatible signs, the diet and feeding practices should be evaluated.

Hypervitaminosis D. Hypervitaminosis D has been reported to occur occasionally in domestic

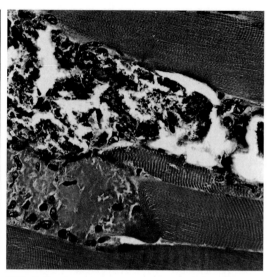

FIG. 6.65—Section of skeletal muscle from a spontaneous case of nutritional myopathy due to vitamin E–selenium deficiency. Note the degeneration of myofibers, with concurrent mineralization.

rabbits fed an improperly formulated diet. Histologic changes include medial degeneration and mineralization of major arteries. Mineralization of the glomerular tufts, basement membranes, and tubules of the kidney may also occur. In the long bones, there is deposition of basophilic material (presumably osteoblasts) on the periosteal and endosteal surfaces, medullary trabeculae, and haversian systems (Fig. 6.66). For additional information on nutritional requirements and disorders, see Cheeke (1987 and 1994).

Disorders Associated with Hypo- or Hypervitaminosis A. The clinical manifestations of vitamin A deficiency or toxicity are similar in domestic rabbits and are characterized by poor conception rates, congenital anomalies, fetal resorptions, abortion, and weak, thin kits. Congenital defects associated with hypervitaminosis A include microencephaly, hydrocephalus, and cleft palate.

Pregnancy Toxemia. This is a poorly characterized and understood condition that occurs in does, usually during the last week of pregnancy or the immediate postpartum period. Obesity and fasting are important predisposing factors. The dis-

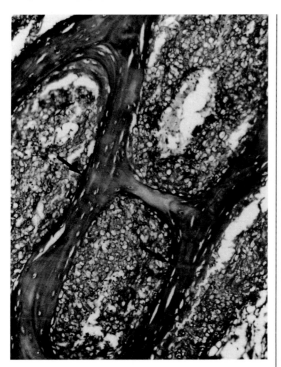

FIG. 6.66—Section of femur from case of hypervitaminosis D. There is deposition of basophilic material
(*arrows*) on the endosteal surfaces. (Courtesy N.C.
Palmer)

ease is characterized by low morbidity and high
mortality. Multiparous does are especially at risk,
and metabolic toxemia also may occur on occasion in obese, "stressed," nonpregnant rabbits.
Obesity, hereditary predisposition, impaired
blood flow to the uterus, and pituitary dysfunction are examples of factors implicated in this disease. There is one report of pregnancy toxemia
and concurrent pancreatitis in a New Zealand
White doe. Clinical manifestations of the disease
are variable and may include incoordination,
abortions, and coma. Most does fail to respond to
treatment. In the typical case of pregnancy toxemia, mobilization of fat deposits for energy
result in metabolic acidosis and ketosis, depression, and death. At necropsy, animals are usually
obese, with marked fatty infiltration of the liver
and adrenal glands.

Lead Toxicosis. With the propensity of some
rabbits to chew foreign items including painted

objects, it is not surprising that there have been
isolated reports of lead poisoning in this
species. Clinical signs observed have included
mild anemia, tremors, and posterior ataxia. In
fatal cases of lead toxicosis, myocardial degeneration, multifocal hepatic necrosis, renal tubular degeneration, and hemoglobin casts in renal
tubules are typical microscopic findings. In
cases diagnosed antemortem, removal of all
lead from the gastrointestinal tract is recommended prior to the administration of chelating
agents, since chelation will enhance the absorption of any lead present in the gastrointestinal
tract.

BIBLIOGRAPHY FOR NUTRITIONAL, TOXIC, AND METABOLIC DISEASES

Bergdall, V.K., and Dysko, R.C. 1994. Metabolic,
    traumatic, mycotic, and miscellaneous diseases of
    rabbits. In *The Biology of the Laboratory Rabbit*,
    ed. P.J. Manning et al., pp. 236–353. New York:
    Academic.
Cheeke, P.R. 1994. Nutrition and nutritional diseases.
    In *The Biology of the Laboratory Rabbit*, ed. P.J.
    Manning et al., pp. 321–35. New York: Academic.
———. 1987. Vitamins. In *Rabbit Feeding and Nutri-
    tion*, pp. 136–53. New York: Academic.
DiGiacomo, R.F., et al. 1992. Hypervitaminosis A
    and reproductive disorders in rabbits. Lab. Anim.
    Sci. 42:250–54.
Greene, H.S.N. 1937. Toxemia of pregnancy in the rab-
    bit. Clinical manifestations and pathology. J. Exp.
    Med. 65:809–32.
Harcourt-Brown, F.M. 1996. Calcium deficiency, diet
    and dental disease in pet rabbits. Vet. Rec.
    139:567–71.
Harkness, J.E., and Wagner, J.E. 1995. *The Biology and
    Medicine of Rodents and Rabbits*. Philadelphia: Lea
    and Febiger.
Hood, S., et al. 1997. Lead toxicosis in 2 dwarf rabbits.
    Can. Vet. J. 38:721–22.
Hurley, R.J., et al. 1994. Evaluation of detomidine
    anesthetic combinations in the rabbit. Lab. Anim.
    Sci. 44:472–78.
Leland, S., et al. 1995. Pancreatitis and pregnancy tox-
    emia in a New Zealand White Rabbit. Contemp.
    Top. 34:84–85.
Ringler, D.H., and Abrams, G.D. 1971. Laboratory diag-
    nosis of vitamin E deficiency in rabbits fed a faulty
    commercial ration. Lab. Anim. Sci. 21:383–88.
———. 1970. Nutritional muscular dystrophy and
    neonatal mortality in a rabbit breeding colony. J.
    Am. Vet. Med. Assoc. 157:1928–34.
Stevenson, R.G., et al. 1976. Hypervitaminosis D in
    rabbits. Can. Vet. J. 17:54–57.
Swartout, M.S. et al. 1987. Lead-induced toxicosis in
    two domestic rabbits. J. Am. Vet. Med. Assoc.
    191:717–19.

Yamimi, B., and Stein, S. 1989. Abortion, stillbirth, neonatal death, and nutritional myodegeneration in a rabbit breeding colony. J. Am. Vet. Med. Assoc. 194:561–62.

Zimmerman, T.E., et al. 1990. Soft tissue mineralization in rabbits fed a diet containing excess vitamin D. Lab. Anim. Sci. 40:212–14.

HEREDITARY DISORDERS

Congenital Glaucoma (Buphthalmia). This condition occurs most frequently in New Zealand White rabbits. Buphthalmia is characterized clinically by enlargement of one or both eyes, with subsequent corneal opacity. Abnormalities may occur within the first few weeks of life, but usually they are first evident by 3–5 mo of age. The primary defect has been identified as an absence or underdevelopment of the outflow channels, with incomplete cleavage of the iridocorneal angles. Thus with impaired drainage of aqueous humor from the anterior chamber, the increased intraocular pressure results in megaloglobus, increased corneal diameter, and protrusion of the corneal contours (Fig. 6.67). The sclera is relatively immature at this stage and thus expands to accommodate the increased volume of aqueous humor within the globe. The defect is inherited as an autosomal recessive, with incomplete penetrance. Therefore some animals homozygous for the *bu/bu* gene may show no evidence of the disease. Buphthalmia does not appear to cause discernable discomfort in affected animals.

Malocclusion. In lagomorphs, normal occlusion brings the lower incisor teeth into apposition against the upper secondary incisors ("peg teeth") located behind the large upper incisors. In rabbits with malocclusion, usually the mandible is abnormally long relative to the maxilla. The overshot lower jaw results in misalignment, failure of the incisors to wear normally, and impaired mastication. In domestic rabbits, combined lengths of growth of both the upper and lower incisors has been shown to be over 20 cm/yr. Thus malocclusion will cause overgrowth of the incisors in a relatively short period of time (Fig. 6.68). The defect appears to be inherited as an autosomal recessive. Although not as evident as malocclusion of the incisors, overgrowth of the premolar and molar teeth also occurs in this species. Dietary deficiencies may also be a contributing factor. Overgrowth with ridging of the incisors and distortion of the cheek teeth has been observed in rabbits fed a diet deficient in calcium and vitamin D. For additional information on other inherited conditions, see Lindsey and Fox (1994).

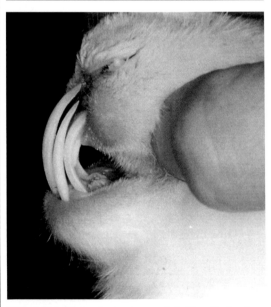

FIG. 6.68—Malocclusion in an adult New Zealand White rabbit. Note the concurrent overgrowth of the accessory incisor teeth.

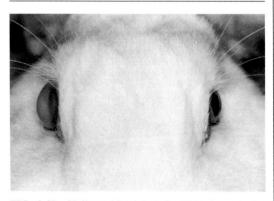

FIG. 6.67—Unilateral buphthalmia. There is marked coning of the cornea of the affected eye.

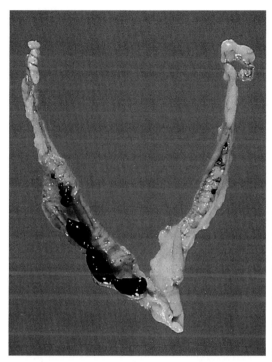

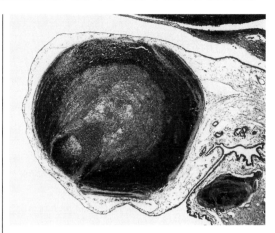

FIG. 6.70—Histologic section of uterus from animal in Figure 6.69. Note the marked dilation of the endometrial vessels (endometrial venous aneurysms) with thrombus formation. (Courtesy M. Savic)

FIG. 6.69—Reproductive tract from Californian breed doe with a history of intermittent vulvar bleeding due to rupture of endometrial venous aneurysms. Blood clots are present in the lumen of the opened uterine horns.

Endometrial Venous Aneurysms. Multiple endometrial venous aneurysms have been associated with persistent urogenital bleeding. At necropsy, clotted blood is present in the uterine lumen (Fig. 6.69), and there are multiple blood-filled endometrial varices that consist of dilated, thin-walled veins (Fig. 6.70). These varices apparently rupture and bleed periodically into the uterine lumen, with subsequent hematuria. They have been observed in nonpregnant multiparous does. The aneurysms are considered to be a congenital defect, and there is no evidence that predisposing factors, such as trauma or bleeding disorders, play a role in the disease.

BIBLIOGRAPHY
FOR HEREDITARY DISORDERS

Bray, M.V., et al. 1992. Endometrial venous aneurysms in three New Zealand White rabbits. Lab. Anim. Sci. 42:360–62.

Burrows, A.M., et al. 1995. Development of ocular hypertension in congenitally buphthalmic rabbits. Lab. Anim. Sci. 45:443–44.

Fox, R.R., and Crary, D.D. 1971. Mandibular prognathism in the rabbit: Genetic studies. J. Hered. 62:23–27.

Hanna, B.L., et al. 1962. Recessive buphthalmos in the rabbit. Genetics 47:519–29.

Harcourt-Brown, F.M. 1996. Calcium deficiency, diet and dental disease in pet rabbits. Vet. Rec. 139:567–71.

Lindsey, J.R., and Fox, R.R. 1994. Inherited diseases and variations. In *The Biology of the Laboratory Rabbit,* ed. S.H. Weisbroth et al., pp. 293–319. New York: Academic.

Shadle, A.R. 1936. The attrition and extrusive growth of the four major incisor teeth of domestic rabbits. J. Mammal. 17:15–21.

Tesluk, G.C., et al. 1982. A clinical and pathological study of inherited glaucoma in New Zealand White rabbits. Lab. Anim. 16:234–39.

Zeman, W.V., and Fielder, F.G. 1969. Dental malocclusion and overgrowth in rabbits. J. Am. Vet. Med. Assoc. 155:1115–19.

NEOPLASMS

Uterine Adenocarcinoma. This is the most commonly encountered spontaneous neoplasm occurring in *Oryctolagus cuniculi.* The relatively low incidence of this tumor seen in most commercial rabbitries and research facilities is due to the fact that these animals are usually relatively young. In one study, the incidence of uterine adenocarcinoma in does 2–3 yr of age was around 4%, and in does 5–6 yr of age, around 80%. A variety of breeds are affected. Thus there is a striking

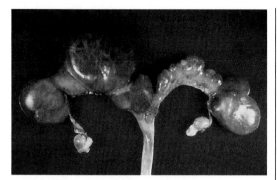

FIG. 6.71—Uterine adenocarcinoma in an aged New Zealand White doe. Note that the typical multicentric nature of the neoplastic process. (Courtesy C.G. Bihun)

increase in the incidence of uterine tumors with increasing age.

PATHOGENESIS. The carcinogenic effects of estrogens have been implicated in the evolution of uterine cancer in this species. However, the evidence is conflicting. In another study, the administration of estrogens to female Dutch rabbits actually reduced the incidence of endometrial adenocarcinomas.

PATHOLOGY. On gross examination, the tumors appear as nodular, frequently multicentric enlargements and usually involve both uterine horns (Figs. 6.71 and 6.72). On the cut surface, masses are firm, frequently with a cauliflower-like surface and central ulcerations. Serosal implantation and metastases to the lung and liver may occur. Typical microscopic changes are those of an adenocarcinoma, with invasion of the underlying layers forming acinar and tubular structures (Fig. 6.73). In rapidly growing tumors, necrotic areas are frequently observed. Metastases and tumor implants usually are similar to the primary neoplasm, often with a prominent stromal component.

Lymphosarcoma. Lymphoreticular neoplasms are the most common malignancy encountered in juvenile and young adult domestic rabbits. Anemia, depressed hematocrit, and terminally elevated BUN are typical changes seen clinically. Affected animals are usually aleukemic, but leukemia occasionally occurs. Although lymphoproliferative disorders have been associated with

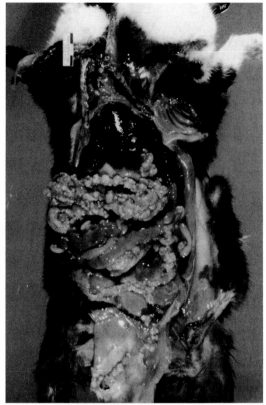

FIG. 6.72—Uterine adenocarcinoma in 6-yr-old Dutch Belted doe. There are multiple implants in the peritoneal cavity.

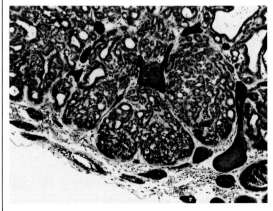

FIG. 6.73—Histological section of uterine wall from spontaneous uterine adenocarcinoma in aged New Zealand White doe. The neoplastic process extends into the myometrium and to the serosal surface of the uterus. Note the acinar structures lined by anaplastic epithelial cells.

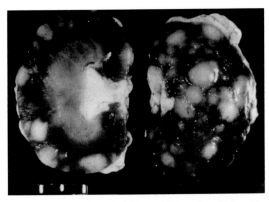

FIG. 6.74—Kidneys from young domestic rabbit with spontaneous lymphosarcoma. There are multiple raised, pale, nodular masses on the cortices, a frequent finding in lapine lymphoma.

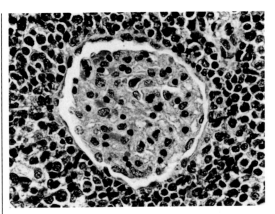

FIG. 6.75—Lymphosarcoma in New Zealand White rabbit. This section of kidney illustrates marked neoplastic lymphocytic infiltrate in the interstitium adjacent to a glomerulus.

Herpesvirus sylvilagus infections in the cottontail rabbit, there is no convincing evidence that viral agents are associated with the disease in domestic rabbits. An autosomal recessive gene has been implicated as an important factor in susceptibility to the disease.

PATHOLOGY. At necropsy, the typical findings are as follows: The kidneys are enlarged and pale gray to tan, with irregular cortical outlines. On the cut surface, the changes are usually confined to the renal cortices (Fig. 6.74). The liver is enlarged, pale, and swollen. Splenomegaly, enlarged lymph nodes, and prominent intestinal lymphoid tissue are typical features seen grossly. The wall of the stomach may be markedly thickened, with irregular surface plaques and mucosal ulceration. On histopathology, there are diffuse infiltrates of lymphoblastic cells in the interstitial regions of the renal cortex, with distortion of the normal architecture and relative sparing of the glomeruli (Fig. 6.75). In the liver, there are periportal to diffuse sinusoidal infiltrates of neoplastic cells. Diffuse infiltration occurs in the spleen, and infiltrates are also usually present in lymph nodes and in lymphoid tissue of the alimentary tract and stomach. Neoplastic cells may also be present in the uveal tract, adrenal gland, and ovary. Neoplastic lymphocytes range from 5 to 35 μm in diameter, with prominent nucleoli. There is usually a high mitotic index.

Thymoma. Thymomas are uncommon in domestic rabbits. Aside from the thymic involvement, there may be variable lymphocytic infiltrates in other organs, including lymph nodes, liver, heart, and lungs. In one case, concurrent hypercalcemia was attributed to the paraneoplastic syndrome.

Prolactin-Producing Pituitary Adenomas with Associated Mammary Dysplasia. Teat and mammary gland enlargement have been observed in older primiparous New Zealand White does with concurrent pituitary gland tumors. Clinically, there is swelling of one or more mammary glands, with enlargement and dark discoloration of the teats. At necropsy, affected mammary glands are discolored and firm, and fluid exudes from the cut surface, and there is variable thinning of the hair coat (Fig. 6.76). Microscopic findings in the affected mammary glands are consistent with dysplastic change. Dilated cystic ducts are lined by flattened to cuboidal epithelium with papillary projections into the cystic areas. Prolactin-producing acidophil pituitary adenomas are present in these animals, resulting in the hormone-responsive dysplastic changes in the mammary glands. Compared with other mammalian species studied, rabbit mammary tissue has proven to be particularly responsive to prolactin. This is the likely explanation why similar

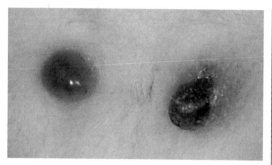

FIG. 6.76—Mammary dysplasia associated with pituitary adenoma in an adult New Zealand White doe. Note the enlargement, loss of hair, and increased pigmentation. (Courtesy J.G. Fox)

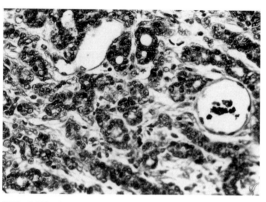

FIG. 6.77—Mammary adenocarcinoma in an aged New Zealand White doe. There was marked local infiltration with multiple metastases to the lung. There was no uterine involvement. (Courtesy M.L. Brash)

mammary changes have not been associated with pituitary gland tumors in the laboratory rat.

Other Neoplasms. Bile duct adenoma, bile duct carcinoma, osteosarcoma, embryonal nephroma, leiomyoma, leiomyosarcoma, testicular tumors, basal cell adenoma, squamous cell carcinoma, melanoma, mammary adenocarcinoma (Fig. 6.77), and papillomatosis are other spontaneous tumors that occur in this species.

BIBLIOGRAPHY FOR NEOPLASMS

Anderson, W.I, et al. 1990. Bilateral testicular seminoma in a New Zealand White rabbit (*Oryctolagus cuniculus*). Lab. Anim. Sci. 40:420–21.

Baba, N., and Von Haam, E. 1972. Animal model: Spontaneous adenocarcinoma in aged rabbits. Am. J. Pathol. 68:653–56.

Baba, N., et al. 1970. Nonspecific phosphatases of rabbit endometrial carcinoma. Arch. Pathol. 90:65–71.

Fox, R.R., et al. 1970. Lymphosarcoma in the rabbit: Genetics and pathology. J. Natl. Cancer Inst. 45:719–30.

Greene, H.S.N. 1958. Adenocarcinoma of the uterine fundus in the rabbit. Ann. N.Y. Acad. Sci. 75:535–42.

Greene, H.S.N., and Newton, R.I. 1948. Evolution of cancer of the uterine fundus in the rabbit. Cancer 1:88–99.

Hotchkiss, C.E., et al. 1994. Malignant melanoma in two rabbits. Lab. Anim. Sci. 44:377–79.

Lipman, N.S., et al. 1994. Prolactin-secreting pituitary adenomas with mammary dysplasia in New Zealand White rabbits. Lab. Anim. Sci. 44:114–20.

Sawyer, D.R., et al. 1997. Basal cell adenoma in a rabbit. Contemp. Top. 36(1):90.

Toth, L.A., et al. 1990. Lymphocytic leukemia and lymphosarcoma in a rabbit. J. Am. Vet. Med. Assoc. 197:627–29.

Vernau, K.M., et al. 1995. Thymoma in a geriatric rabbit with hypercalcemia and periodic exophthalmos. J. Am. Vet. Med. Assoc. 206:820–22.

Weisbroth, S.H. 1994. Neoplastic diseases. In *The Biology of the Laboratory Rabbit,* ed. P.J. Manning et al., pp. 259–82. New York: Academic.

INDEX

GERBIL

Acariasis, 203
Adenocarcinomas, 208
Adrenocortical tumors, 207–208
Aging, diseases associated with, 206–207
Amyloidosis, 205
Anatomic features, 197
Aural cholesteatoma, 206

Bacterial infections, 198–203
Behavioral diseases, 204
Bordetella bronchiseptica, 202

Cardiovascular disease of breeding gerbils, 205
Chronic nephropathy, 206
Cilia-associated respiratory (CAR) bacillus infection, 202
Clostridium piliforme, 198–199
Cutaneous tumors, 207

Demodex aurati, 203
Demodex criceti, 203
Demodex meriones, 203
Dental caries, 204
Dentostomella translucida, 203–204
Dermatitis
    nasal, 201–202
    staphylococcal, 201
Diabetes, 205

Ectoparasitic diseases, 203
Endoparasitic diseases, 203–204
Epilepsy, 204

Focal myocardial degeneration, 206

Genetic disorders, 204–205
Giardiasis, 203
Glomerulonephropathy, 206
Granulosa cell tumors, 207

Heart, focal myocardial degeneration, 206

Helminth infections, 203–204
Hematology, 197
Hepatitis, Tyzzer's disease, 199
Hymenolepis diminuta, 204
Hymenolepis nana, 204
Hyperadrenocortism, 205

Ileum, Tyzzer's disease, 200

Kidneys, chronic nephropathy, 206

Lead toxicity, 205
Leptospirosis, 202
Liponyssoides sanguineus, 203

Malocclusion, 204
Meriones unguiculatus (Mongolian gerbils), 196
Mite infestations, 203
Mongolian gerbils *(Meriones unguiculatus),* 196
Myocarditis, Tyzzer's disease, 200

Nasal dermatitis, 201–202
Neoplasms, 207–208

Obesity, 205
Ocular proptosis, 207
Ovarian tumors, 207
Ovaries, cystic, 206–207
Oxyuriasis, 203–204

Parasitic diseases, 203–204
Peridontal disease, 204
Pinworms, 203–204

Salmonella infection, 199–201
Salmonellosis, 199–201
Staphylococcus aureus, 201
Streptomycin toxicity, 205

Tapeworms, 204
Toxic disorders, 205
Tyrophagus castellani, 203
Tyzzer's disease, 198–199

Viral infections, 198

GUINEA PIG

Acariasis, 228–229
Acute staphylococcal dermatitis, 222
Adenoviral infections, 213–214
Adenoviral pneumonitis, 213–214
Adjuvant-associated pulmonary granulomas, 239
Aging, diseases associated with, 240–244
Alopecia, 237
Anatomic features, 209–217
Antibiotic-associated dysbacteriosis, 217–218
Arenaviral infections, 215–216

Bacterial infections, enteric, 217–219
Balisascaris procyonis, 231
Behavioral diseases, 239
Biliary cirrhosis, 238
Bordetella bronchiseptica, 219–221
Bumblefoot, 222

Calcification, metastatic, 235–236
Cardiovascular system, tumors of, 246
Cavian leukemia, 215, 244–245
Cecal torsion, 238
Chirodiscoides caviae, 228
Chlamydial infections, 221
Cholangiofibrosis, chronic idiopathic, 238
Citrobacter freundii, 221–222
Clostridial infections, 217–218
Clostridium difficile, 218
Clostridium perfringens, 218
Clostridium piliforme, 218
Coccidiosis, 230–231
Conjunctivitis
    bacterial, 225
    GPIC, 221
Coronavirus-like infections, 216
Cryptosporidium wrairi, 229–231
Cystic rete ovarii, 242–243
Cystitis, 242
Cytomegaloviral (CMV) infection, 214–215